Cerebral Aneurysms

Robert R. Smith Yuri N. Zubkov
Yahgoub Tarassoli

Cerebral Aneurysms

Microvascular and Endovascular Management

With 135 Illustrations, 27 Pieces in Color

Lucia Griffin
Project Coordinator

Springer-Verlag
New York Berlin Heidelberg London Paris
Tokyo Hong Kong Barcelona Budapest

Robert R. Smith, M.D.
Department of Neurosurgery
The University of Mississippi Medical Center
Jackson, MS 39216-4505,
USA
and
Methodist Neurological Institute
1850 Chedwick Drive
Jackson, MS 39204
USA

Yuri N. Zubkov, M.D.
Department of Cerebrovascular Surgery
A.L. Polenov Neurosurgical Research Center
St. Petersburg,
Russia

Yahgoub Tarassoli, M.D.
Mehr Hospital
Zartosht Avenue 14157
Tehran
Iran

Library of Congress Cataloging-in-Publication Data
Smith, Robert R.
Cerebral aneurysms: microvascular and endovascular management/
Robert R. Smith, Yahgoub Tarassoli, Yuri Zubkov.
p. cm.
Includes bibliographical references and index.

1. Intracranial aneurysms. 2. Intracranial aneurysms—Endoscopic surgery. I. Tarassoli, Yahgoub. II. Zubkov, Yuri. III. Title.
[DNLM: 1. Cerebral Aneurysm—surgery. 2. Cerebral Aneurysm—diagnosis. WL 355 S668c 1994]
RC693.S64 1994
616.8'1—dc20
DNLM/DLC 93-23192

Printed on acid-free paper.

Production coordinated by Scientific Publishing Services (P) Ltd., Bangalore, India, and managed by Natalie Johnson; manufacturing supervised by Rhea Talbert.
Typeset by Asco Trade Typesetting Ltd., Hong Kong.

9 8 7 6 5 4 3 2 1

ISBN-13: 978-1-4613-9534-8 e-ISBN-13: 978-1-4613-9532-4
DOI: 10.1007/978-1-4613-9532-4

Preface

During middle age, the most common cause of intracranial hemorrhage is rupture of an aneurysm. Prior to the time of rupture, good health has usually prevailed. The onset is sudden and unexpected, causing devastation in the life of the individual whom it affects. The physician who cares for these patients must be prepared to pursue aggressively the workup, the diagnosis, and treatment.

Despite the many gains that have been made in direct surgical care, aneurysmal subarachnoid hemorrhage still carries high mortality and morbidity. Only one-fifth of all patients escape to return to their premorbid condition. The remainder either die of their disease or are left disabled. Much progress has been made in treating aneurysms during the so-called "cold" period, one month or longer after SAH has occurred. However, the propensity of intracranial aneurysms to rupture and rebleed and the fact that major morbidity and mortality occurs during this one-month interval make early obliteration of the aneurysm, prior to rupture, a significant therapeutic goal. The complications that arise after hemorrhage may even be compounded in the first few postoperative days and weeks, making surgical treatment during this interval heavy with risk. It is not only our task to exclude the aneurysm from the arterial circulation but to manage all of the complications of the acute period effectively, thus achieving a better life for the patient.

The purpose of this book is to provide both direct and indirect methods for excluding aneurysms from the arterial circulation. The authors recognize that few gains are to be made on total morbidity and mortality by these technical maneuvers. Thus, an attempt has also been made to outline the many pathological entities that complicate the course of the patient with a recent SAH. The effect of brain edema, hydrocephalus, immediate ischemic deficits, delayed ischemic deficits, and the hypothalamic and endocrinological reactions that appear during the acute phase are presented.

Twenty-five years ago, Charles Drake said, "It is probably true that if we could learn how to keep a patient safe from rebleeding for a week or longer in obtunded patients with cerebral symptoms, the problems of surgery of ruptured intracranial aneurysms would nearly be solved." Ten years ago, Bengt Lundjgren et al. stated, "If we could learn how to keep a patient safe from developing delayed ischemic dysfunction, then the problem of surgery of ruptured aneurysms would be nearly solved." In 1994, it is possible to say that if we could gently assist the patient through the many complications that arise from an SAH, then the surgical treatment of intracranial aneurysms would be nearly solved. Otherwise, the prevention of SAH must be our goal. The early recognition of aneurysms that almost certainly will rupture must be high on our agenda. We await only the development of safe and effective screening methods for the recognition of these lesions.

The authors believe that they bring a unique perspective to the management of the patient with an aneurysm. Working together closely over many years has brought about some consensus in our thinking concerning the application of treatment methods: balloons, microscopes, coils, and clips. For the first time, this book brings together these technologies for the neurosurgeon.

Robert R. Smith, Jackson, MS
Yuri N. Zubkov, St. Petersburg
Yahgoub Tarassoli, Tehran

Acknowledgments

The authors are indebted to many people for making this book possible. Our Dean and Vice-chancellor for Health Affairs, Norman C. Nelson, MD, supported the project and made it possible for three neurosurgeons from different countries and with different backgrounds and talents to come together in this effort. Our wives, Helen Smith, Susan Tarassoli, and Julia Zubkov, sacrificed and supported our work. Some extra domestic measures were required from them during this time also. Our families were without paternal and grandpaternal guidance but survived intact, no worse and perhaps even a little better for it.

We had much guidance from Bill Day and his associates at Springer-Verlag in New York and help from our neurosurgical colleagues in Mississippi. George Benashvili offered suggestions and checked references. Lon Alexander read and made corrections. Andrew Parent and Louis Harkey often saw our patients for us when we were writing. The residents did more than their share also. The Learning Resource Center at the University of Mississippi offered suggestions as well as service.

Lucia Griffin was the project coordinator. She was tremendously capable and organized, and she assisted with editing the manuscript. She was assisted by Mary Jackson. Many others contributed time, effort, and enthusiasm.

Contents

Figure Credits

Figure 1.1. By permission of WL Fox. *Dandy of Johns Hopkins*, Williams & Wilkins, Baltimore, 1984; ii.

Figure 9.2. Modified by permission of AA Zeal and AL Rhoton, Jr. *J Neurosurg.* 1978; 48:541.

Figure 12.3. By permission of M Ono, M Ono, AL Rhoton, Jr, and M Barry. *J Neurosurg.* 1984; 60:382.

Figure 12.4. Modified by permission of RG Martin et al. *Neurosurgery.* 1980; 6:489.

Figure 12.5. Modified by permission of G Hardy, DA Peace, AL Rhoton, Jr. *Neurosurgery.* 1980; 6:11.

Figure 12.6. By permission of AA Zeal and AL Rhoton, Jr. *J Neurosurg.* 1978; 48:537.

Figure 12.7. Modified by permission of AA Zeal and AL Rhoton, Jr. *J Neurosurg.* 1978; 48:538.

Figure 12.8. Modified by permission of AA Zeal and AL Rhoton, Jr. J Neurosurg. 1978; 48:544.

Figure 12.9. By permission of M Ono et al. *J Neurosurg.* 1984; 60:381.

Figure 12.10. Modified by permission of AA Zeal and AL Rhoton, Jr. *J Neurosurg.* 1978; 48:548.

1
The History of Aneurysm Surgery

Early in the eighteenth century, suggestions of intracranial aneurysms began to appear in the medical literature, largely through the work of prosectors. Morgagni of Padua[1] described dilatation of the posterior branch of both carotid arteries in 1761. Ruptured aneurysms were first reported in 1765 by Biumi of Milan.[2] In 1814, Blackall[3] published the report of a patient with subarachnoid hemorrhage (SAH) related to an intracranial aneurysm. This set the stage for recognition of the most common manifestation of the disorder. Wilks, who was also from Guy's Hospital, described a sanguinous meningeal effusion, again linking the clinical features associated with the anatomical lesion.[5] Perhaps the connection had been made centuries earlier.[6] Prior to the development of angiography, few aneurysms could be defined prior to the onset of hemorrhage. Occasionally, they presented as a neoplasm or mass lesion that could be seen on the pneumoencephalogram. In 1890, Keen[7] described Victor Horsley's operation on a patient with a large pulsating blood cyst. Much debate has taken place about whether this was an aneurysm or pituitary apoplexy with a capsule. Harvey Cushing[8] may have discovered a cerebral aneurysm in approaching what he perceived to be a pituitary tumor. In his description of the pituitary body and its disorders, he lists the case of an individual with bitemporal visual problems, hypopituitarism, and a probable interpeduncular aneurysm. In 1917, Cushing[9] ligated an internal carotid artery (ICA) intracranially after an aneurysm burst during surgery. The patient died shortly thereafter. In 1926, Cushing packed an aneurysm of the ICA with muscle, leading to hemiplegia; the patient subsequently died. At autopsy, however, the aneurysm was thrombosed. The preoperative diagnosis had been an intracerebral cyst.[10]

Church and Peterson[11] outlined the difficulty of diagnosing a cerebral aneurysm before the days of angiography. "Occasionally, a patient with a cerebral aneurysm is conscious of his pulsations and hears a bruit. Bruit may also sometimes be heard by auscultation of the cranium, but vascular murmurs have also been heard in the case of extensive softening and in vascular tumors."[11] The chief symptoms of aneurysms at this time resulted from pressure upon the cranial nerves and brain. Clinical symptoms were present in only about one third of the patients before rupture.

Egas Moniz[12] of Portugal demonstrated the first radiographic features of the cerebral vessels in 1927 by injecting contrast material, and, not long afterward, the use of cerebral angiography became commonplace. After Moniz's early description, aneurysms were demonstrated on angiograms by Dott[13] and again by Moniz.[14] Thus began the surgical history of intracranial aneurysms.

In 1939, McDonald and Korb[15] reviewed the old subject of intracranial aneurysms with a renewed interest that was important to surgeons. They reported 1125 cases of saccular aneurysms at the base of the brain verified by operation or autopsy. The youngest patient was $1\frac{1}{2}$ years old; the oldest, 87. Fifty-four percent were over 40 years old when they died. Ruptured aneurysms were three times as frequent on the anterior part of the circle of Willis as on the posterior part.

In 1933, Dott[13] described surgical approaches based on "arterioradiography." He is believed to be one of the first surgeons to operate on an aneurysm and to provide protective coatings to the vessel wall. By 1944, Walter Dandy[16] had operated on 64 verified intracranial aneurysms (Fig. 1.1). His observations concerning surgical treatment carry warnings that would hold for half a century:

> The surgical treatment of arterial aneurysms is exceedingly dangerous and so far, at least, has been unproductive of results. Complete ligation of the arteries of the neck is attended with gravity even in younger individuals. Once a hemorrhage occurs from an aneurysm, subsequent recurrence is almost certain. It is surprising, however, how many patients survive one of several ruptures before death finally results.[16]

Early Operations for Aneurysms

The first aneurysm case imaged antemortem was reported by Speiss and Pfeiffer.[17] A large calcified lesion was imaged on the skull roentgenogram and was con-

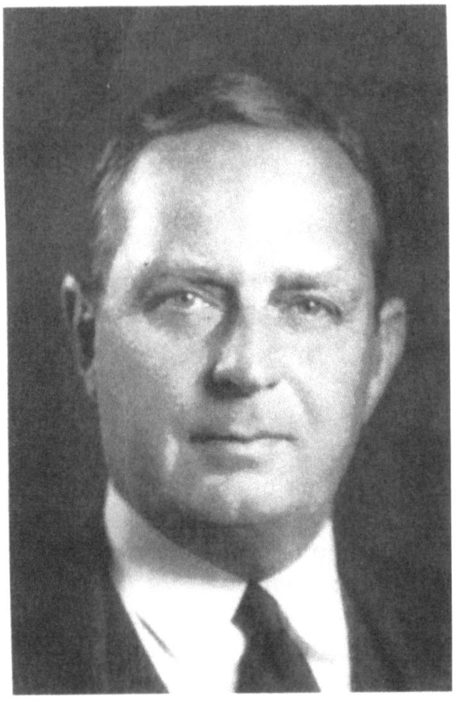

FIGURE 1.1. Walter Dandy (1886–1946) practiced neurosurgery at John's Hopkins Hospital and was the first to intentionally approach an intracranial aneurysm with direct surgery.

firmed later by autopsy. The authors concluded that this was not a rare condition, and it was possible to make an antemortem diagnosis from the clinical and radiographic findings. At this time, no definite therapy had been established. In 1939, Dandy[18] noted that the surgical attack upon aneurysms was just beginning. The first two successful direct attacks were recorded by McConnell.[19] Dott[13] also placed silver clips on both sides of an aneurysm, and Tonnis[20] exposed a cherry-sized aneurysm of the anterior communicating artery (AComA) shown by arteriography.

Others had used indirect attacks on intracranial aneurysms. Dott[13] reported his first cure in 1933, ligating the ICA in the neck. Walsh and Love[21] also reported a treatment whereby the ICA in the neck was tied. Subsequently, the oculomotor nerve palsy disappeared, and the patient returned to work. Jefferson[22] also cured a carotid cavernous aneurysm by this method. In one of his cases, however, contralateral motor weakness developed 36 hours after ligation of the ICA.[23] Dandy[18] equated subarachnoid bleeding with aneurysms of the circle of Willis. He also called attention to the large round hemorrhages that develop in the optic discs. As a result of these early descriptions, this clinical picture of SAH and of intracranial aneurysms became widely known.

Dandy[18] questioned the use of arteriography, which had been introduced in 1927 by Moniz. He feared thrombosis of the big arterial trunk and wondered if a negative arteriogram would confirm the absence of an aneurysm. He stated, "I can see little if any reason for its employment if the history and localizing neurological evidence is so convincing." He employed the Matas test to evaluate the safety of carotid ligation.[18] He recognized that late complications could still develop, but, if the patient failed the Matas test, carotid ligation was very likely to be followed by hemiplegia and probably death.

In 1946, Gardner[24] had introduced deliberate systemic hypotension for brain procedures by withdrawing large quantities of blood into a reservoir, a form of hypovolemic shock. Ganglionic blockade became available soon after and was used for aneurysm surgery in the early 1950s.

By the 1950s, surgical treatment had been well established. Pool[25] stated that bed rest without surgical intervention could no longer be regarded as effective treatment except for those who were very ill, elderly, or comatose. The combined mortality was at least 80% and had been reported as high as 87% for those who were treated nonsurgically. Technical developments made direct surgery safer and easier because small removable clips were available and hypothermia, used by Botterell et al.[26] in Toronto, had been introduced. It was believed that hypothermia protected the brain from the effects of temporary circulatory interference.

Pool[25] regarded the use of temporary clips advantageous in approaching aneurysms of the AComA complex. He was the first to employ early surgery. By the time he reported to the New York Academy of Medicine in 1959, he had operated 23 intracranial aneurysms by direct approach.[25] Five of these patients had died. Nineteen aneurysms had been approached early, less than 12 days after hemorrhage. Vasospasm was one of the most frequent causes of unfavorable results. Sencer[27] reviewed the Mount Sinai Hospital experience in 1963, noting 18 surgically treated patients, 15 of whom survived well beyond hospitalization.

Pool et al.[28] described two kinds of vasospasm. One was produced by stretching or manipulating vessels and would usually respond to 2% procaine or 3% papaverine. However, vasospasm already present as a result of a hemorrhage from an aneurysm would not respond to these agents. They attributed the vasospastic response that could be relieved by papaverine to trauma.[23]

From the earliest observations, it was recognized that aneurysms must be protected from the pressures of the arterial circulation. This concept led surgeons to develop techniques of proximal occlusion of parent artery feeders, wrapping, trapping, and, finally, neck ligation or clipping.

Wrapping

Wrapping, or investment, was first used by Norman Dott[13] in 1933. In this procedure, he reinforced the artery wall with a strip of muscle, and the patient was alive 4 years after the procedure. Others, including Dandy[16] and Logue,[29] however, questioned these methods. Drake,[30] Hamilton,[31] and Falconer,[32] on the other hand, reported many successful investment procedures, but, always, death due to rebleeding was a disappointing feature of this treatment.

Jaeger[33] was the first to use sheets of cotton to stimulate the development of a new fibrous coat to reinforce the lesion (30). Gillingham[34] also wrapped an aneurysm using sterile surgical gauze.

Several surgeons reported the use of surgical foam and plastic resins to invest aneurysms.[10,35–37] Oxyresins, silicone, rubber, and other tissue adhesives have all been employed. In many cases, however, complications occurred. The rate of early rebleeding (within less than 6 months) was 8.6% in the series of 60 cases reported by Todd et al.[38] Late rebleeding (within up to 10 years) was about 1.5% per year. Investment is less effective than occluding the neck of the aneurysm. Additionally, in cases of rebleeding, investment interferes with a secondary operative clipping. Nevertheless, in certain cases, it may be the only alternative to sacrificing a primary vessel that arises from the dome of an aneurysm. Some of the pioneer neurosurgeons had considerable difficulty with both clipping and ligation techniques.

Thrombosing Aneurysms

Theoretically, if a thrombus completely fills the aneurysm and a new endothelium proliferates along the parent vessel to occlude the neck, the aneurysm would be excluded from the cerebral circulation. Theory aside, it is still not clear that thrombosis of an aneurysm necessarily leads to permanent cure or that this method excludes the lesion from the arterial pressure or that the risk of rebleeding is actually reduced.

A muscle tamponade was the first method used to occlude an aneurysm. This type of occlusion was usually employed when, accidentally, the wall of the aneurysm was entered. Gallagher[39] tried placing mammalian hairs within aneurysms using a pneumatic gun. Mullan and co-workers[40] thought it possible to produce thrombosis with electrical current. They used a very small electrical current (200–2000 μA) applied over a course of several hours. At the time of his report in 1965, one of 12 patients had died, but none had rebled during the follow-up interval. Alksne and co-workers[41–43] used delicate iron filings to induce thrombosis. They held these in place with a powerful electric magnet introduced stereotactically near the aneurysm. Zubkov[23] introduced objects directly into the dome of aneurysms using stereotactic methods. Delicate latex balloons were also introduced by these methods to occlude the dome of the aneurysm and block the orifice.[23,44]

Ligatures

Dott[13] and Norlen and Olivecrona[45] were early proponents of ligating aneurysms. Generally, a relatively coarse ligature was selected because of its strength and to avoid damaging the fragile aneurysm during tying. Passing the ligature was less of a problem than the tying itself. Special instruments were developed to permit the passage of a ligature through a carrier that was then passed behind the aneurysm. A hollow tube of some kind was the most effective means. Since the ligature could not be tied with fingers, instruments were necessarily employed. As the era of microsurgery of aneurysms began, ligature passage was revived. A drawback of this technique, however, is that it is not always possible to know that the ligature is securely tied. An aneurysm that is turgid or pulsating after tying is an unfavorable sign.

Clipping

Clipping involves closing off the neck of an aneurysm with some type of metallic clip or clamp. Originally, V- or U-shaped clips were applied with forceps that would permit closure around the neck of the aneurysm. Once the clamps were closed, removal was virtually impossible. The U-shaped clamp had the advantage because it did not force the neck of the aneurysm forward during closure.

Removable clips, probably first introduced by Norlen and Olivecrona,[45] simply added wings to the apex of the V-clip, allowing it to be sprung open for removal. Eventually, it became apparent that some kind of spring-action clip was needed to reduce the stress and torsion of application and for safe removal. Mayfield[46] produced the first removable spring clip that could be implanted. Many sizes and shapes were developed and the clip became the mainstay of aneurysm surgery for many years. The smooth blades, however, allowed the Mayfield clip to migrate away from an aneurysm with pulsation, and the clip was modified by many surgeons to produce abrasions or scores on the blades to keep them from slipping. Heifetz's[47] clips were a further improvement, offering scored blades and small proximal wings for attachment to a special applicating forceps.

The development of aneurysm clips progressed parallel to that of the metallurgical sciences. In the beginning, all clips were fashioned from stainless steel. None of these, however, are currently acceptable for surgical implantation, because of corrosion. Presently, most clips are made from high-strength alloys of cobalt, nickel, molybdenum, and chromium. The same qualities that make a clip safe and compatible for magnetic resonance imaging (MRI) also make it corrosion-resistant. Clips that contain iron are not corrosion-resistant and also distort on exposure to high magnetic fields.[48]

The McFadden clip offered multiangle positioning using special applicators.[48] Yasargil and Fox[49] and Yasargil et al.[50] further refined the blades, making them more rounded so that they would slip smoothly through the microsurgical plane of the aneurysmal neck. The Sugita clip further refined the torsion and scissoring effect that seem to be inherent in small-bladed clips.[51] This superbly engineered clip included reinforcement at the crossing to increase its stability, allowing the blades to be even more delicate.[52] The delicate Sundt clips, which come in many configurations, are engineered to overcome the scissoring tendency and provide various closing pressures. They may be reinforced with other clips and the clip grafts may be used for torn vessels or aneurysms.[53]

As microsurgeons proliferated, the need for less obtrusive applicators and aneurysm clips became important. Solomon and Fukushima[54] reported the advantages of a small clip they developed for small craniotomy openings. The shaft of the applying forceps measures only 4.5 mm in width and has no angles to obstruct the surgeon's view of the operating field.

The History of Endovascular Surgery

The first attempts to exclude an aneurysm from the arterial circulation by thrombosis of the sac began in the early 1960s. Two landmark reports appeared in 1964. Gallagher[39] described a treatment in which a special gun was used to inject hog hair into an aneurysm, causing thrombosis of the sac. The operation was carried out by craniotomy rather than stereotaxically. Of 15 aneurysms operated using this injection technique, occlusion of the fundus was achieved in nine patients, but two of these subsequently died. In the same year, Luessenhop and Velasquez[55] introduced an artificial embolus into the carotid artery of a young female patient with acute SAH. The embolus was directed into the neck of the aneurysm, closing it with preservation of the ICA. Repeat angiography after 1 hour showed preservation of flow in the ICA and they withdrew the embolus that had been previously attached to a small suture. Repeat angiography showed thrombosis of the aneurysm with preservation of flow in the ICA. Unfortunately, after 10 hours, the patient died.[39] At postmortem examination, however, thrombus was found occluding the neck of the aneurysm.

In 1974, Mullan[56] described the stereotaxic introduction of copper wire and electrodes into an intracranial aneurysm. The results of 61 patients treated by this method were published. In 47 patients, complete thrombosis of the aneurysm had taken place with four deaths. In 1967, Bulgakov and Khilko[57] described their results in four patients using methods similar to Mullan's. They employed stainless steel electrodes measuring 0.1–0.2 mm in diameter. The electrodes were introduced stereotaxically. Electric currents of 2 mA were applied to the electrodes for periods ranging from 90 min to $3\frac{1}{2}$ hours. They also used coagulants in the form of ε-aminocaproic acid (EACA) to promote coagulation, but thrombosis was incomplete in all. However, all were large aneurysms, 1.5–2.0 cm in diameter. Of these four patients, two remained in good condition through 15 years of follow-up examination. One died from rebleeding 4 months after introduction of the coils, and, at postmortem examination, the aneurysm was found to be two-thirds thrombosed. However, rupture had occurred at the aneurysm neck in the remaining one-third without thrombosis.[57]

Bulgakov and Khilko[57] published their method of artificial thrombosis of intracranial aneurysms in 1968. These investigators employed coagulants and stasis of arterial blood flow to produce thrombosis in aneurysms. One week prior to operation, the patients were placed on a regimen consisting of EACA and calcium chloride while monitoring venous coagulation factors. After 1 week on this therapy, surgical stenosis of the cervical ICA was carried out, producing stasis in the arterial territory bearing the aneurysm. During the perioperative period, these authors administered large doses of EACA, fibrinogen, or dried plasma. Control of the coagulating factors was monitored carefully and angiography was carried out at repeated intervals during the course of treatment. The therapy was extended an additional week following operative stenosis of the ICA. They concluded that thrombosis occurred much more propitiously in aneurysms arising from long thin necks and less often in those with wide orifices. Among 33 patients subjected to this treatment, complete or near-complete thrombosis occurred in 20 patients. Partial thrombosis occurred in six patients, and two died from either their disease or treatment. In five patients, there was no effect on the aneurysm. Over an interval of 4 to 14 years, and in patients who had complete and incomplete thrombosis, there was no recurrent bleeding from the aneurysm.[57]

In 1965, Alksne and co-workers[41] described the use of iron carbonate to promote thrombosis in intracranial aneurysms. These authors used an electromagnet stereotaxically positioned against the dome of the aneurysm. Afterward, particulate iron particles were injected through an adjacent needle. The magnet was held in place during several days to maintain the iron particles in position. In 1977, Alksne and Smith[43] combined iron carbonate with methylmethacrylate as a hardening material. Only one patient was operated with good result using this method. In 1977, Kikut[58] stereotaxically focused an electromagnet on an intracranial aneurysm. Using 3000 erstadt, there was no evidence of brain injury caused by the intense magnetic fields. After preliminary use in 50 animals with synthetic aneurysms, Kikut employed this method in nine patients harboring recently ruptured intracranial aneurysms. In eight patients, he was able to demonstrate shrinkage of the luminal size as thrombus occluded the fundus.

These preliminary experiments in which thrombosis was induced in an intracranial aneurysm formed the basis for the development of the field of endovascular neurosurgery. The developments in this early period were necessarily hindered by inadequate imaging, inadequate control of the coagulation process, and incomplete methods for maintaining hemostasis in the aneurysm.

The development of modern endovascular surgery awaited the development of the balloon catheter.

Luessenhop and Velasquez[55] were perhaps the first to use embolization techniques for cerebral aneurysms. In 1964, they described a technique for catheterization of intracranial arteries and observations upon the vessels of two patients, one with an arteriovenous malformation (AVM) and the other with a bleeding saccular aneurysm.[55] They used catheters made from delicate flexible Silastic tubing upon which an enlarged inflatable tip was introduced. Using Polaroid films, the catheter tip was maneuvered into the luminal orifice of the saccular aneurysm and inflated with 50% Hypaque to its maximum capacity of 6 mm[55] (Fig. 1.2).

These experimental and clinical observations suggested that intraluminal manipulations within the circle of Willis were possible technically and that the arteries tolerated the procedures when the forces involved approximated those of systolic arterial pressure. These authors concluded that these catheterization techniques and embolization of intracranial arteries might have possible therapeutic uses in the treatment of AVMs and possibly arterial aneurysms. They further suggested that a variety of tips might be fashioned for the balloon catheter to allow them to be introduced into the aneurysm and held within the orifice or impacted there. Alksne[59] and Yodh et al.[60] attempted to improve upon the delivery of the balloon using electromagnetic systems. The method, however, has never realized clinical fruition.

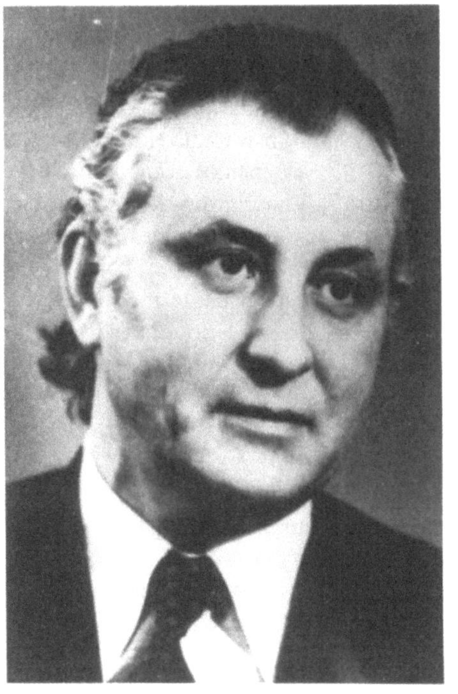

FIGURE 1.3. Fedor Serbinenko is Professor of Neurosurgery at the Burdenko Neurosurgical Institute in Moscow. He put into practice endovascular techniques and was the first to prepare and use a detachable balloon for the treatment of intracranial lesions, in this case, a carotid–cavernous sinus fistula.

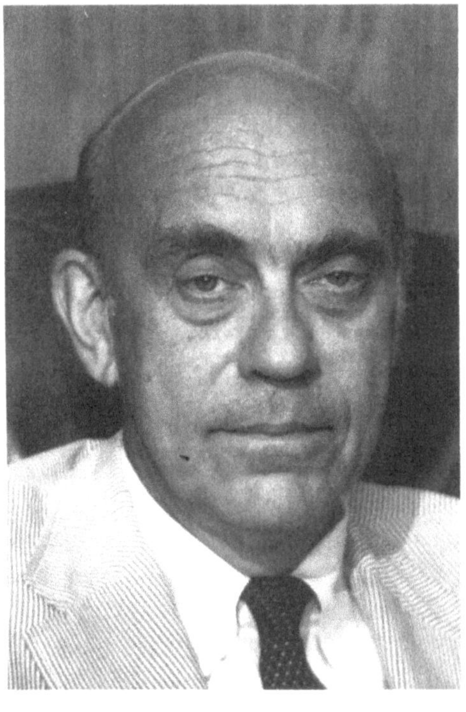

FIGURE 1.2. Alfred Luessenhop, MD, is Professor of Neurosurgery at Georgetown University. He introduced a balloon into an intracranial aneurysm in 1965, opening the way for endovascular surgery of intracranial aneurysms.

A more sophisticated concept of endovascular surgery was connected with the name of F. Serbinenko from the Burdenko Neurosurgical Institute in Moscow when he developed and applied clinically the method of catheterization and artificial occlusion of brain vessels.[61–64] He devised microballoons and catheters containing detachable balloons. Because blood flow and the nutrient arteries to vascular lesions were preserved, these methods fundamentally changed the operation for occluding aneurysms and AVMs (Fig. 1.3).

The Soviet experience can be summarized along two

lines: those that developed from artificial embolization and those that were based on catheter control of the embolus.[64] The former method depended on blood flow for determining the final path of the embolus. Catheter-guided embolization was developed only in the past 20 years. In 1972, Serbinenko and Filatov[64] described new techniques for manipulating the embolus. These authors used a helper balloon to guide the detachable balloon into the ideal site for permanent detachment. The helper balloon was used to occlude the middle cerebral artery (MCA), which diverted flow into the anterior cerebral artery (ACA), thus carrying the balloon for detachment into the aneurysm. Serbinenko[62] also reported the successful treatment of a basilar artery aneurysm by a detachable latex balloon.

In 1973, Zubkov[65] reported the obliteration of a supraclinoid aneurysm of the ICA that had not hemorrhaged. The aneurysm was safely occluded with a detachable balloon, preserving circulation in the ICA. This approach was via the carotid artery in the neck using a Teflon catheter and homemade latex balloon of original construction. The patient did well and was discharged. By 1980, Zubkov and co-workers[66–68,81] had operated on 24 patients for the occlusion of cerebral aneurysms using a detachable balloon catheter; some aneurysms were large or giant. Reconstructive operations, in which the parent artery was preserved, could be carried out in only nine of these patients.

In 1974, Khilko and Zubkov[44] first reported the use of silicone to occlude an aneurysm of the cervical portion of the ICA. In this case, a balloon was inflated proximally to protect the parent artery, while a second catheter was introduced into the aneurysm, which was filled with hardening silicone. In 1976, Zozulia and Shcheglov[69] reported their first series of endovascular procedures for intracranial aneurysms, eventually extending the results to 137 intravascular interventions performed in 119 patients. In 93 of these, aneurysms were occluded with preservation of the parent artery. In 11 cases, failure occurred and seven patients died.

Debrun and coauthors[70] presented their clinical series and careful approach to establishing the indications for endovascular procedures. Their critical analysis of their own cases led the way for further development of this emerging field. Debrun et al. showed that favorable results were obtained in seven of 10 patients treated for aneurysms of the carotid siphon. Reconstructive surgery in which the artery was preserved could be performed in only five patients.[70]

Several newer types of detachable balloon catheters have been developed and used experimentally over the last 15 years.[71–73] Higashida and co-workers[74] reported the results of endovascular treatment of aneurysms that were difficult to reach surgically, such as those that occupy the cavernous portion of the ICA. Between 1981 and 1987, 87 patients were subjected to this treatment. Preservation of the parent artery was achieved in only 19 cases (22%). Of these, 63% had total occlusion of the aneurysm and subtotal occlusion was achieved in 37%. In four cases, there were stroke-related embolic complications. Higashida[75] reported his results in 25 patients with 26 aneurysms involving the distal, vertebral, basilar, and posterior cerebral arteries. In 65% of these aneurysms, a balloon was placed directly into the aneurysm with preservation of the parent vessel. In nine of these, primary occlusion of the parent vessel was performed following test occlusion. Twenty (77%) of the cases had good-to-excellent angiographic results, and 15 (60%) of the patients continued to remain functionally intact and neurologically stable. This was encouraging since these aneurysms were considered difficult and also carried a high risk for surgical treatment.[75]

Berenstein et al.[76] published the results of their percutaneous embolization of intracranial aneurysms using detachable balloon techniques. In nine of these, the aneurysm resided on the cavernous portion, three on the petrous portion, one on the vertebral artery, and one on the posterior–inferior cerebellar artery. Before definitive treatment, these investigators used a double-lumen balloon catheter to evaluate the tolerance to acute occlusion of the carotid and vertebral arteries.

Since the beginning of endovascular surgery in 1964, many surgeons have turned to endovascular surgery for definitive treatment of cerebral aneurysms, and series of cases are currently being reported in the literature. As yet, many of these represent case reports, but no investigatory clinical trials have been carried out. In this first phase, however, the safety and effectiveness of the procedure has been demonstrated. In 1991, Moret and co-workers[77] reported treatment of 124 patients using balloon catheter techniques. In 22 of these cases, there had been acute SAH. In 1991, Shcheglov's aneurysm series included 867 cases treated by detachable balloon techniques.[78] In more than 90% of these patients, the parent artery had been preserved.

The investigation of both catheters and balloon materials continues. Presently, endovascular procedures are being carried out by physicians in several medical specialties. In addition to the anatomical achievements made in directing the balloon catheters into the cerebral lesion, a new field seems to be emerging for physiological testing of the effects of endovascular mechanisms. Currently, investigations are being carried out to learn how balloon techniques affect the cerebral vessels and what the long-term significance might be. Also, cerebral blood flow studies are being carried out along with other means of cerebrovascular testing to improve the safety of the methods.

The pioneering work for the treatment of cerebral vasospasm was carried out by Zubkov at the Polenov

Neurosurgical Institute in St. Petersburg. In 1980, while attempting to place a balloon into a supraclinoid aneurysm of the ICA, he noted that dilatation of the balloon relieved vascular constriction that was proximal to the aneurysm.[68] After vasodilatation, the constriction did not recur. Later, clinical improvement in grade was noted to be associated with radiographic relief of constriction.[4] He noted that dilatations carried out early (before patients developed fixed deficits and before arteriopathy had advanced) yielded much better results than when applied late (after fixed neurological deficits had appeared).[82] The method is currently being applied in many clinics and the results of the treatment for early cerebral vasospasm are encouraging.

In 1975, Gianturco and coauthors[79] apparently were the first to use coils to thrombose a vessel. They used detachable wire coils to occlude the renal artery in patients with hypernephroma. Hilal and co-workers[80] employed platinum microcoils introduced via an endovascular route into intracranial lesions. Since this time, numerous case reports have appeared in the literature in which platinum microcoils have been introduced into intracranial aneurysms and other vascular lesions. To some of these, silk material is attached to promote stasis and thrombosis. Up to the present time, however, there is no substantial series describing results and complications of treatment. Cases have remained largely anecdotal but encouraging to the individual surgeons who have used these methods.

Summary

The history of direct intracranial aneurysm surgery and the history of endovascular surgery tread the same ground. At first, the procedures were carried out during the cold period; the first attempts made required sacrifice of the parent artery supplying the arterial lesion. Later, both techniques accomplished the feat of preserving the parent artery. Still later, both methods turned to the acute hemorrhagic period, when most loss occurs.

The history of endovascular neurosurgery began with the propagation of a thrombus in the wall of an aneurysm. The methods have progressed as technology and imaging have advanced. Recent years have seen a return to the idea of using metallic microcoils to promote thrombosis. However, all treatments suffer from limitations, mainly ischemic and hemorrhagic complications. Incomplete obliteration of an aneurysm sac allows growth at the orifice and late rebleeding due to incomplete separation of the thin arterial wall from the dynamic forces of the intracranial circulation. Problems arising for the endovascular neurosurgeon are similar to those confronting the direct aneurysm surgeon: the fusiform aneurysm, the aneurysm that has important perforating arteries that exit from the fundus and dome, and the aneurysm with a wide orifice that will neither retain the materials placed within it nor effectively accept a clip.

At the present time, intravascular approaches versus conventional operative approaches and clipping are being evaluated. It is perhaps relevant at this time that some patients with some aneurysms respond best and most safely to intracranial operative clipping, whereas in others, endovascular approaches using balloons, coils, or other methods are preferred. The physician who cares for a patient with an intracranial aneurysm must often choose which approach is best suited for the patient and the aneurysm that he is treating. Much depends on facilities available and local technical expertise. Some patients may not be transportable to centers where endovascular methods are generally available. Likewise, certain aneurysms are not clippable by direct methods and must be managed with other operative techniques. To provide the best and safest treatment, the surgeon must be familiar with microvascular procedures such as end-to-end repair, endoaneurysmorrhaphy, and bypass procedures for cerebral protection, as well as with the endovascular approaches.

References

1. Morgagni JB. *De Sedibus et Causis Morborum per Anatomen Indagatis*, Book 1, letters 3 and 4. Venetis, ex typog. Remodiniana, 1769. Alexander B, trans. *The Seats and Causes of Diseases Investigated by Anatomy*. New York: Hafner; 1960;42–43, 77–78.
2. Biumi F. *Observations Anatomicae, Scholiis ilustratae*. Observatio V. In: Sandifort E (ed): Thesaurus Dissertationum, Vol 3. Milan, S & J Luchtmans, 1765 (reprinted 1778); 373.
3. Blackall J. *Observation on the Nature and Cure of Dropsies*. 2nd ed. London: Longman, Hurst, Rees, Orme and Brown; 1814.
4. Zubkov YN, Nikiforov BM, Shustin VA. First experience of dilatation of constricted cerebral arteries after aneurysmal SAH. *Vopr Neirokhir*. 1983;5:17–23.
5. Wilks A. Sanguineous meningeal effusion (apoplexy); spontaneous and from injury. *Guy's Hosp Rep*. 1859;5:119–127.
6. Wiseman R. *Eight Chirurgical Treatises*, 3rd ed. London: Tooke & Meredith; 1696.
7. Keen WW. Intracranial lesions. *Med News (New York)* 1890;57:439–449.
8. Cushing H. *The Pituitary Body and Its Disorders. Clinical States Produced by Disorders of the Hypophysis Cerebri*. Philadelphia: Lippincott; 1912:97–99.
9. Sosman MC, Vogt EC. Aneurysms of the internal carotid artery and the circle of Willis, from a roentgenological viewpoint. *Am J Roentgenol*. 1926;15:122–134.
10. Pool, JL, Potts DG. *Aneurysms and Arteriovenous Anomalies of the Brain. Diagnosis and Treatment*. New York: Harper and Row; 1965:45.
11. Church A, Peterson F. *Nervous and Mental Diseases*. Philadelphia and London: WB Saunders Co; 1922:260.

12. Moniz E. L'encephalographie arterielle, son importance dans la localisation des tumeurs cerebrales. *Rev Neurol.* 1927;2:72–90.
13. Dott NM. Intracranial aneurysms: cerebral arterioradiography: surgical treatment. *Edinburgh Med J.* 1933;40 (section on Trans Med Chir So Edinburgh): 219–234.
14. Moniz E. Aneurysme intra-cranien de la carotide interne droite rendu visible par l'arteriographic cerebrale. *Rev Oto-Neuro-Ophthal.* 1933;11:746–748.
15. McDonald CA, Korb M. Intracranial aneurysms. *AMA Arch Neurol Psychiat.* 1939;42:298.
16. Dandy WE. *Intracranial Arterial Aneurysms.* Ithaca, NY: Comstock Publishing Co, Inc; 1945:133.
17. Speiss and Pfieffer. Ref In: Grodel FM. Roentgendiagnostik in der innern Medizin und der Grenzgfbieter. In: Lehmann, JF ed. *Lehmann's Med. Atlanten,* 3rd ed. Munich: 1921, VII:132 (atlas pl. 58).
18. Dandy WE. The treatment of internal carotid aneurysms within the cavernous sinus and the cranial chamber. *Ann Surg.* 1939;109:689–711.
19. McConnell AA. Subchiasmal aneurysm treated by implantation of muscle. *Zentralbl F Neurochir.* 1937;5–6:269.
20. Tonnis W. Erfolgreiche Behandlung eines Aneurysma der Art. commun. ant. cerebri. *Zentralbl Neurochir.* 1936;1:39–42.
21. Walsh MN, Love JS. Intracranial carotid aneurysm—successful surgical treatment. *Proc Staff Meeting Mayo Clinic.* 1937;12:81–88.
22. Jefferson G. On the saccular aneurysms of the internal carotid artery in the cavernous sinus. *Br J Surg.* 1938;26: 267–302.
23. Khilko VA, Zubkov YN. *Endovascular Neurosurgery.* Leningrad: Medicina; 1982:216.
24. Gardner WJ. Clinical notes, suggestions and new instruments: the control of bleeding during operation by induced hypotension. *JAMA* 1946;132:572–574.
25. Pool JL. Early treatment of ruptured intracranial aneurysms of the circle of Willis with special clip technique. *Bull NY Acad Med.* 1959;35:357–369.
26. Botterell EH, Lougheed WM, Scott JW, Wandewater SL. Hypothermia and interruption of carotid or carotid and vertebral circulation in the surgical management of intracranial aneurysms. *J Neurosurg* 1956;13:1–42.
27. Sencer W. A study of subarachnoid hemorrhage and intracranial aneurysm. *J Mt Sinai Hosp.* 1963;30:302–323.
28. Pool JL, Jacobson S, Fletcher TA. Cerebral vasospasm—clinical and experimental evidence. *JAMA.* 1958;167:1599–1601.
29. Logue V. Surgery in spontaneous subarachnoid haemorrhage: Operative treatment of aneurysms on anterior cerebral and anterior communicating artery. *Br Med J* 1956;1: 473–479.
30. Drake CG. Further experience with surgical treatment of aneurysms of the basilar artery. *J Neurosurg.* 1968;29:372–392.
31. Hamilton JG, Falconer MA. Immediate and late results of surgery in cases of saccular intracranial aneurysms. *J Neurosurg.* 1959;16:514–541.
32. Falconer MA. Progress in the surgical treatment of spontaneous cerebral hemorrhage. *Proc R Soc Med.* 1956;49:166–169.
33. Jaeger R. Aneurysm of the intracranial carotid artery. syndrome of frontal headache with oculomotor nerve paralysis. *JAMA.* 1950;142:304–309.
34. Gillingham FJ. The management of ruptured intracranial aneurysm. *Ann R Coll Surg.* 1958;23:89–117.
35. Hamby WB. *Intracranial Aneurysms.* Springfield, IL: Charles C Thomas; 1952.
36. Selverstone B. Coating of intracranial aneurysms with nontoxic adherent plastics. In: Schmidek HH, Sweet WM, eds. *Current Techniques in Operative Neurosurgery.* New York: Grune and Stratton; 1977:31–40.
37. Steelman HF, Hayes GJ, Rizzoli HV. Surgical treatment of saccular intracranial aneurysms. *J Neurosurg.* 1953;10: 564–576.
38. Todd EM, Crue BL Jr. The coating of aneurysms with plastic materials. In: Fields WS, Sahs AL, eds. *Intracranial Aneurysms and Subarachnoid Hemorrhage.* Springfield, IL: Thomas; 1965:357–371.
39. Gallagher JP. Pilojection for intracranial aneurysms: report of progress. *J Neurosurg.* 1964;21:129–134.
40. Mullan S, Raimondi AJ, Dobben G, Vailati G, Hekmatpanah J. Electrically induced thrombosis in intracranial aneurysms. *J Neurosurg.* 1965;22:539–547.
41. Alksne JF, Fingerhart AG. Magnetically controlled metallic thrombosis of intracranial aneurysms: a preliminary report. *Bull Los Angeles Neurol Soc.* 1965;3:154–155.
42. Alksne JF, Rand RN. Current status of metallic thrombosis of intracranial aneurysms. *Prog Neurol Surg.* 1969;3: 212–274.
43. Alksne JF, Smith RW. Iron-acrylic compound for stereotaxic aneurysm thrombosis. *J Neurosurg* 1977;47:137–141.
44. Khilko VA, Zubkov YN. Intravascular surgery in pathological states vascularized by the external carotid artery, and stenotic and occlusive processes of cerebral arteries [in Russian]. In: *Endovascular Neurosurgery.* Leningrad, Russia: Medicina; 1982:173–174.
45. Norlen G, Olivecrona H. The treatment of the aneurysms of the circle of Willis. *J Neurosurg.* 1953;10:404–415.
46. Mayfield FH, Kees G Jr. A brief history of the development of the Mayfield clip. *J Neurosurg.* 1971;35:97–100.
47. Heifetz MD. A new intracranial aneurysm clip. *J Neurosurg.* 1969;30:753.
48. McFadden JT. Evolution of the crossed-action intracranial aneurysm clip: technical note. *J Neurosurg.* 1989;71:293–296.
49. Yasargil MG, Fox JL. The microsurgical approach to intracranial aneurysms. *Surg Neurol.* 1975;3:7–14.
50. Yasargil MG, Vise WM, Bader DCH. Technical adjuncts in neurosurgery. *Surg Neurol.* 1977;8:331–336.
51. Sugita K, Hirota T, Iguchi I, Mizutani T. Comparative study of the pressure of varios clips. *J Neurosurg.* 1976;44: 723–727.
52. Sugita K, Kobayashi S, Kyoshima K, Nakagawa F. Fenestrated clips for unusual aneurysms of the carotid artery. *J Neurosurg.* 1982;57:240–246.
53. Sundt TM Jr, Nofzinger JD. Clip-grafts for aneurysm and small vessel surgery. 1: repair of segmental defects with

clip-grafts; laboratory studies and clinical correlations. 2: clinical application of clip-grafts to aneurysms; technical considerations. *J Neurosurg*. 1967;27:477–489.
54. Solomon RA, Fukushima T. New aneurysm clip appliers for "key-hole" neurosurgery. *Neurosurgery*. 1991;28:474–476.
55. Luessenhop AJ, Velasquez AC. Observations on the tolerance of the intracranial arteries to catheterization. *J Neurosurg*. 1964;21:85–91.
56. Mullan S. Experiences with surgical thrombosis of intracranial berry aneurysms and carotid cavernous fistulas. *J Neurosurg*. 1974;41:657–670.
57. Bulgakov NP, Khilko VA. Artificial thrombus formation like method of treatment of some arterial aneurysms of brain vessels. In *Clinical Diagnostic and Surgical Treatment Vascular Pathology of Brain*. Leningrad, Russia: 1968:157–159.
58. Kikut RP. *Using of magnetic-biological effects in treatment of arterial aneurysms of brain vessels*. Moscow, 1977. Thesis.
59. Alksne JF. Magnetically controlled intravascular catheter. *Surgery* 1968;64:339–345.
60. Yodh A, Pierce N, Weggel R. A new magnetic system for intravascular navigation. *Med Biol Engl*. 1968;6:143–147.
61. Serbinenko FA. Catheterization and occlusion of brain magistral vessels. First Congress of Neurosurgeons USSR. Moscow; 1971;1:114–119.
62. Serbinenko FA. Catheterization and occlusion of major cerebral vessels and prospects for the development of vascular neurosurgery. *Vopr Neirokhir*. 1971;35:17–27.
63. Serbinenko FA. Balloon catheterization and occlusion of major cerebral vessel. *J Neurosurg*. 1974;41:125–126.
64. Serbinenko FA, Filatov YM. Method of catheterization of anterior cerebral artery. Proceedings of the Third Neurosurgical Conference of the Baltic Republics, Riga: 1972: 160–162.
65. Serbinenko FA. Possibilities of catheterization and occlusion of cerebral vessels. In: *Materials of Plexus of Problem-commission Neurosurgical and Neurologist*. Sverdlovsk: 1973:91–102.
66. Ugrjumov VM, Kesaev SA, Zubkov YN. Endovascular operations in system of surgical treatment of brain vessel pathology. In: *Clinics and Surgical Treatment of Brain Pathology* [in Russian]. Leningrad, Russia: 1979;15–19.
67. Zubkov YN. *Treatment of Patients with Intracranial Arterial Aneurysms in Hemorrhagic Period*. Leningrad, Russia; 1990:297. Thesis.
68. Zubkov YN, Matsko DE. Some clinico-anatomical peculiarities of large and giant cerebral vessel arterial aneurysms. *J Neurol Psychiatry*. 1980;12:1809–1812.
69. Zozulia YA, Shcheglov VI. Intravascular operations with balloon catheter in cerebrovascular disease and brain tumors [in Russian] *Vopr Neirkhir*. Jan–Feb 1976:7–12, English abstract.
70. Debrun G, Lacoun P, Caron J, Hurth M, Comoy J, Keravel Y. Detachable balloon and calibrated-leak balloon techniques in the treatment of cerebral vascular lesions. *J Neurosurg*. 1978;49:635–659.
71. DiTullio MV, Rand RW, Frisch E. Detachable balloon catheter: its application in experimental arteriovenous fistulae. *J Neurosurg*. 1978;48:717–723.
72. Laitinen L, Servo A. Embolization of cerebral vessels with inflatable and detachable balloons: technical note. *J Neurosurg*. 1978;48:307–308.
73. Taki W, Handa H, Yamagata S, Matsuda I, Yonekawa Y, Ikada Y, Iwata H. Balloon embolization of a giant aneurysm using a newly developed catheter. *Surg Neurol*. 1979;12:363–365.
74. Higashida RT, Halbach VV, Dowd C, Barnwell SL, Dormandy B, Bell J, Hieshima GB. Endovascular detachable balloon embolization therapy of cavernous carotid artery aneurysms: results in 87 cases. *J Neurosurg*. 1990;72:857–863.
75. Higashida RT. Detachable balloon embolization therapy of posterior circulation intracranial aneurysms. *J Neurosurg*. 1989;71:512–519.
76. Berenstein A, Ransohoff J, Kupersmith M, Flamm E, Graeb D. Transvascular treatment of giant aneurysms of the cavernous, carotid and vertebral arteries: functional investigation and embolization. *Surg Neurol* 1984;21:3–12.
77. Moret J, Boulin A, Mowad M, Castaings L. Endovascular treatment of berry aneurysms by endovascular balloon occlusion. *Neuroradiology*. 1991;33(suppl):135–136.
78. Fox AJ. Highlights of the First Congress of the World Federation of Interventional and therapeutic Neuroradiology; October 11–13, 1991; Zurich, Switzerland. *AJNR* 1992;13:1021–1024.
79. Gianturco C, Anderson JH, Wallace S. Mechanical devices for arterial occlusion. *Am J Roentgenol*. 1975;124:428–435.
80. Hilal SK, Khandji AC, Chi TL, Stein BM, Bello JA, Silver AJ. Synthetic fiber-coated platinum coils successfully used for the endovascular treatment of arteriovenous malformations, aneurysms and direct arteriovenous fistulas of the CNS. *AJNR*. 1988;9:1030.
81. Zubkov YN. Catheterization of cerebral vessels. *Annals of the Polenov Neurosurgical Institute*. 1973;5:228–233.
82. Zubkov YN, Nikiforov BM, Shustin VA. Balloon catheter technique for dilatation of constricted cerebral arteries after aneurysmal SAH. *Act Neurochir*. 1984;70:65–79.

2
Pathology and Classification of Cerebral Aneurysms

Debate continues over whether environment, stress factors, or congenital defects are the most important contributors to the pathogenesis of cerebral aneurysm. Anatomically, the cerebral arteries are quite different from their counterparts outside the cranium. In general, their intima and media are much thinner, and they have a much more conspicuous internal elastic lamina. The media, consisting primarily of a thin layer of smooth muscle cells, is occasionally absent at bifurcations, thus leading to the idea that, since aneurysms develop at these locations, the two are interrelated.

In 1887, Eppinger[1] described defects in the elastic layer of vessels and related them to "congenital aneurysms." Degenerative and atheromatous processes also were given some credit.

Forbus[2] believed that the intima bulged through a weak medial defect and then underwent secondary degeneration. Forster and Alpers[3] observed defects in the medial layer and concluded that congenital rather than traumatic factors were more important. In the 1950s, Bremer[4] favored the idea of a congenital origin for aneurysms.

Forbus[2] found medial degeneration and fragmentation of the internal elastic membrane due to continued overstretching. Stehbens,[5-7] on the other hand, questioned the role of medial defects. He found medial defects in all animal species that he studied, but in only one animal, an 8-year-old chimpanzee, could he identify an intracranial aneurysm that had been responsible for subarachnoid hemorrhage (SAH). Glynn[8] concluded that the medial defect may play no part in the development of an aneurysm. He found these defects not only in 10 cases in which aneurysms were present, but also in 13 of the 15 control cases. Forster and Alpers[3] reviewed anatomical defects and pathological changes in the arteries of eight patients who died of aneurysms. Connective tissue plays a role in maintaining the integrity of the vessel wall.[9]

Wilson and co-workers[10] concluded that anomalous formations of the circle of Willis could contribute to the development of aneurysms. Hyperplasia of one or more segments or persistence of channels was significant. Vessels that perform maximum work, such as those that supply an arteriovenous malformation (AVM), are often those from which cerebral aneurysms arise. Likewise, when hypoplasia occurs in one segment, the A_1 segment, for example, the opposite vessel supplies both anterior cerebral arteries and usually harbors the aneurysm when it is present. Both Alpers and Berry[11] and Riggs and Rupp[12] also noted that the configuration of the cerebral circulation was important. In patients having aneurysms, the basal circulation was "normal" in 21%; some type of deformity occurs in 79%.

Most investigators believe either congenital or degenerative factors are involved in aneurysm formation. Proponents of the congenital hypothesis accept the view that there is some inherent weakness in the wall of the artery, either in the muscular layers or in the collagen structure. Proponents of the degenerative theory accept the view that the arterial wall partly degenerates, leading to a weakness through which the intimal layers gradually herniate. The weakness is the progenitor, and other factors such as arterial hypertension further lead to herniation of the sac. The third hypothesis encompasses both theories. Proponents believe that there must be inherent weakness in the vessel wall, but, later, the degenerative changes accelerate this weakness. Recently, many investigators have recognized that the age of onset, between 50 and 60 years of age, favors some degenerative condition.[13]

Classification Based on Pathogenesis

Intracranial aneurysms may be broadly classified into fusiform and saccular types. Saccular aneurysms, generally, arise near bifurcations of vessels, and are probably caused by focal weaknesses or degenerative processes in a portion of the arterial wall. Anatomically, they consist of a neck, a body, and a dome. Fusiform aneurysms arise diffusely and may involve most of the vessel wall but not necessarily all of it. They have a long and often tortuous course but may be quite asymmetrical in form.

Recently, the underlying mechanism for the formation of at least some intracranial aneurysms has become known. This has led to investigators proposing a number of classification schemes based upon these factors.[14,15] The classification of Medvedev and Matsko[16] details the many pathological processes that have been identified as directly relating or contributing to aneurysm development (Table 2.1).

There are, no doubt, other direct causations or contributing factors to aneurysm formation; in pregnancy, in childhood, and in families, the causes may be multifactorial.

TABLE 2.1. Classification of pathological processes contributing to aneurysm development

1. Bifurcation-hemodynamic aneurysms (BHA), formerly the so-called congenital
   - 1.1 Systemic arterial hypertension
     - 1.1.1 Hypertensive disease (essential hypertension)
     - 1.1.2 Polycystic renal dysplasia
     - 1.1.3 Aortic coarctation
     - 1.1.4 Other types of systemic arterial hypertension
   - 1.2 BHA in regional hemodynamic disorders
     - 1.2.1 Arteriovenous malformation
     - 1.2.2 Fibromuscular dysplasia
     - 1.2.3 Nishimoto–Takeushi–Kodo disease (moyamoya)
     - 1.2.4 Craniocerebral trauma (see 4.2.1 Hemodynamic stress)
     - 1.2.5 Malformations of cerebral arterial circulation
   - 1.3 BHA with unidentified hemodynamic component
2. In certain hereditary mesenchymopathies
   - 2.1 Marfan's syndrome (dystrophia mesodermalis congenital)
   - 2.2 Ehlers–Danlos syndrome (fibrodysplasia generalisata)
3. Degenerative necrotic
   - 3.1 Atherosclerotic
   - 3.2 Hypertensive (intracerebral military)
   - 3.3 Radiational (see 8.2 Postradiational)
4. Traumatic (in craniocerebral trauma)
   - 4.1 Direct (primary) lesion area
   - 4.2 Outside the direct lesion area
     - 4.2.1 Hemodynamic stress (see 1.2.4 Craniocerebral trauma)
     - 4.2.2 Secondary arterial lesions
5. Inflammatory aneurysms (see 6.1 and 6.2)
6. Embolic aneurysms
   - 6.1 Bacterial (microbial)
   - 6.2 Mycotic (fungal)
   - 6.3 Oncogenic
     - 6.3.1 "Benign" (in atrial myxomas)
     - 6.3.2 "Malignant" (in malignant tumors)
7. Dysembryogenetic aneurysms and aneurysm-like formations
   - 7.1 "Childhood"
   - 7.2 From the so-called residual vessels
   - 7.3 Infundibular widening of posterior communicating artery ostium
   - 7.4 Dolichoectasia
8. Iatrogenic Aa
   - 8.1 Postsurgical
   - 8.2 Postradiational (see 3.3 Radiational)
9. Others
   - 9.1 Friedreich syndrome (ataxia herediatrica)
   - 9.2 Blum syndrome (telangiectasia faciales)
   - 9.3 Pompe disease (systemic glycogenesis type II)

Aneurysmal rupture has been associated with pregnancy and the puerperium and probably is the most common presentation. The location(s) on the arterial tree in pregnancy is not unique, and they occur in approximately the same proportion as seen in nonpregnant patients. The treatment must be individualized, however, to take into consideration labor and delivery. Aneurysms seem prone to rupture during the seventh and eighth months of pregnancy and at delivery. There are a number of reasons why the pregnant patient is more susceptible to SAH. Increased blood volume, increased generalized edema, and increased arterial pressure occur during pregnancy, labor, and delivery.[17]

In Cannell and Botterell's[18] series, some patients were sectioned and others were delivered vaginally. The series was small, but there was no clear advantage for caesarean section, according to these authors. Hypotensive anesthesia was used in two patients at 18 and 33 weeks' gestation. Both infants survived, showing no cerebral damage attributable to hypoxia. There is considerable theoretical risk. According to Pedowitz and Perell,[19] SAH is the most common cerebral vascular complication encountered during pregnancy. They reviewed 79 cases and reported two others. It appears that the risk of rupture of cerebral aneurysms parallels the hemodynamic changes, reaching an apex in the third trimester in concert with blood volume changes. One percent of the cases reported occurred near or at term. However, hemorrhage was recorded in 25% of those who bled either during labor or in the first 24 postpartum hours. They concluded that the hemodynamic changes of pregnancy were a much greater precipitating factor for hemorrhage than the stress of labor, when vaginal delivery was undertaken. Diaz and Sekhar[17] reviewed the records of 154 pregnant patients with verified intracranial hemorrhage. One hundred and eighteen (77%) of these were due to intracranial aneurysms. The 30th through 34th weeks seemed to be a particularly risky period for intracranial hemorrhage but the method of delivery was not significantly important. Eleven patients died before delivery. The fetal mortality was 11% for cesarean and 20% for vaginal delivery.

The surgical treatment of cerebral aneurysms has advanced considerably since these reports were published, and anesthetic methods have become much safer. Therefore, it is our present belief that if the mother is in fair neurological condition and surgery can be performed early for clipping of the aneurysm then immediate cesarean section should be undertaken if a viable infant is to be expected. Then, without delay, the aneurysm should be surgically managed.

Aneurysms are rare in both infants and children. The incidence in patients under 20 years of age makes up only

1.5% to 4.6%. The sites of origin are somewhat different from those in adults, and the configuration may be unusual. Heiskanen[20] reviewed the children's cases encountered among 1346 aneurysm patients in Helsinki. Sixteen were under 20 years of age (1.2%). In this series, the most common sites, were the anterior communicating artery (AComA) and the internal carotid artery (ICA) at the posterior communicating junction. Multiple aneurysms were rare. One case was associated with coarctation of the aorta. Heiskanen feels the results of microsurgery on aneurysms in childhood are perhaps better than in adults, provided that good clinical grade patients are seen. Overall management mortality, however, is still high—39–46%.

A familial relationship in the development of intracranial aneurysms has been established. Ayer[21] mentioned cases among cousins of ages 6 and 10. Chambers et al.[22] were the first to emphasize intracranial aneurysm development in a father and son (11). Hemorrhage occurred in this family within a few months of each other. Phillips[23] reported aneurysms in sisters, both of whom presented with SAH due to aneurysms at the ICA.

Arterial aneurysms are also found in patients with moyamoya disease. Aneurysms occur in 10% to 15% of patients in whom a diagnosis of moyamoya disease is established angiographically. Aneurysms occur both on the diseased segment and on the counterpart normal vessels. Since the hemorrhagic form of moyamoya disease is characterized by spontaneous hemorrhage, the differential diagnosis becomes especially complex in the patient harboring an aneurysm. There are two forms of moyamoya disease. In the childhood type, the ischemic symptom prevails. However, in the adult type or in those who survive childhood and carry their disease into the adult situation, intracranial hemorrhage becomes a factor to be considered. The prognosis in patients with cerebral aneurysm and moyamoya disease is quite unfavorable.

Cerebral aneurysms develop in patients with sickle cell disease or occur coincidentally in this lesion. Multiple aneurysms have been described in some patients with this disease. In our series, aneurysms were found in children and in young adults.[24] Widespread arterial lesions have been observed in patients with sickle cell anemia. The vessels of the conjunctiva are similarly affected, showing more profound changes in those afflicted with the homozygous entity.[25] The arterial lesions, at least in children, may be demonstrated with magnetic resonance angiography (MRA), which shows an intraluminal defect in the vascular distribution of the affected territory and correlates well with the arterial lesions observed on conventional angiography.[26] Since patients with sickle cell anemia undergo arteriography with great risk, they should be subjected first to studies that do not necessitate the injection of contrast materials.

Intracranial arterial aneurysms arise commonly in patients with anomalies of the basal cranial vessels and in those with diseases or structural abnormalities of these vessels. It is now possible to recognize many of these anomalies and variations in anatomical structure using ultrasound, magnetic resonance, and selective angiography. Abnormal embryogenesis results in the retention of primitive vessels and peculiarities in collateralization and anastomotic patterns.

The primitive trigeminal artery is the first branch of the primitive ICA and usually is obliterated in the embryo stage (Fig. 2.1). It persists into the adult stage in approximately 0.6% of the population who undergo angiography. Usually, this artery originates as the ICA enters the cavernous sinus. It originates also from the cavernous portion of the ICA at the apogee of the first forward curve. It passes extradurally and posteriorly, near the roots of the trigeminal nerve, to connect with the basilar artery (BA). The most frequent site of connection is between the superior cerebellar artery (SCA) and the anterior inferior cerebellar artery (AICA). Caudal to the anastomotic site, the BA is usually hypoplastic. This anomaly is associated with intracranial hemorrhage,

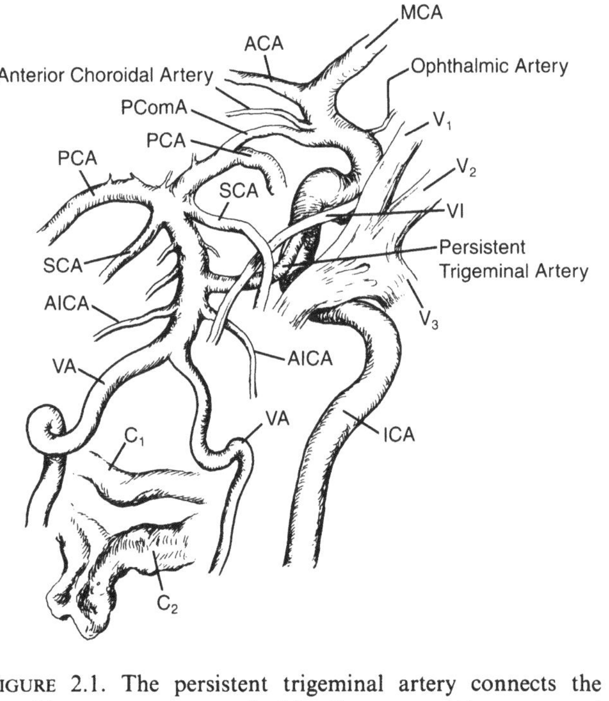

FIGURE 2.1. The persistent trigeminal artery connects the carotid system to the vertebral basilar system. The most usual location is shown. The relationship of the artery to the superior cerebellar artery and the sixth cranial nerve is shown in its typical form. ACA, anterior cerebral artery; AICA, anterior inferior cerebellar artery; ICA, internal carotid artery; MCA, middle cerebral artery; PCA, posterior cerebral artery; PComA, posterior communicating artery; SCA, superior cerebellar artery; VA, vertebral artery.

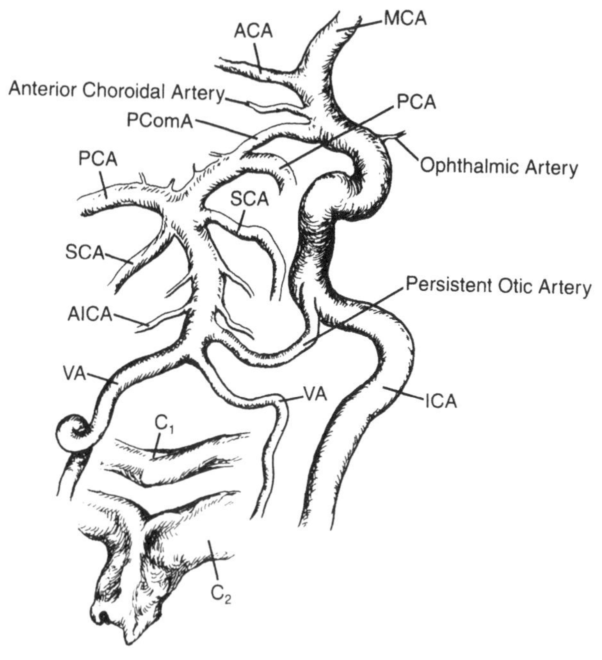

FIGURE 2.2. The relationship of the persistent otic artery is shown.

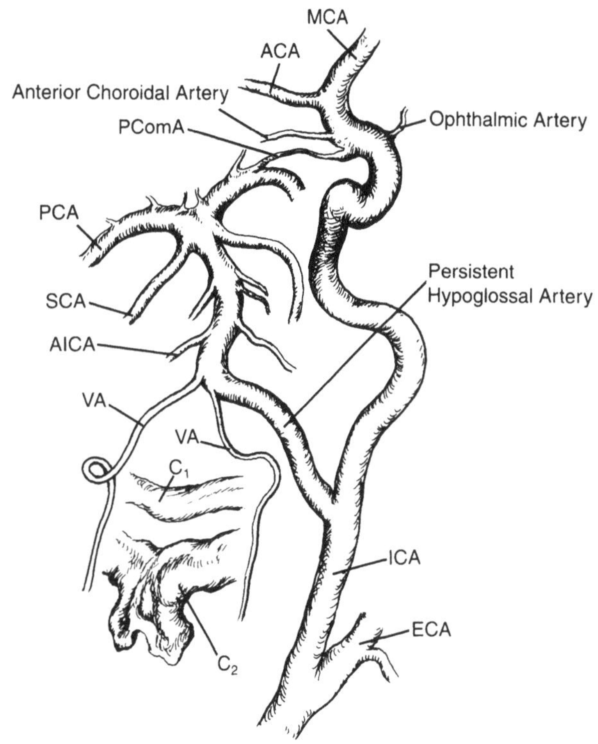

FIGURE 2.3. The persistent hypoglossal artery. The branch connects the internal carotid artery to the basilar artery. Both vertebral arteries are hypoplastic. ECA, external carotid artery.

from both aneurysms and AVMs. Although some aneurysms arise near the anastomotic site, they appear throughout the intracranial arterial tree as well. George and co-workers[27] reported that 14% of patients who have persistence of the primitive trigeminal artery also have intracranial aneurysms.

Persistence of the primitive otic artery is very rare (Fig. 2.2). This artery persists as the remnant of the hyaloid artery of the embryo. The primitive otic artery arises from the ICA in the pyramidal portion. It leaves the ICA at the superior and medial curve and passes through the internal auditory canal with the seventh and eighth cranial nerves entering the posterior cranial fossa. The primitive otic artery joins the caudal portion of the basilar trunk at this level beneath the pons. There is usually an associated aplasia or hypoplasia of the ipsilateral vertebral artery.

The primitive hypoglossal artery arises from the ICA in the cervical portion, between C_1 and C_3 (Fig. 2.3). It passes into the posterior cranial fossa through the hypoglossal canal with the hypoglossal nerve. It connects with the BA near the vertebrobasilar junction. It also occurs in association with other anomalies, the most common of which is aplasia or hypoplasia of the ipsilateral vertebral artery. There may be absence or aplasia of the ipsilateral posterior communicating artery as well.

The proatlantal intersegmental arteries arise due to maldevelopment of the vertebral arteries (Fig 2.4). The intersegmental artery originates from the carotid artery at the level of C_2 and C_3 and passes posteriorly to connect with the horizontal portions of the vertebral artery within the arch of C_1. Thereafter, the course follows that of the absent vertebral artery. It passes into posterior cranial fossa through the foramen magnum to join the opposite vertebral artery. The proatlantal intersegmental artery may also originate from the external carotid artery (ECA) proper or from the external carotid artery branches. Aplasia or agenesis of the ipsilateral vertebral artery is the most common associated anomaly.

One or both ICAs may fail to develop or may develop in a hypoplastic state. Most commonly, this anomaly is discovered incidentally during angiography in patients who have no vascular symptomatology. The primary collateral channels providing blood flow to the intracranial compartment are the vertebral and basilar arteries. In these cases, the BA becomes large and tortuous, and when the course leads the BA into contact with cranial nerves, the presenting signs may be associated with cranial nerve loss (usually the lower cranial nerves). Collateral channels also develop from the opposite ICA and from the opposite vertebral artery (VA). These anomalies, however, are quite rare, and only a few cases of each variation have been described.

Transsellar anastomoses usually develop with aplasia

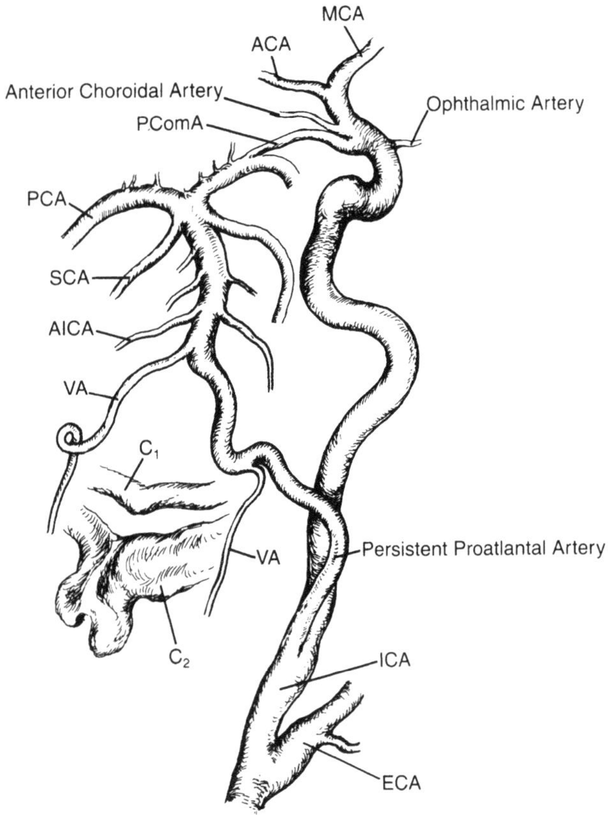

FIGURE 2.4. The persistent proatlantal artery connects the circulation of the internal carotid artery to the aplastic vertebral artery.

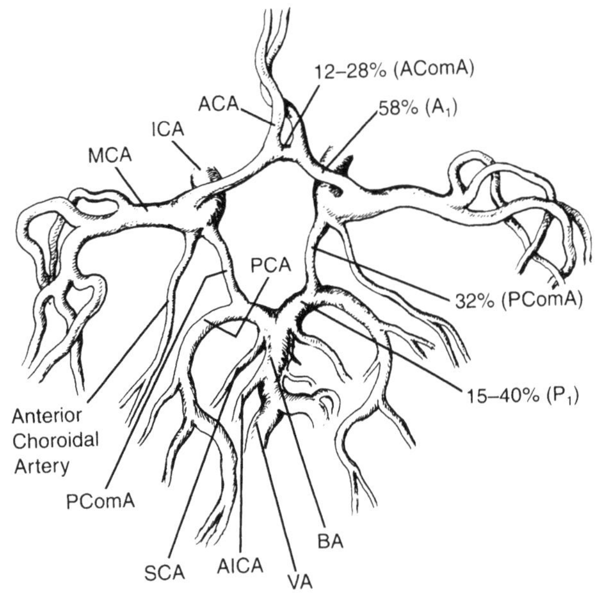

FIGURE 2.5. The ideal normal configuration of the circle of Willis is shown. The number in brackets indicates the incidence of abnormal anatomical configurations.

or hypoplasia of one ICA as a collateral channel. They pass through the base of the brain, probably extradurally to anastomose with the ICA of the opposite side intracranially. Intracranial intracarotid anastomoses also occur. The carotid artery may anastomose directly with the anterior cerebral artery (ACA) on the opposite side. The carotid artery may also anastomose with the AICA or SCA. An anastomosis may develop between the BA and the middle meningeal artery. All of these variations are quite rare, but they are mentioned here because intracranial aneurysms have been associated with these variations. They may occur at sites distant to the anastomosis or at the junction.

Abnormalities of the Circle of Willis

Located at the base of the brain, the circle of Willis provides blood flow via a collateral network (Fig. 2.5). The AComA connects the blood supply from the two separate hemispheres anteriorly. The posterior communicating arteries (PComAs) connect the anterior circulation to the vertebrobasilar system posteriorly and thereby interconnect the hemispheres. From dissection studies, it is known that the ideal circle of Willis, in which each vessel is made up of its average size, occurs rarely in any single individual. More often, hypoplasia and asymmetry occur in the circle of Willis of any individual patient. This occurs even more frequently in patients with intracranial arterial aneurysms. In 1966, Kirgis and coauthors[28] studied 1000 Willesian circles, 7% of which harbored aneurysms. Of the 26 patients with AcomA aneurysms, 58% also had hypoplasia of one A_1 segment. Hypoplasia was found overall in only 14% of the 1000 cases. Rhoton et al.[29] found a normal circle of Willis in 54% of their cases. The most common variation was hypoplasia of one PComA, and this occurred in 32% of the cases examined. In 26% of the cases, the anomaly was unilateral, but in 6% there was bilateral hypoplasia of the PComA segment. Kayembe and coauthors[30] studied 44 patients with intracranial arterial aneurysms and found asymmetry of the PComA in 36% and asymmetry of the A_1 in 23%. In only 11% was the pattern "normal" for the circle of Willis. In 148 circle of Willis studies, without aneurysm, the incidence of PComA asymmetry was 16%, A_1 asymmetry was absent in 11%, and no variations occurred in 46%.[31] More variations are encountered in the recurrent artery of Heubner. Yasargil and Smith[32] analyzed the variations in 283 AComA aneurysms operated in their clinic. Asymmetry of the A_1 segment was found in 78%. Aplasia of the A_1 was found in 4% and duplication of the A_1 in 2%. Hyperplasia of the A_1 was found in 71%

and a normal pattern in 29%. Interestingly, a triple A_2 was found in 6% of the cases, and a network, representing the AComA, in 3%. Partial duplication of the ACA occurred in 7% and duplication in 10%.

Five groups of diseases have been identified that lead to the development of intracranial aneurysms. Arteriosclerosis, infection, other inflammatory diseases, disorders of connective tissue, and tumors have all been implicated. The role that arteriosclerosis plays in the formation of aneurysms is unclear. Some aneurysms originate within an area of atheroma that involves the parent artery and extends into the neck. Courville[33] described pyramidal, fusiform, spherical, and multiple small outpouchings on arteries containing atheroma. Arteriosclerotic aneurysms may develop after the atheroma has destroyed the medial layer, allowing herniation of the intima (Fig. 2.6). They commonly originate at the bifurcation of an intracranial artery, also the most common site of atheroma formation. These also occur at the bifurcation of arteries in patients over 50 years of age who have arterial hypertension. Classification is made more complex by the fact that atheroma forms in the wall of some aneurysms secondarily, much like it forms in the artery wall.

The association of intracranial aneurysms with bacterial endocarditis was made early. In the series of 1125 aneurysms reported by McDonald and Korb,[34] 70 were thought to be definitely linked to mycotic origin (6.2%).

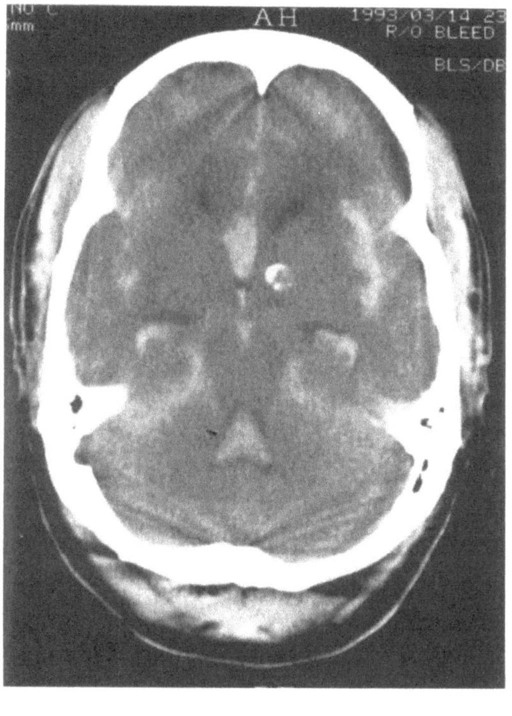

FIGURE 2.6 Severe diffuse subarachnoid and intraventricular hemorrhage associated with an arteriosclerotic aneurysm arising at the bifurcation of the left internal carotid artery.

In the series reported by Roach and Drake,[35] they made up 2.6%. Bacterial endocarditis fosters aneurysms quite infrequently, less than 5%. They postulated that a microscopic infected embolus lodges in the vasa vasora. However, in our studies, vasa vasora were found only on the first segment of the ICA; this is not the usual site for the development of bacterial aneurysms. The middle cerebral arteries (MCAs) and their branches are frequently involved, but the site is usually where an embolus impacts with the orifice of a small central perforating branch.

Intracranial arterial aneurysms develop in 2% to 10% of patients with subacute bacterial endocarditis (SBE).[36] Most of these aneurysms subsequently lead to intracranial hemorrhage. Fox,[37] summarizing the available data, found 175 arterial aneurysms in 140 patients with SBE. Eleven percent were on the ICA, 64% were on the MCA, 11% were on the AComAs, 8% on the PComA, and 6% to 7% were on the vertebrobasilar system. Usually, the bacterial aneurysm is peripherally placed and may be both saccular and fusiform in type. In 25 cases, Fox found more than one bacterial aneurysm. Typical SAH occurred in 18% of the patients. Ischemic disorders occurred in 11%, and tumor and epilepsy were encountered rarely. In 12%, the aneurysm was discovered incidentally. Seventy-one percent of the cases were associated with endocarditis, 11% had meningitis, 10% septicemia; rarely, thrombophlebitis of the cavernous sinus osteomyelitis, and skin abscess were also encountered. The bacterial origin in most cases was β-hemolytic streptococcus and *Staphylococcus aureus*. Pneumococcus and corynebacteria also were encountered. Fungal, syphilitic, spirochetal, and amoebic aneurysms also occur, but occur quite rarely.

Bacterial aneurysms seem to localize upon peripheral branches intraparenchymally. The predilection for these sites is determined apparently by the course of the infected embolus. After embolization, the organisms flourish, causing injury to the internal elastic membrane and endothelial layers. Later, the muscular layers and medial collagen network are broken through, allowing herniation of the newly formed endothelial layer through the defect produced. The microembolus apparently lyses and passes on, preserving blood flow in the vessel.[38]

Bacterial aneurysms have unpredictable bleeding rates, and while waiting for antibiotic treatment to be effective, rebleedings have occurred among our patients. In those cases in which the aneurysm is embedded in eloquent brain areas and significant resection would be required in order to obliterate the aneurysm, a course of antibiotic therapy is still warranted. When the lesion can be excised or clipped at low risk, this treatment should prevail.

Connective tissue disorders cause aneurysms by contributing to early degeneration of connective tissue layers. Among the causes listed are fibromuscular dysplasia, Ehlers–Danlos syndrome, Marfan's syndrome, pseudoxanthoma elasticum, lupus erythematosus, and the Osler–Weber–Rendu syndrome. Rubinstein and Cohen[39] reported the first association of an intracranial aneurysm with Ehlers–Danlos syndrome. The patient had defective collagen tissue and skin, hyperelastic skin, and elastic joints. An aneurysm developed on the ICA and caused SAH. At operation, the surgeon described the intracranial carotid artery as flimsy, virtually falling to pieces when touched. Other vessels seemed to be defective in collagen content. Neil-Dwyer et al.[40] studied type III collagen to type I collagen ratios in 17 patients undergoing surgery for ruptured cerebral aneurysms. In this group, 11 of the 17 were type III collagen deficient. All controls had normal collagen ratios. Type IV for Ehlers–Danlos syndrome is caused by a type III collagen deficiency, and these patients are known to harbor more intracranial aneurysms with increased frequency.[41,42]

Weir[43] listed the aneurysms associated with systemic tumors. Metastatic carcinoma of the arterial wall leads in frequency. Cardiac myxoma, choriocarcinoma, and carcinoma are the most likely offending neoplasms (Fig. 2.7). Aneurysms also develop from invasions by contiguous neoplasms such as carcinoma, glioma, or lymphoma; some aneurysms are associated with primary central nervous system (CNS) tumors such as meningiomas (29%), adenomas (26%), and gliomas (22%). In some

A

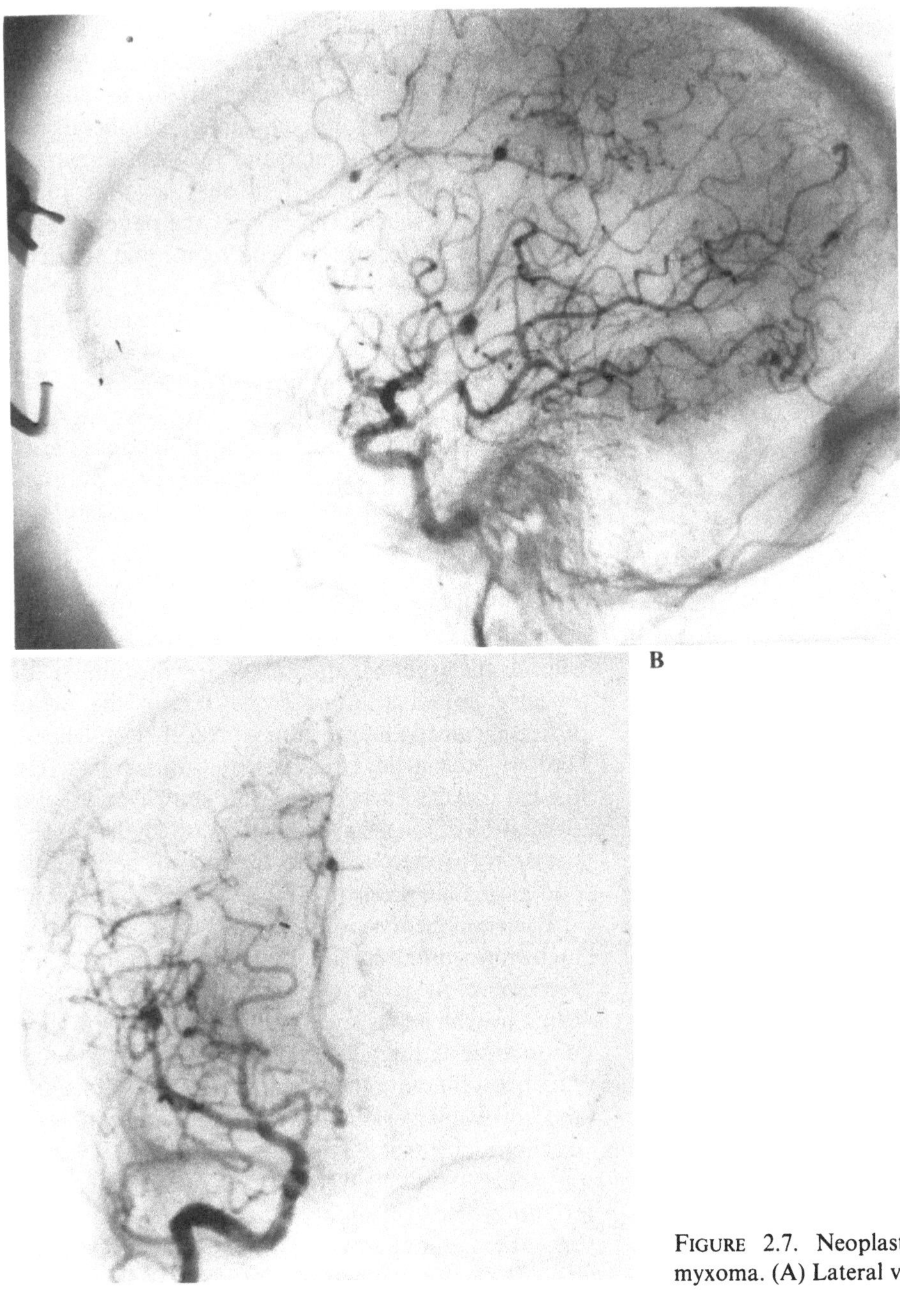

B

FIGURE 2.7. Neoplastic aneurysms associated with atrial myxoma. (A) Lateral view. (B) Anterior–posterior view.

cases, these aneurysms grow to giant size and present clinical features similar to intracranial tumors.

Neoplastic aneurysms develop where implantation of a malignant tumor occurs in a penetrating vessel. This occurs most often from tumors arising in the heart that embolize to the peripheral intracranial circulation. Other neoplastic aneurysms evolve from the invasion of adjacent vessels by nearby malignant tumors. In each case, however, the neoplastic cells penetrate the vessel wall, causing destruction of the internal elastic membrane.

In addition to the known etiological agents responsible for intracranial aneurysms, there are a number of conditions that have been poorly linked to the development of arterial aneurysms and yet, by association, must be included.

The coexistence of an intracranial aneurysm and an AVM is widely appreciated. However, the exact relationship between the aneurysm and the AVM has never been completely established. In general, the aneurysm occurs on vessels supplying the angioma. Whether both lesions represent an underlying defect in vascular development is unclear. Perhaps, and more likely, arteries supplying angiomas are subject to more flow and stress that somehow weakens the vessel wall.

AVMs often harbor intracranial arterial aneurysms, both on their feeding arteries and on adjacent normal arteries elsewhere. Arterial aneurysms are found in about 5% of the patients harboring AVMs, and, likewise, about 5% of patients with aneurysms harbor AVMs. The diagnosis of the source of an intracranial hemorrhage in the patient who has both an aneurysm and an AVM may create a diagnostic dilemma. In addition to hemorrhages, patients harboring both aneurysms and AVMs have only seizures as a first manifestation.

Over a period of time, the development of aneurysms seems to be logarithmic. Stehbens[44] identified two other anomalies in which intracranial arterial aneurysms have been found. Coarctation of the aorta and polycystic kidney disease are both congenital disorders associated with intracranial arterial hypertension, which may place additional stress upon the cerebral vessel. Stehbens found that, although many patients with coarctation also have bacterial endocarditis, the intracranial aneurysms almost invariably arise due to mechanical factors.

There are other conditions that seem to predispose to aneurysms or at least to make the presence of an aneurysm more difficult to manage. Bigelow[45] reviewed and commented on 32 acceptable cases of aneurysm associated with polycystic renal disease. By 1953, at least 20 patients with polycystic renal disease had suffered intracranial hemorrhage, and perhaps more had demonstrated aneurysms that had ruptured. The underlying problem leading to the development of both lesions is not entirely clear. Hypertension commonly accompanies polycystic renal disease and could be the underlying factor. Also, defects in connective tissue deposition may be present in both disorders. The link to hypertension, however, has been made in other instances. Coarctation of the aorta is a well-known progenitor of intracranial aneurysms, and we have observed stenosis of the renal artery as the etiology of hypertension in one case. Wright[46] collected 304 cases of coarctation of the aorta and found 16 intracranial aneurysms, causing death in 11 instances. Other vascular lesions have also been associated with polycystic renal disease, notably angioblastoma of the cerebellum and elsewhere in the CNS.

Traumatic aneurysms may be subcategorized into spontaneous and iatrogenic arterial wall injury. These may also be further classified into true aneurysms in which part of the arterial wall is present and false aneurysms in which a remnant of the blood clot forms the outer wall. Traumatic aneurysms occur on virtually any artery but more often on those susceptible to external trauma. The ACA in its relationship to the falx is a favorite site. The carotid artery in relation to the clinoid processes and the MCA as it becomes peripheral are also susceptible sites. Aneurysms may also arise from surgical manipulation along the tract of needle puncture sites or at the site of arterial anastomoses.

Traumatic aneurysms have been reported almost since the cause of SAH became known.[21] These are of several types. Pseudoaneurysms form when a major artery is torn and hematoma forms about it. If only the elastic lamina is torn, the intima bulges through the defect, producing a true traumatic aneurysm. These are found on susceptible vessels, such as the ACA in juxtaposition to the falx, the carotid artery adjacent to the tentorium, or the MCA near a bone flap or depressed fracture. As reported by Benoit and Wortzman,[47] the course of these lesions is treacherous. Over 50% have resulted in death due to hemorrhage.

Histology of the Aneurysm Wall

Recently, connective tissue deformation as a causative factor in aneurysm development has received more attention. In some patients with aneurysms of the aorta, defective collagen formation and deposition have been confirmed. In the case of cerebral aneurysms, the case is less clear. Patients with Ehlers–Danlos syndrome, in whom collagen type III formation is impaired, show a propensity toward cerebral aneurysm formation. In others, a pattern of type III abnormality has been shown in as many as 50%. However, when fibroblasts are grown in tissue culture from patients with intracranial aneurysms, they seem to produce normal amounts of this protein. Perhaps deposition could be at fault.[29]

Before the use of scanning electron microscopy and digestive techniques, most studies were aimed at the cellular structure of vessel walls, which is best observed under light microscopy. More recent studies in our laboratory have indicated that the structural integrity of any blood vessel is derived not from its cellular makeup but from its connective tissue. Multiple layers of intersecting collagen fibers are deposited during a vessel's development, but defects at major arterial junctions may occur. The multiple plies of a collagen fiber give integrity to the vessel wall and the muscle and cellular layers probably contribute little.

Hassler[48] constructed Plexiglas models of vessels. He found pits in areas corresponding to those where medial defects had been seen at bifurcations. Stehbens[5] also recognized abnormalities in collagen, and noted that medial defects, which are recognized as common, increase with age. He attributed these defects primarily to mechanical factors.

The role of the atheroma in the pathogenesis of cerebral aneurysms has received little attention. Walker[9] called attention to the areas of proliferation that develop around cerebral aneurysms. Since this time, however, few reports have been devoted to this subject.

Histologically, the wall of a cerebral aneurysm contains three layers: the endothelium, a tight connective tissue layer, and a loose adventitial layer. The internal elastic membrane fragments at the orifice of an aneurysm and the muscle layer thins dramatically, contributing to the thin structure and making rupture more likely. When aneurysms continue to grow without rupturing, there is increased turbulence and stasis, and the tendency to spontaneous thrombosis is increased. Matsko and Bogachenko[49] outlined the special structures of giant aneurysms. The outer layer consists of combinations of pia mater and a friable connective tissue. The middle layer consists of calcification, small fragments of bone, and more dense collagen-like connective tissue. The inner layer consists of thrombus with organized fibrosis alternating with layers of friable nonorganized thrombus. No endothelium is present and no internal elastic membrane can usually be found in aneurysms measuring greater than 20 mm. The literature contains inferences that large aneurysms and giant aneurysms are immune from rupture but this may not be true. Even large aneurysms and giant aneurysms may be a source of SAH. Zubkov and Matsko[50] reported that two-thirds of their giant aneurysms (measuring greater than 20 mm) had already bled by the time they were diagnosed.

Many investigators have looked at the concept of spontaneous thrombosis occurring in intracranial aneurysms. In 1945, Dandy[51] described a single case among 133 patients harboring intracranial aneurysms. Khilko,[52] Nikiforov,[53] and Zlotnik[54] also described spontaneous thrombosis in intracranial aneurysms. Thrombosis occurs not only in the aneurysm, but also in the parent artery from which the aneurysm arises as well as distally. Many factors may be important in initiating spontaneous thrombosis in aneurysms but the hemodynamics of aneurysms may be the most important factor. Flow within an aneurysm may be smooth or turbulent, and stasis may be present; much of this depends on the size of the orifice, the artery from which the aneurysm arises, and the angle of takeoff between the aneurysm and the parent vessel. Near the dome of an aneurysm, stasis is most likely to be present, and the washout of contrast material may occur here last. This is also the area in which spontaneous thrombosis most likely often occurs. Kikut[55] studied blood flow in intracranial aneurysms using diaphanoscopy. He described three distinct zones in an intracranial aneurysm using this technique. In one zone, blood flow was nearly normal. In another zone, turbulence was identified. In the third zone there was a silent area in which little movement of the blood cells could be appreciated. If the proximal portion of the parent artery was narrowed either by arteriosclerosis or vasospasm, the flow pattern in intracranial aneurysms was altered. In some cases, little or no flow in an aneurysm might be observed. Kikut[56] postulated that low blood flow may be one of the most important factors that are responsible for spontaneous thrombosis in aneurysms. Zubkov and Matsko[50] also demonstrated that in a large proportion of patients with giant aneurysms there is preexisting narrowing of the parent artery, perhaps leading to the high incidence of thrombosis in these aneurysms.

Hematological factors are no doubt also responsible for thrombosis in aneurysms. As with thrombosis elsewhere in the vascular system, intimal damage may play an important role in spontaneous thrombosis. Kudrjashov[57] demonstrated that stimulation of the cervical sympathetic chain could add to local coagulation response in the intracranial tree. In large and giant aneurysms, the increased presence of fibrin breakdown products characterizes the local intravascular coagulopathy. Spontaneous thrombosis in aneurysms may have some protective and curative effect. However, this effect may also lead to complication through distal thrombosis or embolism. Soon after the use of antifibrinolytic agents came into popularity, several reports appeared in which spontaneous thrombosis in aneurysms had occurred. Shortly thereafter, however, other reports also appeared describing increased thrombosis of small adjacent arteries. Crompton[58] studied 159 cases in which an intracranial aneurysm had been responsible for the patient's death. Although the incidence of ischemic cerebral vascular lesions in this group of patients was 75%, in only 2% of the cases was thrombosis of a vessel identified. Crompton concluded that microemboli were not significant factors in the high incidence of ischemic lesions seen after rupture of an aneurysm. Antunes and Correll[59] and Auld and Shafey[60] also identified thrombosis of vessels adjacent to large unruptured aneurysms. Suzuki et al.[61] also carefully studied the brain sections in patients dying of vasospasm and found evidence of microembolic phenomena. The embolization distal to an aneurysm must always be considered during manipulation of the artery or the aneurysm because thrombi may be dislodged back into the parent artery.

Little is known about the rate of growth and the events leading to the rupture of intracranial aneurysms. They begin at major branchings of the basal cerebral vessels as small outpouchings. Weakness of the collagen and connective tissue layers probably occurs concurrently. Continual stress must play a predominant role. Bjorkesten and Troupp[62] described 19 cases in which aneurysms were followed serially with repeat angiography. In 10 of these 19 cases (52.6%), the aneurysm had definitely grown between the two imaging procedures. In eight patients, examined from 4 to 88 months after the original study that identified the lesion, the size of the aneurysm was unchanged. Aneurysms that had enlarged did so in the interval between one-half month and 125 months (an average of 32 months). Six (31.6%) of these had also caused a recurrent hemorrhage on average 32 months after the first hemorrhage. Spontaneous thrombosis occurred in one instance in which an ICA aneurysm had been identified on the first study. In summary, the chance of an aneurysm growing is 53%, the chance of hemorrhage is 32%, and the chance of it remaining the same is 47%. Those remaining the same size rarely rupture.

Multiple Intracranial Aneurysms

Publications describing multiple intracranial aneurysms began to appear in the 1840s. Thompson[63] described a patient with three intracranial aneurysms who subsequently died of SAH.

The incidence of multiple aneurysms has varied between 3% and 24%. In the Cooperative Study, Sahs[64] reported an incidence of 20% in over 3000 patients. From autopsy data the aneurysms occur in 22% and from angiographic data, 19%. Yasargil[65] reported 203 patients with AComA aneurysms. In 11% of these, a second aneurysm was also found. Eight percent harbored two aneurysms and 3% three or more. In over 1000 patients, Yasargil later found an incidence of 24%. In 488 patients, Fox[37] found over 1200 aneurysms. The incidence of multiple aneurysms was 13.5% in this series. Some investigators have noted that the incidence of multiple intracranial aneurysms rises with systemic arterial hypertension. From 128 patients with multiple aneurysms, Franks found that those having hypertension accounted for 44% of these. In those without arterial hypertension, multiple aneurysms were found in only 19%.[66]

The rupture of more than one intracranial aneurysm simultaneously must be quite rare. Turnbull and Dolman[67] described a single case in which four aneurysms apparently ruptured simultaneously. McKissock and co-workers,[68] in 1964, described the courses of 251 patients with multiple aneurysms; 166 of these patients were conservatively managed, and the mortality in this group was 63%. In 34 patients with multiple aneurysms in which direct surgery was carried out, there was a mortality of 48%. Heiskanen[20] found that 14% of his cases had multiple aneurysms. The most common location was the MCA (24%), then the ICA (21%), and the rest were scattered throughout the arterial tree. Thirteen percent harbored three aneurysms and 1% had more than three.

Multiple aneurysms are commonly discovered during the angiographic evaluation of a patient with a recent SAH. Usually, one of these has been the source of SAH and the other is discovered incidentally. The clinical features associated with multiple aneurysms depend usually on the aneurysm that has bled, the amount of hemorrhage present, the onset, and its dissection into cerebral substance and subarachnoid spaces. A primary rule in the investigation of patients with SAH, therefore, is complete cerebral angiography. If more than one aneurysm is discovered, the tactics of surgical treatment must be decided.

Surgical Classification

Along with the underlying pathology that leads to aneurysm development, the morphology, size, and location are also important to the surgeon in planning treatment. Morphology determines not only the kind of surgical approach needed but also whether the aneurysm in question requires any treatment or whether the treatment will produce successful outcome. The size of aneurysms has been previously designated as small, medium, and giant, if they exceeded 2.5 cm in the greatest dimension. According to the work of Matsko[69] and Benashvili,[70] when an aneurysm reaches 2 cm in size, the histology of its wall changes. The wall thickens and clots adhere to the fundus. Aneurysms smaller than 10 mm may have lesser tendency to rupture but there is conflicting data on this subject. In the cooperative study, those that were 6 mm in size had already bled when they were discovered. Whether measurements were made angiographically or on postmortem (when they were not expanded with blood) is also important. There is convincing evidence that minute aneurysms 2 to 4 mm in size, may also be benign. Many of these are found in postmortem studies of older hypertensive patients and rarely cause hemorrhage. They may be found in as many as 5% to 6% of autopsies.

In the classification that follows, location was considered to be of paramount consideration because it dictates surgical approach. Aneurysm location has been designated previously according to the artery of origination of the orifice, artery nearest to the takeoff, or by the proximity to cranial or cerebral structures.

To organize this confusing matter, the authors have elected to classify aneurysms first on the basis of their major vessel of origination. These are further subdivided as to the artery nearest their site of origin.

I. Morphology
   A. Saccular
   B. Fusiform
   C. Infundibular
   D. Dissection
   E. False
II. Size
   A. Minute or infundibulae
   B. Small, less than 10 mm
   C. Large, 10–20 mm
   D. Giant, 20 mm and greater
III. Location
   A. Internal carotid artery aneurysms
      1. Cavernous
      2. Ophthalmic
      3. Supraclinoid
         a. Posterior communicating artery aneurysms
         b. Anterior choroidal artery aneurysms
         c. Bifurcation aneurysms
   B. Anterior cerebral and anterior communication artery aneurysms
      1. A_1 anterior cerebral aneurysms
      2. Anterior communicating artery aneurysms
      3. Distal anterior cerebral artery aneurysms
   C. Middle cerebral artery aneurysms
      1. M_1 main trunk aneurysms
      2. Middle cerebral artery bifurcation aneurysms
      3. Distal middle cerebral artery aneurysms
   D. Vertebrobasilar artery aneurysms
      1. Vertebral artery aneurysms
         a. Posterior inferior cerebellar artery aneurysms
         b. Main trunk vertebral artery aneurysms
      2. Basilar artery aneurysms
         a. Junction aneurysms
         b. Basilar trunk aneurysms
         c. Anterior inferior cerebellar artery aneurysms
         d. Superior cerebellar artery aneurysms
         e. Aneurysms of the basilar artery apex
         f. Distal branch aneurysms
      3. Posterior cerebral artery aneurysms
         a. P_1 posterior cerebral artery aneurysms
         b. Distal posterior cerebral artery aneurysms

Conclusions

The above classification ties together pathological, surgical, and clinical significance. The preceding discussion was not intended to present all the available pathology material concerning cerebral aneurysms to the reader. To the neurosurgeon providing care to the patient with a SAH, a basic understanding of the underlying vascular disease is vital, however. SAH is rarely an isolated event in the life of a patient but is a manifestation of a disease process. It may occur also as a complication of another disorder such as those described in this chapter. The effects of SAH always have devastating consequences on the patient's future life and work.

References

1. Eppinger H. Pathogenesis (Histogenesis und Aetiologie) der Aneurysmen einschliesslich des Aneurysma equi verminosum. Pathologisch-anatomische Studien. *Langenbecks Arch Klin Chir*. 1887;35(suppl):1–563.
2. Forbus WD. On the origin of miliary aneurysms of the superficial cerebral arteries. *Bull Johns Hopkins Hosp*. 1930;47:239–284.
3. Forster FM, Alpers BJ. Anatomical defects and pathological changes in congenital cerebral aneurysms. *J Neuropathol Exp Neurol*. 1945;4:146–154.
4. Bremer JL. Congenital aneurysms of the cerebral arteries. *Arch Pathol*. 1943;35:819–831.
5. Stehbens WE. Medial defects of the cerebral arteries of man. *J Pathol-Bacteriol*. 1959;78:179–185.
6. Stehbens WE. Histopathology of cerebral aneurysms. *Arch Neurol*. 1963;8:272–281.
7. Stehbens WE. Cerebral aneurysms of animals other than man. *J Pathol Bacteriol*. 1963;86:161–168.
8. Glynn LE. Medial defects in the circle of Willis and their relation to aneurysm formation. *J Pathol Bacteriol*. 1940; 51:213–222.
9. Walker AE, Allègre GW. The pathology and pathogenesis of cerebral aneurysms. *J Neuropathol Exp Neurol*. 1954;13: 248–259.
10. Wilson G, Riggs HE, Rupp C. The pathologic anatomy of ruptured cerebral aneurysms. *J Neurosurg*. 1954;11:128–134.
11. Alpers BJ, Berry RG. Circle of Willis in cerebral vascular disorders: the anatomical structure. *Arch Neurol*. 1963;8: 398–402.
12. Riggs HE, Rupp C. Variation in form of circle of Willis. *Arch Neurol*. 1963;8:8–14.
13. Housepian EM, Pool JL. A systematic analysis of intracranial aneurysms from the autopsy file of the Presbyterian Hospital, 1914 to 1956. *J Neuropathol Exp Neurol*. 1958;17: 409–423.
14. Stehbens WE. Aneurysms and anatomical variations of cerebral arteries. *Arch Pathol*. 1963;75:45–64.
15. Weir BKA. The management of intracranial aneurysms – prospects for improvement. *Clin Neurosurg*. 1988;34:154–160.

16. Medvedev YA, Matsko DE. Classification of brain aneurysms based on etiological and pathogenetic principles. In: *Pathological Anatomy of Brain Surgical Diseases*. St. Petersburg, Russia: 1991;32–104.
17. Diaz MS, Sekhar LN. Intracranial hemorrhage from aneurysms and arteriovenous malformations during pregnancy and the puerperium. *Neurosurgery*. 1990;27:855–866.
18. Cannell DC, Botterell EH. Subarachnoid hemorrhage and pregnancy. *Am J Obstet Gynecol*. 1956;2:844–855.
19. Pedowitz P, Perell A. Aneurysms complicated by pregnancy: II: Aneurysms of the cerebral vessels. *Am J Obstet Gynecol*. 1957;73:736–749.
20. Heiskanen O. Ruptured intracranial arterial aneurysms of children and adolescents. Surgical and total management results. *Childs Nerv Syst*. 1989;5:66–70.
21. Ayer WD. So-called spontaneous subarachnoid hemorrhage: a resume with its medicolegal consideration. *Am J Surg*. 1934;26:143–151.
22. Chambers WR, Harper BF Jr, Simpson JR. Familial incidence of congenital aneurysms of cerebral arteries: report of cases of ruptured aneurysms in father and son. *JAMA*. 1954;155:358–359.
23. Phillips RL. Case reports and technical notes: familial cerebral aneurysms case reports. *J Neurosurg*. 1963;20: 701–703.
24. Smith RR, Miller JD. Pathophysiology and clinical evidence of subarachnoid hemorrhage. In: Youmans JR, ed. *Neurological Surgery: A Comprehensive Reference Guide to the Diagnosis and Management of Neurosurgical Problems*. 3rd ed. Philadelphia, PA: WB Saunders Co, 1990;III:1644–1660.
25. Sigueira WC, Figueiredo, Cruz AA, Costa FF, Zago MA. *Acta Ophthalmol (Copenh)*. 1990;68:515–518.
26. Wizniter M, Ruggier PM, Masaryk TJ, Ross JS, Modic MT, Berman B. Diagnosis of cerebrovascular disease in sickle cell anemia by magnetic resonance angiography. *J Pediatr*. 1990;117:551–555.
27. George AE, Lin JP, Morantz RA. Intracranial aneurysm on a persistent primitive trigeminal artery. Case report. *J Neurosurg*. 1971;35:601–604.
28. Kirgis HD, Fisher WL, Llewellyn RC, Peebles EM. Aneurysms of the anterior communicating artery and gross anomalies of the circle of Willis. *J Neurosurg*. 1966;25:73–78.
29. Rhoton AL Jr, Saeki N, Perlmutter D. Microsurgical anatomy of the circle of Willis. In: Rand RW, ed. *Microneurosurgery*. 2nd ed. St. Louis, MO: CV Mosby; 1978; 278–310.
30. Kayembe KNT, Sasahara M, Mazama F. Cerebral aneurysms and variations in the circle of Willis. *Stroke*. 1984;15: 846–850.
31. Ozaki T, Handa H, Tomimoto K, Hazama F. Anatomical variations of the arterial system of the base of the brain. *Arch Jpn Chir*. 1977;46:3–17.
32. Yasargil MG, Smith RD. Management of aneurysms of anterior circulation by intracranial procedures. In: Youmans JR, ed. *Neurological Surgery: A Comprehensive Reference Guide to the Diagnosis and Management of Neurosurgical Problems*. WB Saunders; Philadelphia, PA: 1982;3: 1663–1696.
33. Courville CB. Arteriosclerotic aneurysms of the circle of Willis. Some notes on their morphology and pathogenesis. *Bull Los Angeles Neurol Soc*. 1962;27:1–13.
34. McDonald CA, Korb M. Intracranial aneurysms. *Arch Neurol Psychiatr*. 1939;42:298–328.
35. Roach MR, Drake CG. Ruptured cerebral aneurysms caused by micro-organisms. *N Engl J Med*. 1965;273:240–244.
36. Ziment I. Nervous system complications in bacterial endocarditis. *Am J Med*. 1969;47:593–607.
37. Fox JL. *Intracranial Aneurysms*. New York: Springer-Verlag; 1983;1:418–431.
38. Stehbens WE. *Pathology of the Cerebral Blood Vessels*. St Louis, MO: CV Mosby; 1972:559.
39. Rubinstein MK, Cohen NH. Ehlers–Danlos syndrome associated with multiple intracranial aneurysms. *Neurology*. 1964;14:125–132.
40. Neil-Dwyer G, Bartlett JR, Nicholls AC, Narcisi P, Pope FM. Collagen deficiency and ruptured cerebral aneurysms: a clinical and biochemical study. *J Neurosurg*. 1983;59:16–20.
41. Pope FM, Kendall BE, Slapak GI, Kapoor R, McDonald WI, Compston DAS, Mitchell R, Hope DT, Millar-Craig MW, Dean JCS, Johnston AW, Lynch PG, Sarathchandra P, Narcisi P, Nicholls AC, Richards AJ, Mackenzie JL. Type III collagen mutations cause fragile cerebral arteries. *Br J Neurosurg*. 1991;5:551–574.
42. Pope FM, Limburg M, Schievink WI. Familial cerebral aneurysms and type III collagen deficiency. Letter-to-editor. *J Neurosurg*. 1990;72:156–157.
43. Weir B. *Aneurysms Affecting the Nervous System*. Baltimore, MD: Williams & Wilkins; 1987.
44. Stehbens WE. The pathology of intracranial arterial aneurysms and their complications. In: Fox JL, ed. *Intracranial Aneurysms*. New York: Springer-Verlag; 1983;I:272–357.
45. Bigelow NM. The association of polycystic kidneys with intracranial aneurysms and other related disorders. *Am J Med Sci*. 1953;225:485–494.
46. Wright CJE. Coarctation of the aorta with death from rupture of cerebral aneurysms. *Arch Pathol*. 1949;48:382–386.
47. Benoit BG, Wortzman G. Traumatic cerebral aneurysms. *J Neurol Psychiatry*. 1973;36:127–138.
48. Hassler O. Morphological studies on the large cerebral arteries with reference to the aetiology of subarachnoid haemorrhage. *Acta Psychiatr Neurol Scand*. 1961;36(suppl 154):5–93.
49. Matsko DE, Bogachenko DV. Giant aneurysms of cerebral vessels. *Arch Pathol*. 1981;1:29–35.
50. Zubkov YN, Matsko DE. Some clinical anatomical peculiarities of large and giant arterial aneurysms of brain vessels. *J Neurol Psychiatry*. 1980;80(N12):1809–1813.
51. Dandy WE. *Intracranial Arterial Aneurysms*. Ithaca, NY: Comstock Publishing Co, Inc; 1945.
52. Khilko VA. *About aneurysms of cerebral vessels*. Leningrad, Russia: 1964. Thesis.
53. Nikiforov BM. Thrombosis of anterior circulation saccular aneurysms after cerebral subarachnoid hemorrhage. *J Neurol Psychiatry*. 1970;2:209–212.
54. Zlotnik, ET. *Aneurysms of Cerebral Vessels*. Minsk: 1967.
55. Kikut RP. Experimental investigations of intraaneurysmal blood flow. *Vopr Neurosurg*. 1966;2:17–21.

56. Kikut RP. *Using magnetic-biological effects in the treatment of arterial intracranial aneurysms*. Moscow, Russia: 1977. Thesis [in Russian].
57. Kudrjashov BA. Modern condition knowledge about the antihemostatic system of blood. *Probl Hematol Blood Transfusion*. 1962;12:3–13.
58. Crompton MR. Cerebral infarction following the rupture of cerebral berry aneurysms. *Brain*. 1969;87:263–279.
59. Antunes JL, Correll JW. Cerebral emboli from intracranial aneurysms. *Surg Neurol*. 1976;6:7–10.
60. Auld AW, Shafey S. Transient ischemic attacks not produced by extracranial vascular disease. A plea for complete and early angiographic investigation. *South Med J*. 1978; 69:722–724.
61. Suzuki S, Suzuki M, Iwabuchi T, Kamata Y. Role of cerebral microthrombosis in symptomatic cerebral vasospasm: with a case report. *Neurosurgery*. 1983;13:199–203.
62. Bjorkesten GAF, Troupp H. Changes in the size of intracranial arterial aneurysms. *J Neurosurg*. 1962;19:583–588.
63. Thompson AT. A case of aneurysms, within the skull, terminating in apoplexy and paralysis, with clinical remarks. *Monthly J Med Sci*. (*London, Edinburgh*). 1842;2: 557–563.
64. Sahs AL, Perret GE, Locksley HB, Nishioka H. *Intracranial Aneurysms and Subarachnoid Hemorrhage. A Cooperative Study*. Philadelphia and Toronto: JB Lippincott, Co; 1969.
65. Yasargil MG. Subarachnoid hemorrhage. Diagnosis and therapy. *Praxis*. 1975;64:439–444.
66. Franks AJ. Prognostic factors in ruptured aneurysms of the circle of Willis: the significance of systemic hypertension. *Neuropathol Appl Neurobiol*. 1978;4:61–70.
67. Turnbull F, Dolman CL. Simultaneous hemorrhage from multiple intracerebral aneurysms: a case report. *Can J Surg*. 1962;5:87–92.
68. McKissock W, Richardson A, Walsh L, Owen E. Multiple intracranial aneurysms. *Lancet*. 1964;1:623–626.
69. Matsko DE. Aneurysms of the brain vessels. Pathology and modern surgical treatment. Leningrad, Russia: 1983. Thesis.
70. Benashvili GM. *Treatment of giant intracranial aneurysms*. Leningrad, Russia: 1989. Thesis.

3
Diagnostics: The Clinical and Neurological Examination

Intracranial aneurysms cause half of all intracranial hemorrhages. The remainder are due to arteriovenous malformations (AVMs), hypertension, arteriosclerosis, tumors, blood dyscrasia, substance abuse, and other degenerative diseases of the cerebral vasculature. A presumptive diagnosis can often be made on clinical grounds, before definitive diagnostic tests are performed. Occasionally, patients harboring intracranial aneurysms can be identified by the precursors they carry. Familial factors, arterial hypertension, and arteriosclerosis are known progenitors.

An antecedent history of headaches or hemorrhagic problems is, of course, relevant. Arterial hypertension may be manifest, but an enlarged and displaced left ventricle on the physical examination or accentuation of the second aortic sound may indicate long-standing hypertension. Tortuosity of cerebral vessels may be accompanied by tortuosity of the great vessels of the chest, the neck, or the temporal area. Heart murmurs may indicate subacute bacterial endocarditis, or infection of the liver, kidneys, or spleen may be found, leading to suspicions of aneurysms of infectious origin.

Meningeal irritation from innumerable causes may simulate acute aneurysmal subarachnoid hemorrhage (SAH). Samoilov[1] noted that the diagnosis was apparent from the initial clinical examination in 62% of patients with acute SAH. In the other 38%, the diagnosis was obfuscated by other diseases or nondiagnostic clinical features. In 12%, there was evidence of vascular disease elsewhere. In 11%, infection confused the issue, and, in some, intraventricular hemorrhage was the cause of an inaccurate or delayed diagnosis. In 9% of patients who were unresponsive, a differential diagnosis of coma was necessary. The differential diagnosis of an epileptic seizure was carried out in 2.6%, and, in 2%, there was a question of an intracranial mass. In 10% to 15%, the diagnosis was not apparent.

The neurological manifestations of SAH involve levels of consciousness, the motor system, mental processes, and abnormal motor movements. In examining a patient with acute subarachnoid hemorrhage, the overall neurological picture should be evaluated first. The establishment of speech contact with a patient who is lucid allows questions concerning hearing, vision, movement, and sensory phenomena to be answered. A history should be obtained relating to the event that precipitated onset. The Cooperative Aneurysm Study showed that certain environmental and stress factors are associated with aneurysm rupture more commonly than would ordinarily be expected. Among the conditions of interest are sexual intercourse, straining, micturition, trauma, and perhaps sleep.

Examination of the visual system is especially important in the alert patient. Along with the reaction of the pupils to light and accommodation, extraocular movement should be evaluated. The presence of nystagmus and diplopia or ptosis is especially useful in diagnosing the presence of an aneurysm. In the cooperative patient, the eye grounds may be examined carefully to find the small subhyaloid hemorrhage characteristic of recently ruptured aneurysms. Paresis of upward gaze or skew deviation indicates midbrain dysfunction, perhaps due to herniation or ischemia. The patient with brain stem abnormalities is the one most likely to deteriorate rapidly and unexpectedly and the one who may need special attention to survive this critical phase. Brain stem signs also identify the patient who will progress to higher clinical grades and dictates the therapy necessary in the coming days.

Funduscopic examination and visual field evaluation can be carried out in the patient who is alert and cooperative. Intracranial pressure (ICP) may be estimated by the venous pulse, although papilledema is rarely present in the acute phase. Diabetic retinopathy or hypertensive arteriopathy indicates other potential causes of the hemorrhage. Evaluation of the visual system also gives information relating to the optic nerve, optic chiasm, optic radiation, and occipital lobes. In Samoilov's[1] series of 1700 patients, hypertensive angiopathy was found in the fundus in 43% of the patients examined. Arteriosclerotic changes occurred in 4.7% and preretinal hemorrhages in 26.8%. Edema of the optic nerve was found in only 4.6% and optic neuritis in 0.4%. Disorders of the visual field were found in 207, nearly one third of all visual abnormalities.

Lumbar puncture (LP) and cerebrospinal fluid (CSF) examination should not be carried out without a clear goal in mind. If SAH has been shown on computed tomography (CT) scanning, the LP may be omitted and could lead to herniation if performed. If LP must be carried out in order to establish a diagnosis or to differentiate between meningitis and SAH, then special precautions are needed. A small needle placed accurately in the lumbar subarachnoid space without excessive fluid withdrawal is the method of choice. Measurement of lumbar CSF pressure is always required if LP is performed. The presence of blood in the subarachnoid space not only establishes a diagnosis of SAH, but also indicates the degree of severity of the hemorrhage. If a traumatic tap is suspected, a drop of CSF may be allowed to fall on absorbent tissue. If the hemorrhage has resulted from a traumatic tap, there will be clear separation of blood and CSF in a ring sign. However, if the hemorrhage results from an aneurysm, there will be even distribution of blood throughout the field.

Another useful test is to collect several tubes of CSF and observe clearing in the fluid collected. In the case of a traumatic puncture, the last tubes collected will be clear when compared to the first ones.

The third examination relates to xanthochromia of CSF. After collecting specimens, the CSF sample should be centrifuged and the supernate compared with clear water. If any yellowness is present, spontaneous subarachnoid hemorrhage may be considered over traumatic puncture. The amount of protein in the CSF is also important. High protein has been associated with ischemia and infarction.

Special Examination of the Vascular System

Understanding the pathology of the vascular system may require angiography, CT, magnetic resonance imaging (MRI), cerebral blood flow (CBF) and cerebral blood volume studies, and velocity measurements. The enhanced CT examination allows confirmation of the diagnosis of SAH and, occasionally, even identifies the site of the aneurysm. In conjunction with ^{133}Xe, the CT allows estimation of CBF and differentiates, by virtue of contrast, between aneurysms and tumor.

CT Grading

Fisher and co-workers[2] proposed grading on the basis of the amount of blood visualized in the subarachnoid pathways on CT scans. They recognized that the estimation of the amount of subarachnoid blood was limited because of the irregular dimensions of the cisterns and fissures. Subarachnoid blood accumulates in several forms, including clots and admixture with CSF. However, these investigators found it appropriate to measure the dimensions of the clot both in longitudinal and transverse planes. The volume of subarachnoid blood was categorized in four groups. In group 1 patients, no blood was detected. In group 2, there was a diffuse deposition or thin layers detected within all vertical layers. This would occur in the interhemispheric fissure, the insular cistern or the ambient cistern, and would be less than 1 mm thick. In group 3, there were localized clots and/or vertical layers of blood as thick as 1 mm or more. In group 4, diffuse clotting was seen or there was no subarachnoid blood, but intracerebral or intraventricular clots were present.

In group 1 patients, in whom no subarachnoid blood was detected, seven had no radiographic vasospasm, two had moderate vasospasm, and only two showed severe vasospasm. None, however, developed delayed symptoms or signs of cerebral vasospasm. In group 2 patients where there were some diffuse subarachnoid blood but no clots or vertical layers of more than 1 mm thick, four had no vasospasm, three had slight to moderate vasospasm, and none had severe vasospasm. All these were also free of delayed neurological signs.

In group 3, there were 24 patients whose CT scans showed localized blood clots as thick as 1 mm or more. Twenty-three of the 24 had severe vasospasm and all of these developed delayed symptoms and signs. There were five patients in group 4, but only two had slight vasospasm. Thus, it appeared that the presence of subarachnoid blood was of more importance in causation than was intracerebral or intraventricular bleeding. Clots measuring 1 mm or more are strong predictors of significant clinical cerebral vasospasm[2] (Fig. 3.1).

Hornyak et al.[3] extended Fisher et al.'s report by reviewing the CT scans of 100 patients consecutively operated on for ruptured cerebral aneurysms. Intracerebral or extended intraventricular hematomas were a poor prognostic sign, and acute hydrocephalus had a negative effect. Twenty-two percent of the patients developed ischemic infarction on the postoperative CT scan. Enlargement of the ventricles was observed in 32 patients, but only 15% came to shunting. Nine infarctions were located in the caudate nucleus and putamen, some of which remained clinically asymptomatic. Eleven had infarctions in the temporoparietal and frontotemporal area, and two of these remained asymptomatic. These authors attributed approximately half of the infarctions to intraoperative complications.

The distribution of extravasated blood on CT scans may predicts the site of a ruptured aneurysm but also outlines several more benign conditions associated with SAH, such as nonaneurysmal perimesencephalic SAH.

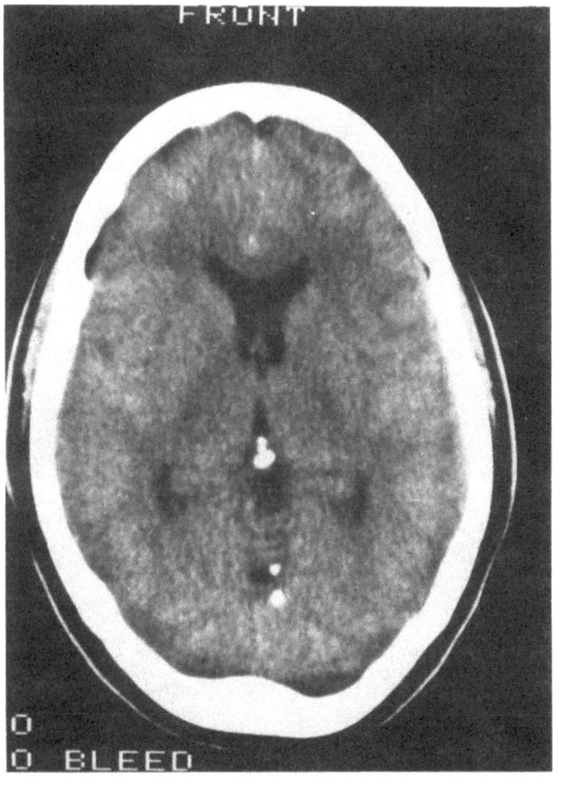

A

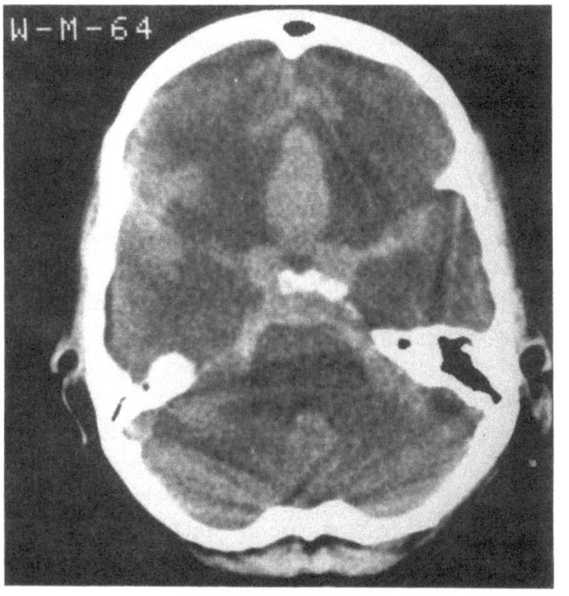

C

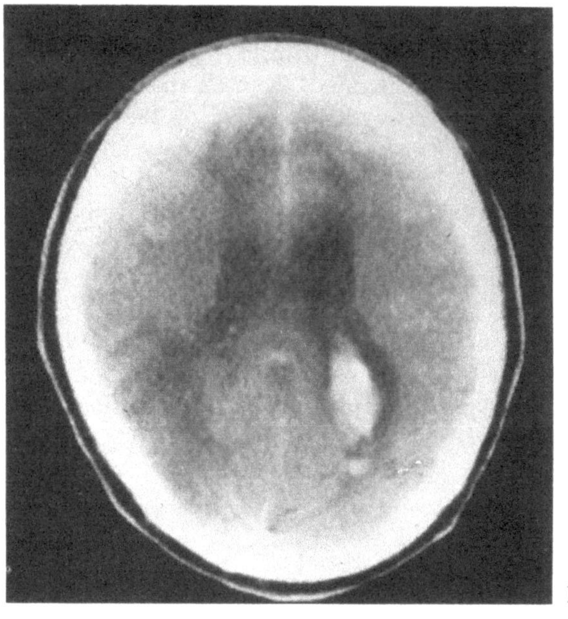

D

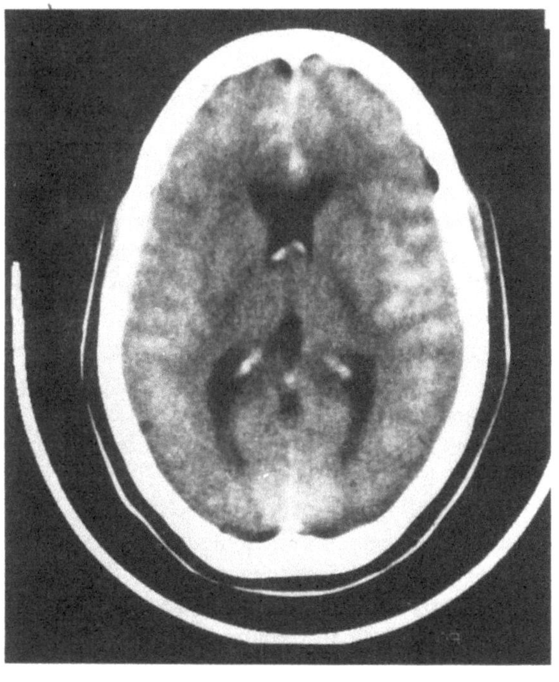

B

FIGURE 3.1A–D. The CT findings in mild (A), moderate (B), and severe (C) subarachnoid hemorrhage and intraventricular hematoma (D) with early ischemic deficit.

Rinkel and co-workers[4] described the characteristic distribution of cisternal blood in 52 patients with this benign disorder confirmed by angiography. These authors thought that the benign perimesencephalic hemorrhage resulted from rupture of one of the anterior longitudinal prepontine veins. An uncomplicated clinical course without rehemorrhage or ischemia with an excellent prognosis describes the clinical course of the disorder.

Magnetic Resonance Imaging and Magnetic Resonance Angiography

Magnetic resonance imaging (MRI) has proven to be of special use in patients with a recent SAH by disclosing aneurysms, blood in the cisterns, the distribution and site of hemorrhage, and the presence of a dilated ventricular system. The MRI also has certain risks in patients containing magnetic compounds in the cranial cavity, such as old aneurysm clips or certain modern clips that contain ferromagnetic minerals. Dujovny and co-workers[5] investigated the magnetic qualities of aneurysm clips using motion measurements during MRI examinations of experimental aneurysms. Scoville clips containing 5% martensite, Mayfield clips, and some others deflected as much as 45°.

The CT, especially the MRI, has made predicting the size of an aneurysm much easier and the estimation of intraaneurysmal clot more dependable.

Magnetic resonance angiography (MRA) relies on the absence of a signal produced by moving particles. Since blood flows rapidly through most of the basal intracranial vessels, early work indicates that this method may have utility in identifying cerebral aneurysms. In a comparison of 164 studies in patients undergoing both MRA and conventional angiography, the overall image quality was excellent in 90% of the MRAs. Eighteen of the 19 (94.7%) aneurysms were detected using MRA. The parent artery, the anatomy of the neck and dome, and the size were correctly shown in 17 of the 19 (89.5%) aneurysms. All vascular malformations were seen on the MRA.

Routine MRI is especially useful for detecting dissection in major extracranial and intracranial arteries. The use of dynamic MRI shows narrowing of the lumen, but the false lumen can also be demonstrated with dynamic imaging. Both the MRI and the MRA are useful in screening patients with SAH from intracranial aneurysms and more benign disorders such as perimesenceph-

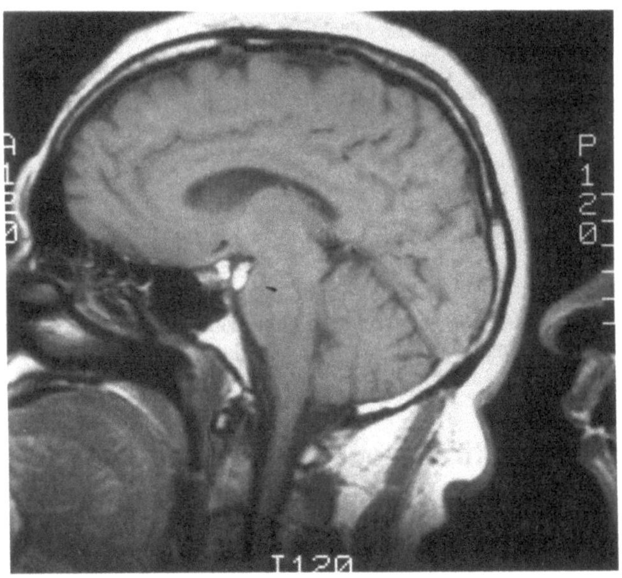

FIGURE 3.2. The MRI in perimesencephalic subarachnoid hemorrhage. This is a benign disorder usually not associated with aneurysm rupture.

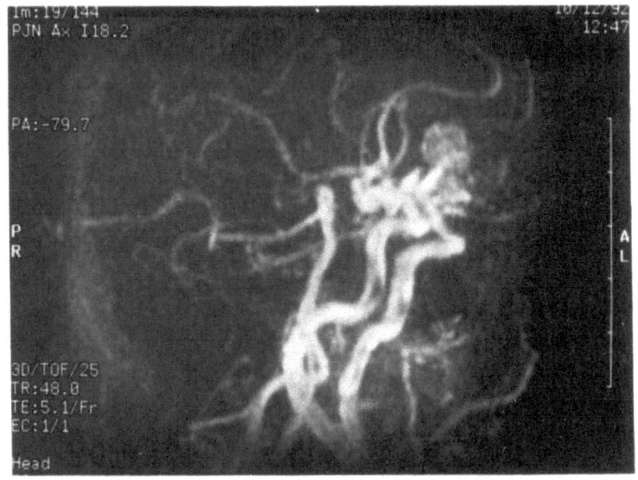

FIGURE 3.3. MRA demonstrating aneurysms arising from the ophthalmic segment.

alic SAH (Fig. 3.2). They may also be used in evaluating the patient with unruptured and asymptomatic lesions (Fig. 3.3).

CBF Measurements and SPECT

^{133}Xe can be used to evaluate dynamic changes following SAH from an intracranial aneurysm and to evaluate treatment (Fig. 3.4). Levels of approximately 40 ml/100 g of brain tissue usually mark the patient who will become symptomatic; at 20 ml/100 g, irreversible lesions appear. A recently available cerebral perfusion imaging agent, ^{99}Tc-HMPAO, is proving useful in measuring cerebral circulation in patients with recently ruptured aneurysms. Using single photon emission computed tomography (SPECT), Hasan and co-workers[6] studied CBF in eight patients who gradually deteriorated after their aneurysms ruptured. Four had cerebral ischemia and four acute hydrocephalus. There were multiple regions of decreased uptake of ^{99m}Tc-PAO, mainly in the watershed areas. In patients with acute hydrocephalus, the decreased uptake was seen mainly in the basal parts of the brain around the third ventricles and in the basal part of the frontal horns. Shinoda et al.[7] evaluated cerebral vasodilatory capacity using ^{123}I-IMD SPECT. Low-perfusion areas corresponded to regions of hematoma seen on the CT. Poor acetazolamide reactivity occurred in 100% of patients in the first postoperative week after aneurysm repair. The method is also useful in evaluating CBF after balloon occlusion or during balloon test occlusion of major intracranial arteries. The method may be used to identify normal pressure hydrocephalus and to identify those who would benefit from shunting.[8] Frontal lobe blood flow increased in comparison to temporal flow after lumbar taps in patients who benefited most

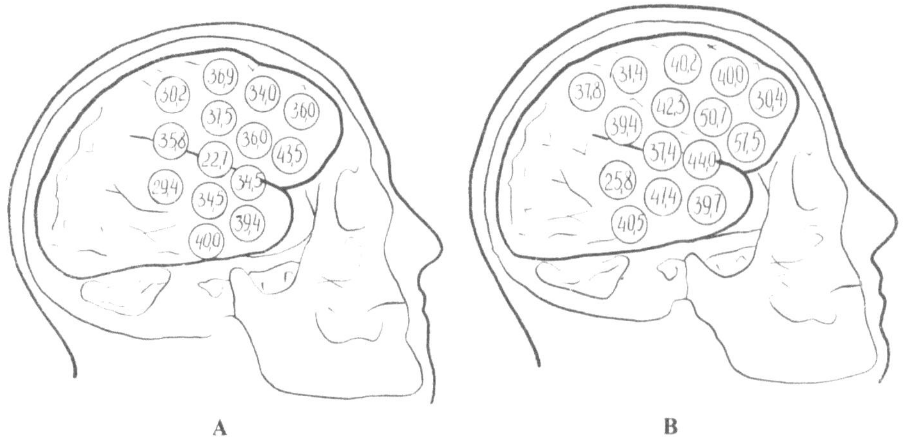

FIGURE 3.4. (A) ^{133}Xe CBF before angioplasty. (B) ^{133}Xe CBF following angioplasty.

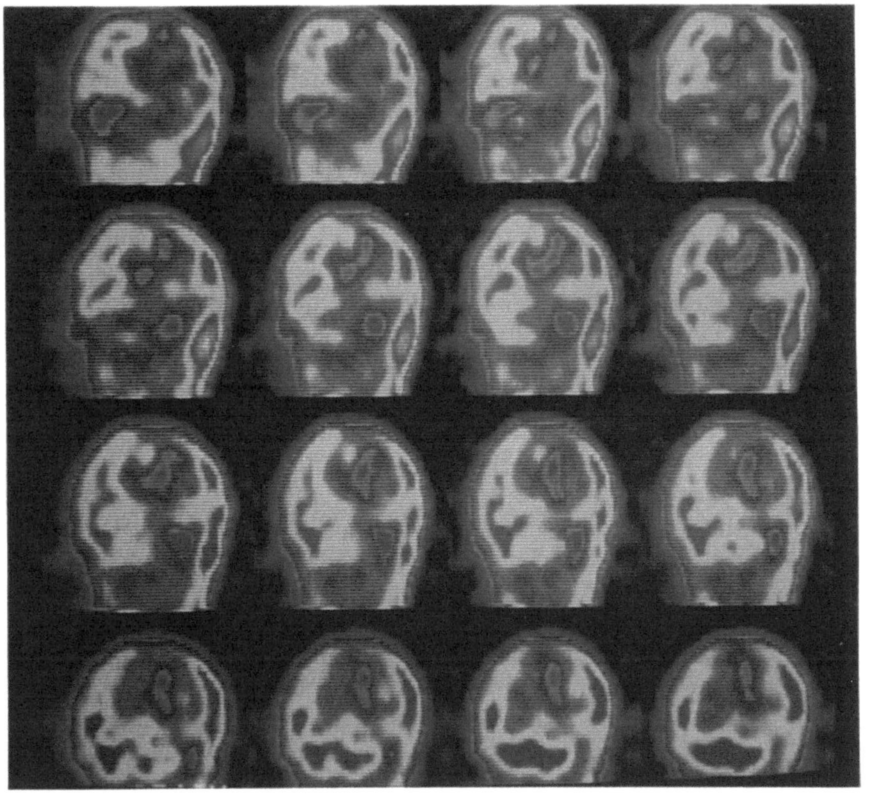

FIGURE 3.5. A SPECT scan showing perfusion defects in the left hemisphere and in the distribution of the anterior cerebral artery. The patient had multiple ischemic infarcts secondary to vasospasm associated with rupture of a left carotid artery bifurcation aneurysm.

from shunting. The method may also be useful in identifying the patient with vasospasm who will become clinically symptomatic and develop infarction (Fig. 3.5).

Transcranial Doppler Sonography in Subarachnoid Hemorrhage

Ultrasound has been a part of the neurosurgical armamentarium for many years. Originally, it was used to evaluate midline structures and to determine if shift had taken place. However, low frequency ultrasound has also been used to detect arteriovenous abnormalities dating back to the mid-1950s. Recently, velocimetry has found significant clinical use in evaluating cerebral vasospasm. Because of the ease of use and repeatability of the noninvasive test, daily examinations can be carried out inexpensively and noninvasively at the bedside.

According to the Doppler principle, sound can be used to measure the velocity of moving objects by calculating the difference in frequency between the transmitted signal and the returning or echo signal if the objects causing deflection are moving parallel with the direction of flow. Since the basal cerebral vessels lie largely in a parallel direction to the cranial base and perpendicular to the temporal bones, they are nearly parallel to the direction of flow, making Doppler measurement of velocity especially accurate for these vessels. By using the temporal window, the angles of insonation can usually be less than 30° and thus highly accurate. The speed of sound propagation through various tissues is known, allowing the depth to be estimated by range gating. This can be performed by having the receiver accept only signals that return in a specific time interval. Several pulsed wave Doppler instruments are available for velocity measurements.

In the patient with SAH, the examination may be done at the bedside. Insonating through thin portions of the cranium permits evaluation of virtually all of the basal vessels. The middle cerebral artery (MCA) may be insonated through the temporal window. Flow is always toward the probe, and velocities are 40 to 80 cm/s. The anterior cerebral artery (ACA) flow is directed away from the probe at a depth of 60 to 80 mm from the temporal surface and velocities range from 35 to 60 cm/s. The ICA bifurcation may be insonated through the temporal window.

Posterior cerebral artery (PCA) flow is found somewhat posterior to the MCA and is directed toward the probe at a velocity of 30 to 50 cm/s. The sound is somewhat coarser than that of the MCA, and the signal disappears at a depth of 50 mm as the vessel becomes perpendicular to the probe. The ophthalmic artery can be insonated via an orbital window at a depth of 40 to 60 mm.

As the lumen of any artery narrows, all other factors being equal, flow velocity rises. Exceptions occur when the heart fails, when the vessel is occluded proximally, or when edema or hematoma shifts the vessel position in relation to the Doppler probe. In our patients, the most important cause for insensitivity has been the presence of proximal vasospasm that reduces flow distally at the point of measurement. Insonating through the orbits to detect spasm in the proximal ICA may eliminate or reduce this artefact. Sloan et al.[9,10] point out, however, that both sensitivity and specificity are not as good when evaluating vertebral or the basilar artery spasm.

Several patterns emerge in evaluating SAH patients. Velocities are increased slightly from unknown causes during the first day or so. On days 4 to 6, velocity begins to accelerate. Mean velocities tend to peak on day 9 or 10 and then return to baseline levels in asymptomatic patients (Fig. 3.6). Symptomatic patients tend to show sustained high velocities weeks after hemorrhage and these are usually associated with CT infarcts (Fig. 3.7). Velocities tend to rise first on the side of the hemorrhage and are thus sometimes helpful in identifying which

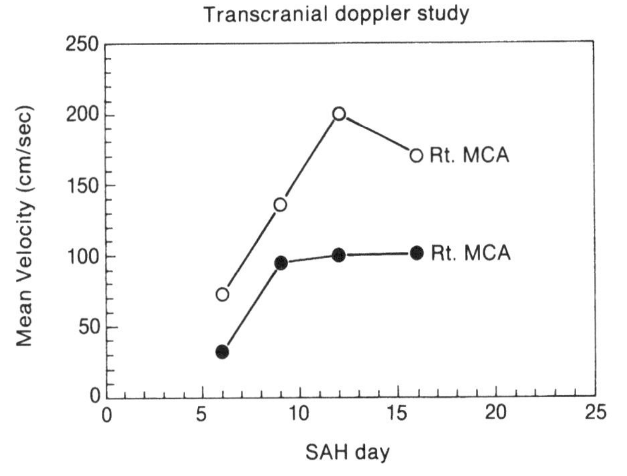

FIGURE 3.6. Serial transcranial Doppler recordings of the right intracranial vessels after SAH. Velocity peaked on the 12th day in the right MCA, the site of the aneurysm.

aneurysm bled in the patient with multiple aneurysms. However, after the initial rise, velocity changes are more diffuse and velocities in both the anterior and middle cerebral arteries usually rise together. There is no significant difference in peak velocities in symptomatic and asymptomatic patients although symptomatic patients' velocities may rise more abruptly. Velocity changes of 25% or greater from one examination to the next forewarns of the onset of clinical ischemia. On average, the shift occurs between the seventh and eighth days, and clinical events are usually recorded between the eighth and ninth days. The velocity shift is highly sensitive and specific for the onset of clinical ischemia.

Turbulence and musical murmurs may be heard in roughly 20% of cases, mostly in patients with symptomatic vasospasm (Fig. 3.8). Thus, a shift of 25% in velocity in any vessel, starting from day 3 may herald the onset of symptomatic vasospasm and may identify the patient who needs more specific therapy, such as balloon angioplasty. In SAH, the velocity equation is complex, and such variables as blood pressure, cardiac output, blood viscosity, volume of the extracellular space, and cerebral autoregulation must all be taken into account. Any single sonographic reading may not be helpful, but daily readings correlated with the angiogram and the clinical condition make this simple noninvasive method indispensable in the management of the patient with an intracranial aneurysm.

Cerebral vascular reactivity may also be of use in distinguishing the patient who will become symptomatic due to vasospasm. Near the ischemic threshold, penetrating cerebral vessels are maximally dilated and do not dilate further when carbon dioxide or acetazolamide is administered. These changes can be identified with both the SPECT scan and with Transcranial Doppler (TCD)

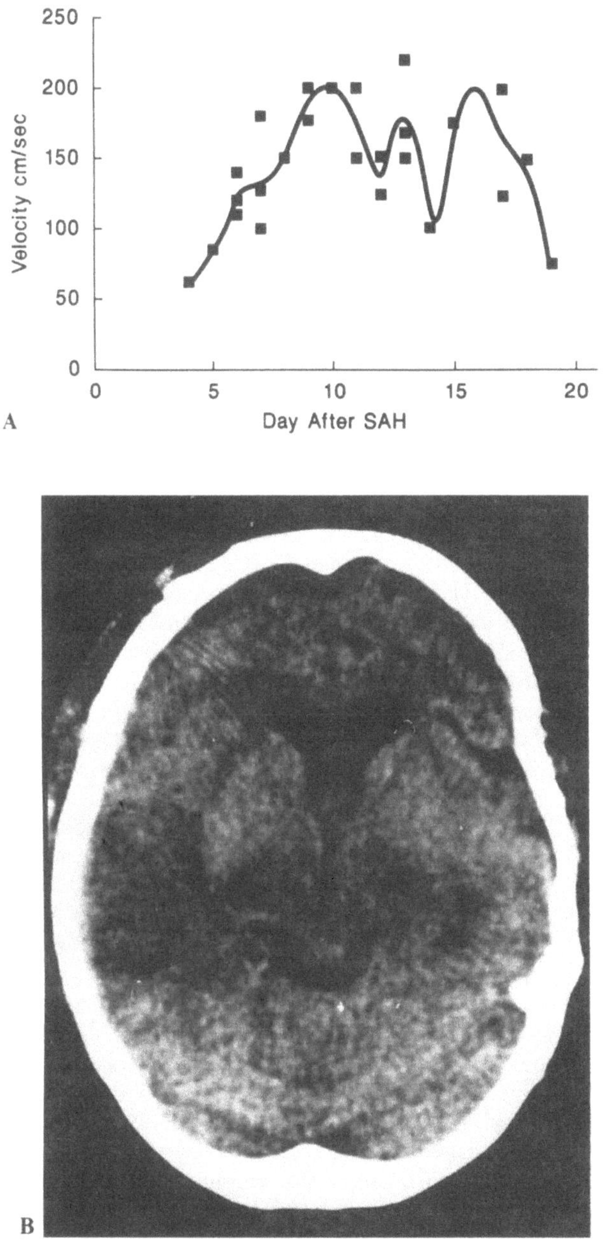

FIGURE 3.7. (A) Initially, velocity reaches a peak on day 8–11 after SAH in most patients. Late velocity elevation is often associated with cerebral infarction. (B) Infarction associated with right MCA vasospasm.

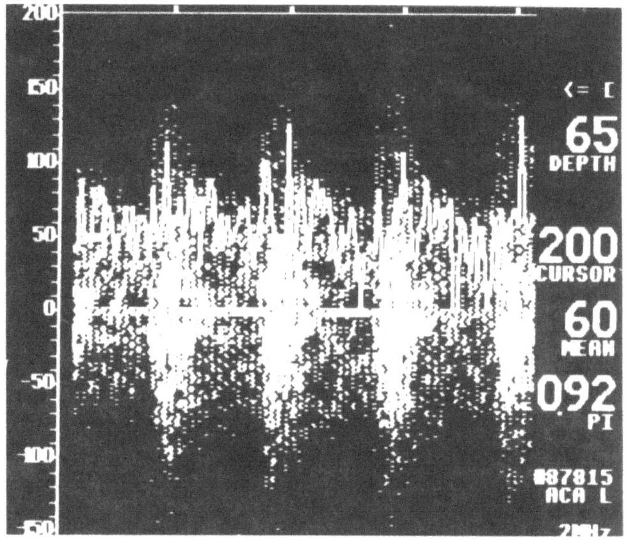

FIGURE 3.8. Transcranial Doppler recording of the anterior cerebral artery in severe vasospasm secondary to SAH from aneurysm of AcomA. "Musical murmurs" and "seagull" sounds may also be detected near the orifice of the aneurysm. They appear as turbulence below the baseline.

sonography. Normally, velocity in the MCA rises 3% to 4% with each mm Hg rise in P_{CO_2}.

Cerebral Angiography

The cerebral angiogram, selected, positioned, and magnified, is still the standard for diagnosis and treatment planning for a patient with a ruptured intracranial aneurysm. Along with the traditional angiography, highly selected digital angiography and MRA may be used supplementarily. In the patient with SAH from an intracranial aneurysm, four-vessel studies are imperative. The vertebral artery must be demonstrated including all of its intracranial branches. The angiographer should be in close contact with the surgeon and should discuss the varying operative approaches so that the aneurysm can be viewed in varying dimensions and projections. Oblique projection for aneurysms rising from the anterior communicating artery (AComA) must be a part of the routine examination. Special views, including the submental vertex position, may be necessary to demonstrate the neck of an aneurysm, and magnification views are sometimes required.

As soon as the diagnosis of SAH is made, the angiogram should be done. The lesion that is being treated and the complications associated with it justify an aggressive approach. The primary contraindication to any angiographic examination is severe systemic disease, such as hypotension, cardiac disease, pulmonary embolism, or severe neurological devastation such as deep coma. In patients in whom the diagnosis has been established and an aneurysm identified, a repeat arteriogram may be required if the condition changes significantly. If the patient deteriorates due to what is presumed to be cerebral vasospasm, then this diagnosis must also be established clearly by angiography as well as with TCD. Repeat angiograms may be necessary one or more times during the patient's course. If the initial angiogram has been made a week or more before the operation, repeat angiography may be needed. If an aneurysm is not demonstrated on conventional angiography immediately following the hemorrhage, the angiograms should also be repeated after 10 to 14 days to identify aneurysms that have been missed on the initial study. Intraoperative angiography is also useful for determining if the aneurysm has been satisfactorily clipped and whether clips have been applied to major nutrient vessels. This also allows the surgeon to prognosticate the outcome and plan rehabilitative strategies.

In the patient with multiple aneurysms, the angiogram is also useful in determining which aneurysm may have been the source of SAH. Aneurysms causing recent hemorrhage usually arise from arteries that are constricted or displaced. Aneurysms that are recently ruptured may be associated with secondary loculations. The larger aneurysm is usually the source of SAH as well. The initial angiogram may fail to disclose aneurysms in 5% to 10% of the cases due to clot within the fundus. Repeating the angiogram in 10 days will disclose another 10% of aneurysms previously missed on the first examination.

Summary

SAH is a serious disorder affecting individuals of all ages and races, of both sexes, and spares no occupation or socioeconomic group. In any one physician's practice, it must occur infrequently because the diagnosis is still missed far too often. Making the diagnosis on purely clinical data is both possible and, in fact, the only reasonable alternative for the large number of people at risk. Ideally, the intracranial aneurysm should be diagnosed just prior to its rupture, but at present this is neither likely nor feasible for most patients. However, once the lesion manifests itself either by its mass effect or a minor hemorrhage, immediate recognition is imperative because of rebleeding and its risks of death and disability. Careful clinical examination combined with the intelligent use of physiologic and diagnostic imaging data provides the answer but conservatism is uncalled for. This lesion must be pursued aggressively.

References

1. Samoilov VI. *Subarachnoid Hemorrhage* [in Russian]. Leningrad, Russia: Medicina; 1990;232.
2. Fisher CM, Kistler JP, Davis JM. Relation of cerebral vasospasm to subarachnoid hemorrhage visualized by computerized tomographic scanning. *Neurosurgery*. 1980; 6:1–9.
3. Hornyak M, Gilsbach J, Harders A. Clinical significance of computed tomography in early aneurysm surgery. *Neurochirurgia*. 1991;34:135–140.
4. Rinkel GJ, Wijdicks EF, Vermeulen M, Ramos LM, Tanghe HLJ, Hasan D, Meiners LC, van Gijn J. Nonaneurysmal perimesencephalic subarachnoid hemorrhage: CT and MR patterns that differ from aneurysmal rupture. *AJNR*. 1991;12:829–834.
5. Dujovny M, Kossovsky N, Kossowsky R, Diaz FG, Ausman JI. Magnetic aneurysm clips – correlation with martensite content and implications for nuclear magnetic resonance (NMR) examination. *Surg Forum*. 1983;34:525–527.
6. Hasan D, Vermeulen M, Wijdicks EFM, Hijdra A, van Gijin JV. Effect of fluid intake and antihypertensive treatment on cerebral ischemia after subarachnoid hemorrhage. *Stroke*. 1989;20:1511–1515.
7. Shinoda J, Kimura T, Funakoshi T, Araki Y, Imao Y. Acetazolamide reactivity on cerebral blood flow in patients with subarachnoid haemorrhage. *Acta Neurochir* (*Wien*). 1991;109:102–108.
8. Hasan D, Vermeulen M, Wijdicks EFM, Hijdra A, Van Gijin JV. Management problems in acute hydrocephalus after subarachnoid hemorrhage. *Stroke*. 1989;20:747–753.
9. Sloan MA, Rigamonti D, Rothman M, Burch C, Permutt T, Bradstreet P, Numaguchi Y. Sensitivity and specificity of transcranial Doppler for detection of basilar artery vasospasm. Abstract. (The 16th International Symposium on Cerebral Hemodynamics, Transcranial Doppler, Cerebral Blood Flow, and Other Modalities; January 27–29, 1992; Phoenix, AZ.). *Stroke*. 1992;23:469.
10. Sloan MA, Rigamonti D, Rothman M, Burch C, Permutt T, Bradstreet P, Numaguchi Y. Sensitivity and specificity of transcranial Doppler for detecting vertebral artery vasospasm. Abstract. (The 16th International Symposium on Cerebral Hemodynamics, Transcranial Doppler, Cerebral Blood Flow, and Other Modalities; January 27–29, 1992; Phoenix, AZ.). *Stroke*. 1992;23:469.

4
Clinical Features

Once an aneurysm ruptures, morbidity and mortality rise sharply. Only about one in five patients escapes unharmed, and even those complain of headache, fatigue, and memory disturbances. Our common goal must be to recognize and assign risks to the unruptured aneurysm in order to apply treatment effectively.

Unruptured Aneurysms

Unruptured aneurysms may be classified in several categories. *Incidental aneurysms* are those that are discovered during a neurodiagnostic procedure such as magnetic resonance imaging (MRI) examination that is carried out for conditions other than the aneurysm. If they are associated with another aneurysm that has recently ruptured, they are accompanied by special risks for bleeding.

Symptomatic unruptured aneurysms present with signs and symptoms unrelated to subarachnoid hemorrhage (SAH), most often due to the effect of their size and relationship to adjacent structures. Perhaps 90% of all aneurysms remain asymptomatic until they rupture, leaving only 10% causing symptoms prior to the onset of hemorrhage. The aneurysm causing symptoms or signs by virtue of enlargement also falls into a special high-risk category.

The incidence of unruptured aneurysms is difficult to determine. Some studies indicate that as many as 8% or as few as 1% of the population show some aneurysmal dilatation along the cerebral arterial tree by the time they die.[1,2] With an annual incidence of SAH cases at 15 to 20 per 100 000 population SAH cases per year, the risk (less than 1%) is thus fairly low for SAH from a single unruptured aneurysm.[3–5]

Clinical Signs of Unruptured Aneurysms

In 1929, Sands[6] recognized the special relationship of carotid artery aneurysms to the third cranial nerve. Dandy[7] described a case in 1938 in which pain in a retroorbital location and third cranial nerve palsy led him to explore the carotid artery area, confirming the association of an aneurysm with paralysis of the third cranial nerve in a living patient. Dandy believed that his case was the first attempt to cure an aneurysm of the circle of Willis by direct approach upon the aneurysm.

The window of opportunity for the manifestation of symptoms without rupture is small but existent. Headache is a common complaint in patients whose aneurysms are increasing in size. The head pain cannot localize the aneurysm, but periorbital pain in patients with carotid artery aneurysms may signal impending rupture.[8]

Anterior communicating artery (AComA) aneurysms and middle cerebral artery (MCA) aneurysms tend not to localize. Diplopia and evidence of third cranial nerve involvement are symptoms that lead most patients with unruptured aneurysms (in the range of 90%) to seek medical attention. These most often occur with aneurysms located at the internal carotid–posterior communicating artery junction. Aneurysms at the junction of the ophthalmic artery and internal carotid artery (ICA) are the second most frequent to produce symptoms prior to rupture. In this group, headache and orbital pain are the most common complaints although disturbance of vision, due to involvement of the optic nerves, occurs in approximately one-third of the patients.

Aneurysms of the vertebral artery may compress multiple nerves of the posterior fossa including the fifth, seventh, and eighth. Tortuous vessels and fusiform dilatations are much more common in the etiology of trigeminal neuralgia than saccular aneurysms. Since no prospective trials have yet been completed, there is little scientific data relating to how patients with unruptured or incidental aneurysms fair. Wiebers et al.[9] noted a hemorrhage rate of 1.5% per year among 81 patients with unruptured aneurysms in the Mayo Clinic series. In one subset, all of these aneurysms that ruptured were greater than 10 mm in diameter.

The matter of size is even more controversial because some of the case reports refer to fixed aneurysms observed at postmortem examination and others compare aneurysms observed angiographically while distended with blood. A critical size must be reached before aneurysms begin to cause symptoms. Almost 75% of patients with symptoms have aneurysms at least 10 mm in size. The critical size for rupture is about 7 mm. Kassell and Torner[10] have operative treatment for lesions of 5 mm or greater in diameter based on the rebleeding rate, but aneurysm size may fluctuate or even change rapidly. There is little data regarding age, hypertension, or other variables on growth and rupture rates of unruptured intracranial aneurysms. However, the incidence of SAH increases linearly up to about age 70; beyond this age, there are many questions as to whether adequate angiographic studies were carried out. For patients older than 60, who harbor an intracranial aneurysm, however, the risk of rupture may be as high as 5% to 6% per year. In the series reported by McCormick and Acosta-Rua,[2] over 80% of aneurysms measuring 6 mm were discovered at autopsy and had already bled. These would have been larger had they been observed on the angiogram.

The symptomatic unruptured aneurysm represents a special risk class. The mechanisms that produce symptoms are enlargement, embolism, and compression of adjacent structures (Fig. 4.1). Their annual risk of bleeding may be as high as 6.25%. Wiebers et al.[11] followed patients with symptomatic but unruptured aneurysm, and 36% of these subsequently bled with an extremely high mortality over 8 years of follow-up.

Even giant asymptomatic aneurysms may have an unfavorable outcome. In Drake's[12] study of 18 patients with giant symptomatic but unruptured aneurysms, 15 either died or became disabled. Thus, the presence of a symptomatic but unruptured intracranial aneurysm carries anything but a benign clinical course, and these lesions must be managed operatively when risks are commensurate with their natural history. This risk must be estimated and measured carefully for each patient. While several series report low operative mortality, there is morbidity.

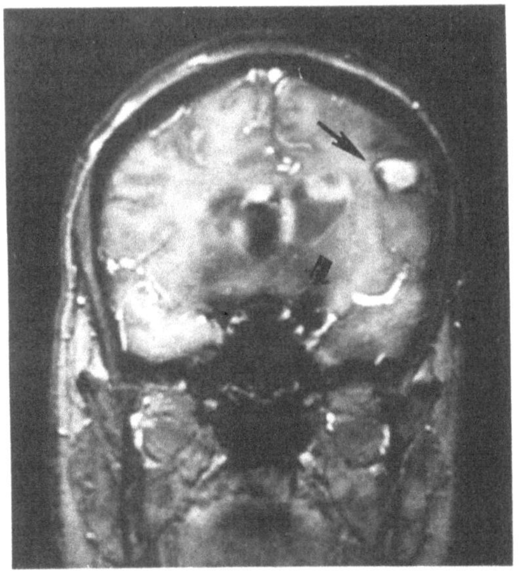

FIGURE 4.1. A large fusiform aneurysm of the internal carotid artery (large arrow) with distal embolization and infarction (small arrow).

Aneurysm size and location influences operative safety. Those less than 5 mm in diameter cause the fewest problems, with less than 2.3% morbidity. Aneurysms 6 to 15 mm in diameter were associated with a 6.8% morbidity and those 16 to 25 mm in diameter caused 14% of the patients to have problems postoperatively.[13]

Unruptured ophthalmic aneurysms are associated with 8% to 11% operative complications, while AComA aneurysms were among the most difficult with a 15.5% risk of operative morbidity. The carotid bifurcation aneurysm had a 16.8% operative morbidity.

No aneurysm should be viewed in a cavalier manner, especially one that is enlarging or causing symptoms when operated.

Ruptured Aneurysms

Worldwide, SAH probably accounts for about 50% of all cases of spontaneous intracranial bleeding. Kessler and Vogt[14] found aneurysms in 52% of over 6000 patients with SAH. Intracranial hemorrhage is the first and the most important sign of aneurysm rupture. The clinical signs depend on the location of the aneurysm, the mass effect of the hemorrhage, and the rate of bleeding. There are two main types of intracranial hemorrhage to be considered. SAH alone accounts for approximately 60% of the hemorrhages seen. Another 40% of the cases with ruptured aneurysm have hematomas either in the ventricular system or in the cerebral substance, based on computed tomography (CT) examination. The extent of the hemorrhage varies from the subtle sentinel hemorrhage that occurs in 25% of patients to the massive and usually fatal hemorrhage that tamponades cerebral blood flow (CBF).[8,15] In patients younger than 50, a rupture has already taken place in over 80% of the cases when the aneurysm is identified. Aneurysms that have secondary loculations have often ruptured while smooth-walled lesions may be asymptomatic. Even giant aneurysms, once believed to be safe, are sources of SAH.[16] Small asymptomatic aneurysms also rupture over time. Although the true incidence of rupture of an asymptomatic aneurysm is currently unknown, perhaps it falls in the range of 0.5% per year.

Aneurysms tend to bleed during times of stress imposed by everyday life and work. Early studies indicated that a large number of hemorrhages occurred during sleep.[17] If more careful histories had been sought, in light of today's freer discussions of sexual matters, perhaps the activity responsible would have been different. Otherwise, it is generally recognized that straining or excessive physical stress may precipitate aneurysm rupture.[18,19] Minor trauma has also occurred extraordinarily frequently in relation to hemorrhage.

Classifying the forms of hemorrhage in over 700 patients has allowed the definition of certain characteristic anatomical patterns of hemorrhage following aneurysm rupture. These are:

1. Subarachnoid hemorrhage
2. Cerebro-subarachnoid hemorrhage with extraventricular hematoma (< 50 ml)
3. Cerebro-subarachnoid hemorrhage with large extraventricular hematoma (> 50 ml)
4. Cerebro-subarachnoid hemorrhage with intraventricular hematoma without occlusion of the cerebrospinal fluid (CSF) pathways
5. Cerebro-subarachnoid hemorrhage with intraventricular hematoma and ventricular blockade

Subarachnoid Hemorrhage

The intensity of subarachnoid bleeding plays a large role in the makeup of the blood that fills the subarachnoid spaces. Small amounts of blood-tinged fluid may fill the subarachnoid pathways or thick clots may fill the subarachnoid cisterns. With large hemorrhages, there is retrograde propulsion of blood through the subarachnoid pathways into the ventricular system, and finally into the sulci overlying the cerebral cortex. The widest dissemination is seen from aneurysms that arise from the basilar apex, the basilar trunk, and the supraclinoid portion of the ICA. These aneurysms lie in large cisterns that communicate and can carry more blood per unit time at higher pressures. For aneurysms occupying the M_1 portion of the MCA, only 50% develop diffuse subarachnoid bleeding, based on the CT scan. Another 50% show hematoma formation in the sylvian fissure or in the surrounding cerebral substance.[20]

In small SAHs, the clinical course may be entirely benign and there may be few signs of brain translocation. Local neurological deficits are minimal or absent in the majority of cases. The hemodynamics remain stable for days and weeks after the hemorrhage. In massive hemorrhage, there may be evidence of acute intracranial hypertension with resulting signs attributable to midbrain or medullary compression secondary to brain herniation. If large clots are not found in the basilar cistern, the outcome is usually one of progressive improvement and stability. In patients with clots either in the basal cisterns or in the ventricles, the course is much more complicated and prolonged. Headache may be more intense, and lethargy, stupor, disorientation, nuchal rigidity, and focal neurological deficits may be noted. Deterioration from many causes can be expected to begin as early as 3 or 4 days after ictus and peak toward the beginning of the second week after onset of hemorrhage. At the end of the second or third week, there may again be stabilization.

The first clinical symptom of aneurysm rupture is usually headache. It is of sudden onset and probably caused by meningeal irritation. It radiates quickly into the occiput, down the cervical spine, and may eventually radiate into the lower extremities. If a clear history is available from the patient who is alert, the headache described is sudden in onset, involves the occiput, and, regardless of the site of the aneurysm, is initially nonlocalizing. Approximately one-fourth describe the so-called sentinel headache.[18] This is a premonitory clue occurring days to weeks prior to the major catastrophic hemorrhage. Headache, nausea, vomiting, and loss of consciousness are described by two-thirds of those who develop SAH. Patients observed during aneurysm rupture tend to develop decerebrate posturing, profuse sweating, pupillary dilatation, and clonic movements suggesting epileptic seizures. Some patients become comatose at onset, and a small percentage develop true grand mal seizures. Patients surviving this major hemorrhage experience violent nausea and vomiting as they awaken. The neck becomes rigid and within a few hours they complain of neck, back, and leg pain. Photophobia quickly ensues, and the patient may become confused or disoriented. Localizing neurological findings are often absent. A rare patient might not notice headache but might describe a loud popping sensation. Others notice loss of hearing or vision. One-fourth of the patients describe relatively minor discomfort due to headache.[21]

Aneurysms that rupture in the sylvian fissure produce intratemporal and sometimes deep hematomas in the frontal lobe that cause contralateral paresis or sensory disturbances. Occasionally, homonymous hemianopsia may be encountered. Although vertigo and balance disturbances have poor localizing value, aneurysms of the posterior cranial circulation are more commonly associated with these symptoms than those of the anterior circulation. An oral apraxia or akinetic mutism is sometimes encountered in patients who have aneurysms of the AComA, especially if they rupture into the septal area. The patient seems alert and responsive but can neither form words nor use the mouth to eat or drink. In other cases, there may be weakness of the lower extremities from secondary ischemia of the anterior cerebral artery (ACA) territory. Another clinical indicator of SAH is nuchal rigidity that develops almost as soon as the examination can be carried out. By the time blood has traversed the CSF pathways, Kernig's and Brudzinski's signs are also positive.

The computerized axial tomogram and lumbar puncture still play an important role in the management and diagnosis of acute aneurysmal SAH. The CT scan should be the first ancillary examination used in the patient who describes acute onset of headache associated with meningeal signs. Coital headache, even without meningeal irritation, is an indication for CT scan and/or lumbar puncture. For the patient with sentinel hemorrhage, the CT may not be diagnostic, however, and only the lumbar puncture is reliable for minor bleeding. Red blood cells, no matter how few, in the patient with acute onset of headache should raise the specter of SAH due to an intracranial aneurysm. It is at this stage that treatment can be applied most efficaciously.[22]

Eye findings may be especially useful in patients with SAH. Quite a number develop large dark pools of blood in the preretinal space or subhyaloid space. These are pathognomonic of acute increased intracranial pressure (ICP) and also occur with acute subdural hematomas. Approximately 50% of aneurysms located on the ICA near the posterior communicating junction develop ipsilateral pupillary dilatation.[23] Pupillary fibers are superficial on the third cranial nerve while medial rectus and levator fibers are quite deep. Without pupillary dilatation, another source, such as diabetes mellitus, should be sought to explain the third cranial nerve palsy.

All of the first symptoms appear abruptly as the aneurysm ruptures and bleeding occurs within the subarachnoid space. During the next few hours and days, other symptoms and signs, such as hydrocephalus, vasospasm, and intracranial hypertension, may appear insidiously due to complications of the hemorrhagic period.

Cerebro-subarachnoid Hemorrhage

In patients with this form of hemorrhage, hematoma forms within the cerebral substance, within the subdural space, within the interhemispheric fissure, in the sylvian fissure, or in the ventricular system. Hematomas making up a volume of 50 ml or less are found in approximately 25% of all of those who have hematomas.[16] Large hematomas with volumes greater than 100 ml make up 22% of the total group. Hematomas occupying the lateral ventricles only, without blockage in the third ventricle aqueduct or foramen Monro, make up 15%. Hematomas occupying all the ventricular chambers and forming casts that tamponade CSF flow unfortunately make up the largest group, accounting for 36% of those with intracranial hemorrhages.[16]

Intracranial hematomas are the most important consideration in patients with acute ICP, brain herniation, and hydrocephalus. The clinical signs produced depend on the volume, location, and the rate of onset of bleeding. Larger hematomas invariably cause greater overall diffuse and focal neurological findings. In patients with small hematomas, compensation is the rule, and an entirely benign clinical course may be encountered. In those with large hematomas greater than 100 ml, the opposite is true.[24] One-third of these patients decompensate due to acute hydrocephalus or acute brain herniation. In patients with major intraventricular hemorrhage, the vast majority deteriorate due to brain stem compression or hydrocephalus. Prompt ventricular drainage may stabilize the clinical course at least for a time. Most often, small hematomas occupy the frontal horns and the anterior aspect of the temporal horns. Rarely, the occipital horns and third ventricles are affected. Large hematomas may tamponade the ventricular system. Following an AComA aneurysm rupture, hematomas dissect into the anterior aspect of the lateral ventricle or temporal horn. However, some present with hematomas in both frontal horns and the third ventricle. In most cases, the entry of the hematoma is apparently through the medial basal frontal lobe and through the lamina terminalis. In patients harboring aneurysms on the MCA, the blood dissects into the ventricles near the temporal lobe but rarely into the frontal lobe. Hematomas occupying the fourth ventricle and the aqueduct of Sylvius are often due to retrograde propulsion of blood through the subarachnoid pathways. In these cases, with retrograde dissection, severe acute hydrocephalus due to tamponade of the cisterna magna and major basal cisterns invariably occurs.

Clinical signs depend on the location of the hematoma, and its size. Commonly, hematomas develop near the central sulcus and thus, motor and sensory disorders, and speech problems arise if the hematoma is in the dominant hemisphere. Normally, the deficits associated with hematomas appear immediately at onset. However, even in patients without hematomas, transient acute vasospasm may produce paresis due to ischemic lesions in the territory of these vessels. In patients with small hematomas, a benign clinical course is possible. However, those with large hematomas often succumb to their disease.

The clinical course of patients with intracranial hematomas due to a ruptured intracranial aneurysm, as observed on CT scanning, can be more or less accurately predicted. SAH causes a distinct clinical pattern that correlates with the amount of blood present in the subarachnoid pathways. Those with cerebro-subarachnoid hemorrhage (Cerebro-SAH) can be separated into two distinct classes based on the volume of the hematoma present in the brain. Those in whom the hematoma dissects into the ventricular system also have predictable clinical courses and outcomes dependent upon tamponade.

Associated Disorders of the Hemorrhagic Period

The causes of the deterioration in SAH relate to vasospasm, hydrocephalus, intracranial hypertension, and coagulation disorders. The expression of these pathological processes varies according to the time of onset of hemorrhage, the intensity of the SAH, and its severity. The pathological events that develop following aneurysm rupture follow a periodicity that can be predicted from patient to patient.

Intracranial Hypertension

Intracranial hypertension develops from a number of causes: the space-occupying lesion in the subarachnoid space, the intracerebral hematoma, the blockage of subarachnoid pathways, ischemic edema, and failure of autoregulation. In its worst form, it results in herniation and death. Intracranial hypertension affects all stages and is the most significant factor in determining outcome. Many cases do not come to the clinical attention of neurologists or neurosurgeons due to the high incidence of sudden death associated with acute aneurysm rupture.

The hypertension–hydrocephalic syndrome is the common term used to describe the increasing ICP of the acute period. All factors combine to produce a common clinical syndrome, and all finally result in involvement and compression of the brain stem. Doshi and Neil-Dwyer[25] looked at the hypothalamus of 12 patients who had died of acute aneurysm rupture. In 92%, there was evidence of hypothalamic damage. Using radioimmunoassay, Alexeev et al.[26] demonstrated the interrelationship with the hypothalamus–hypophysis and suprarenal system in patients with SAH. There was a clear correlation with hyperactivity of this system initially in patients with severe hemorrhage. These authors also demonstrated collapse of the system.

Harden et al.[27] demonstrated high initial levels of dopamine β-hydroxylase, which decreased as the suprarenal system failed. Accompanying this was an acute hypothalamic deficiency syndrome and peripheral epinephrine supersensitivity.

Intracranial hypertension may be of two distinct types. Hypertension may be due to the presence of an intracranial mass lesion such as a hematoma in the cerebral substance or in the subarachnoid pathways. Second, hypertension may result from hydrocephalus due to obstruction of CSF pathways, ischemia, and brain edema. The clinical signs that predominate in patients with intracranial hypertension are headaches of increasing severity, disorders of consciousness and decerebracy. In Zubkov's[24] series of 395 patients, headache was absent only in 1%. Headache was intense in 93%, and moderate in only 5%. Headache is usually described as expansile and associated with nausea and vomiting.

Of greater gravity, disorders of consciousness occur in 55.2% of patients with recent SAH. It is present in 75.4% of those harboring cerebral subarachnoid hematomas, further suggesting the role of intracranial hypertension. Patients harboring large intracerebral or intraventricular hematomas are always unconscious for periods longer than 30 min. Intracranial hypertension may also be associated with signs of brain stem dysfunction. Initially, increased ICP may be so severe as to compromise flow into the cerebral microcirculation resulting in multiple microinfarctions. As swelling develops, the brain stem may be compressed by the herniated uncus, and this may further result in brain stem ischemia.

Herniation syndromes often develop in patients with intracerebral hematomas. Later, herniation syndromes develop due to vasogenic edema and hydrocephalus. Both lateral and axial dislocations occur.

Fundoscopic examination shows edema of the optic nerve in 15% and vitreous hemorrhage (Terson's syndrome) in 8% of those with acute SAH. Terson's syndrome has been seen more often in patients with severe SAH and develops early after the onset.

Three stages of intracranial hypertension may be recognized and identified. Mild intracranial hypertension is characterized clinically by lethargy, moderate headache, and minimal brain stem symptoms such as reduced corneal reflex and gag reflex. No evidence of herniation occurs in this group of patients who have mild meningeal and neurological signs.

In the moderate intracranial hypertension group, headache is severe and agitation is present. The level of consciousness is further decreased and the patient may become hostile and belligerent. More pronounced brain stem symptoms appear. Upward gaze paresis is often present. The blood pressure may be slightly elevated and the pulse diminished. Increased reflexes in the lower extremities and bilateral Babinski signs may also develop. Anisocoria and strabismus may be noted. Among patients showing these signs, over half had SAH only and the remainder had intracerebral hemorrhage.

Severe intracranial hypertension occurs in patients in higher clinical grades, most harboring intraventricular and intracerebral hematomas. The condition is characterized by further decrease in the levels of consciousness and the appearance of brain stem signs such as decerebracy characteristic of herniation.

Hydrocephalus

Many factors may be responsible for hydrocephalus following SAH. Among these, the subarachnoid clot plays a primary role. Julow[28] looked at the arachnoidal granulations following SAH using the electron microscope. He found fibrosis of the basal cisterns correlating well with the amount of blood that was present in the subarachnoid space and the presence of hydrocephalus.

The diagnosis of hydrocephalus is facilitated by the use of MR and CT scanning. Wenig et al.[29] reported hydrocephalus in 69% of the cases that were studied. The use of MRI and CT establishes the diagnosis of SAH and allows the surgeon to differentiate between the communicating and noncommunicating varieties. The dynamics of the CSF circulation can also be tested. The disproportionate size between the lateral, third, and fourth ventricles gives a good estimation of where the obstruction lies. A normal-sized fourth ventricle in the presence of enlargement of the third and lateral ventricles suggests aqueductal stenosis.

Radioisotopic cisternography, once a procedure widely used, is now usually unnecessary. However, when introduced into the subarachnoid pathways, yttrium (Y) finds its way into the ventricular circulation within 24 hours if there is no obstruction. Otherwise, it may pass throughout the subarachnoid pathways to be absorbed without entering the ventricular system.

Two types of hydrocephalus have been recognized clinically, based on the time of onset in relation to the SAH. Acute hydrocephalus developing within hours or days is usually caused by ventricular or outflow obstruction. Hydrocephalus developing days or weeks after the initial hemorrhage and persisting for days or weeks is usually referred to as subacute hydrocephalus. Subacute hydrocephalus may extend into a chronic phase and is often associated with normal ICP. Subacute and chronic hydrocephalus occur more often when antifibrinolytic agents are used.

In 1984, Hayashi et al.[30] described chronic low pressure hydrocephalus, or normal pressure hydrocephalus in 17.6% of their patients. Both CBF and cerebral blood pressure were investigated. These authors separated hydrocephalus into three stages: the acute phase (occurring within one week), a prodromal phase, and a normal pressure hydrocephalus stage. Patients in the prodromal phase and with low-pressure hydrocephalus usually had ventricular dilatation with periventricular edema associated with malabsorption. The third stage, hydrocephalus, resulted in the accumulation of radioactive isotopes in the ventricular system, and ventricular dilatation. Blood flow during the acute phase was 42.9 ml per 100 g/min. During the prodromal phase it is diminished to 35.1 ml/min, and then finally to 23.8 ml/min during the low-pressure hydrocephalus variant. The low CBF correlated closely with the low CSF pressures that were encountered. Shunting operations led to the recovery of patients with normal pressure hydrocephalus if CBF was greater than 25 ml per 100 g brain tissue.

Vassilouthis and Richardson[31] described the clinical signs associated with subacute hydrocephalus. Among these, disturbances of consciousness, moodiness, decreased mentation, gait disorders, and urinary disturbances predominated. In our series, hydrocephalus was found in 76% of patients in grade 1, in 86% in grade 2, and in 95% in grade 3. Graded on the basis of severity, hydrocephalus was severe in only 20% of grade 1 patients, in 25% of grade 2, but in 50% of grade 3 or decompensated patients. From day 4 to day 14 following SAH, hydrocephalus tends to become more frequent and severe. Many factors apparently combine to influence the development of late hydrocephalus including herniation, edema, and organization of the clot within the ventricular system. Dilatation of the temporal horn, as seen on the CT scan, may be the first sign of temporal lobe herniation. Hydrocephalus tends to occur more often in patients with cerebro-SAH than in patients with hematomas localized within the subarachnoid space. The combination of vasospasm, ischemia, and hydrocephalus often leads to increasing ICP and clinical deterioration.

Cerebral Vasospasm

Angiographic constriction of the cerebral circulation after aneurysm rupture was described originally by Ecker and Riemenschneider,[32] who theorized that it was due to compression or traction upon the vascular structures. Later, however, Echlin[33] showed that fresh blood could cause an immediate constriction of cerebral arteries when applied locally. The term *vasospasm* was born in this era from these experiments. Serotonin and a number of blood-related products can also produce this acute constriction. By definition, a spasm is an involuntary but transient contraction of a muscle or group of muscles. There is convincing evidence that long-lasting or propagated spasm is actually due to constriction rather than muscular contraction. Unfortunately, the clinical disorder like that observed in human cases has no counterpart in nature and the pathophysiology of the reaction remains unclear.

In 1964, Crompton[34] studied the vessels of patients who had died of aneurysmal SAH; he described thickening in the medial and subintimal layers of both arteries and veins. More recently, it has been recognized that the term *vasospasm* may have been applied inappropriately. Konovalov[35] emphasized that the condition is a "steady long-lasting reaction of basal arteries due to rupture of the vessel and development of SAH." Wilkins et al.[36] reviewed the response of vasospasm to various dilating drugs, and, although over 100 drugs had been used over the past two decades, none had proven to be consistently effective in relieving the condition. Recently investigators have used other terms to define and describe narrowing of the brain vessels. Clower et al.[37] referred to the condition as *constrictive endarteropathy of SAH*. Ausman et al.[38] used the term *vasculopathy* and Finn et al.[39] termed the condition *vasoconstrictive arteriopathy*. The arterial wall becomes stiffer after SAH, related either to the rearrangement or the further deposition of connective tissue.

The angiopathy that develops after SAH has been characterized by Smith et al.[40,41] The first stage is characterized by intimal edema with reduction in wrinkling of the internal elastic membrane. In the second stage, Sasaki et al.[42] found necrosis in the medial layer and widespread deposition of mucopolysaccharides. In the third stage, atrophy of the medial layers with increase in the subintimal layers occurs. The fourth stage is characterized by opening of the lumen and reduction in the wall thickening. Stage five is characterized by regeneration in the medial layer but with further opening of the vessel lumen. The pathological events occur all along the vessel wall but not necessarily in equal proportion. Although the pathology is much clearer, the mechanisms responsible for contraction and for inciting the morphological alterations are still unknown.

The etiology of cerebral vasospasm is also unknown at present. Many believe that the lysis of the clot with the liberation of iron-containing compounds promotes a cascade of phospholipid peroxidation. The cascade expands from cell to cell, injuring the vessel wall. The resulting injury in some way results in the polymerization of actin and a prolonged type of contraction. One possible mechanism may be compared to that which occurs when a gouged-out wound of skin contracts, pulling the margins together. This is accomplished by a cell known as a myofibroblast, which may be derived from either smooth muscle cells, fibroblasts, or others. The proliferation of myofibroblasts has been observed in the intracranial vessels of virtually every patient dying of vasospasm in our hospitals. Myofibroblasts have been cultured from the cerebral arteries of five patients who died of cerebral vasospasm. No myofibroblasts have been cultured from arteries of patients dying of other causes. Therefore, the presence of these contractile cells suggests that they may be operant in the patient with cerebral vasospasm. The fact that they respond to angioplasty but not to smooth muscle relaxing agents is further suggestive of their role in the chronic or recurrent phase of vasospasm.

Myofibroblasts function quite differently from smooth cells. Since they are migratory cells, they send foot processes through the connective tissue layer and these filopodia attach themselves to collagen fibers at specific binding sites. Then the connective tissue is tightened and woven together in a process that causes constriction (Fig 4.2). Apparently, simultaneous traction and twisting of the fibers occurs as they are contracted. The myofibroblast, being a migratory cell, responds directly to agents in the chemical milieu. Likewise, these cells probably respond to wound hormones such as the platelet-derived growth factor (PDGF) or transforming growth factor–β (TGF-β).[43]

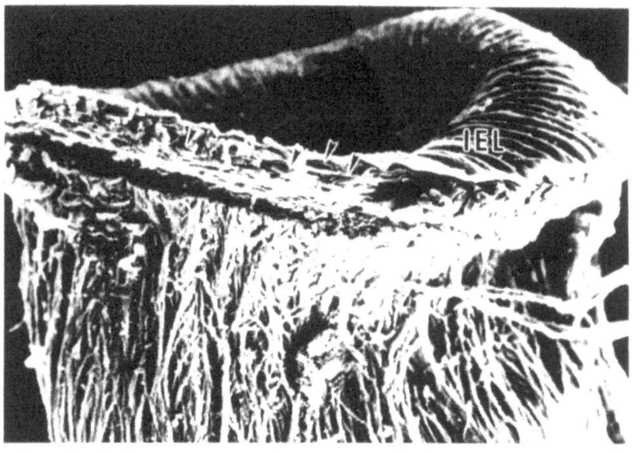

FIGURE 4.2. Middle cerebral artery demonstrating the collagen matrix. The fibers are arranged in layers. The internal elastic membrane runs longitudinally, the medial layers circumferentially, and the adventitial layers are longitudinal. This provides strength to the cerebral vessel. The myofibroblast migrates between the collagen fibrils, binding to them at specific sites, and tightening them to produce constriction of the cerebral artery.

Diagnostic Features of Vasospasm

To the angiographer, vasospasm is seen as a vessel that narrows sequentially on the diagnostic studies performed after SAH. The narrowing may occupy only a segment (segmental vasospasm), the major vessel upon which the aneurysm arises (regional vasospasm), or it may be seen throughout the subarachnoid pathways (diffuse vasospasm). To the angiographer, several types and degrees of vasospasm are easily recognized. In one, if the artery in question is narrowed to only half the diameter of its normal diameter, it may be spoken of as moderate vasospasm. If it is narrowed by more than 50% of its prehemorrhagic state, severe vasospasm is declared.

Hamer and Gotte[44] studied 80 patients who were operated. Three kinds of vasospasm were described in this group: diffuse, multisegmental, and local. These authors also concluded that patients in the highest clinical grades deteriorated not only from vasospasm but for other reasons also. Simeone et al.[45] indicate that ischemic symptoms begin when the diameter of the vessel is less than one-half of normal. In addition, thrombosis in the aneurysm and in the parent vessels, blood viscosity, cardiac output, the status of the penetrating arteries, and many other factors probably play a role. Such variables as ICP, the individual peculiarities of the regional circulation, accompanying hypertension or hypotension, and disorders of microcirculation must also be considered.

Based on the angiogram, vasospasm of different degrees develops in more than half of all patients following aneurysm rupture. However, with transcranial Doppler (TCD) sonography, virtually every patient may have some increase in velocity after aneurysm rupture.[46] In a cooperative study, all studies seemed to indicate that patients who have the most blood in subarachnoid pathways are at greater risk of developing clinical signs of vasospasm.[27] Kassell and co-workers[47] postulated that the clinical events relate not only to the degree of vasospasm but also are tied closely to the presence of collateral vessels in the subarachnoid pathways. The mere presence of angiographic vasospasm should not be assumed, however, to account for the patient's deteriorating state until all other possible factors that might be responsible have been excluded.

Ancillary tests may be useful in prognosticating vasospasm. The EEG often shows focal slowing, correlating well with the radiographic pictures. Xe blood flow studies may also be useful. A poor clinical condition usually correlates with low blood flow and the CBF studies may be of value in localizing ischemic areas. Loss of autoregulation is nearly a constant feature of all extremely ill patients. A reduction in CBF to about half of the normal values is often accompanied by unsatisfactory outcomes.

Clinical Features of Vasospasm

The clinical features of vasospasm usually appear toward the end of the first week after hemorrhage. They may be delayed until the 12th day but rarely longer. Over 50% of patients who have a ruptured intracranial aneurysm develop clinical ischemia. There is, however, a great deal of variability in the incidence. More than 80% of obtunded patients have constricted vessels but fewer than 15% of those who are alert on admission show the angiographic pattern. Based on the TCD measurements, almost all patients with SAH develop some constriction. In our series, almost 65% of the patients developed clinical symptomatic vasospasm.[46]

Thirty-five percent of our patients did not develop angiographic constriction following SAH. Moderate vasospasm was present in 47%, and severe radiographic constriction was present in 18%. Thus, vasospasm, as seen from the angiogram, is present in two-thirds of all patients who have SAH from an intracranial aneurysm. In patients with higher clinical grades, vasospasm is always diffuse. In lower grades, segmental or focal vasospasm may be present. Sixty percent of the patients in whom blood occupies the subarachnoid space have vasospasm on the initial angiogram, 16.8% of a severe nature. In patients with intracerebral and intraventricular hematomas, the incidence of vasospasm is 73% on the initial angiogram.

There are clinical corollaries of angiographic vasospasm. To a large extent, the clinical picture is determined by the clinical grade and the collateral circulation and thereby the expression of ischemic findings. Two types of onset can be defined: gradual and apoplectic.

The gradual type of clinical onset occurs more commonly in patients in lower clinical grades. The primary sign of brain ischemia is deepening of the level of consciousness at the end of the first or beginning of the second week (3–5 days). Signs of midbrain dysfunction, such as upward gaze paresis and divergent strabismus, appear. Mild motor signs, such as a drift of the outstretched extremities, may also appear. The CSF may be hemorrhagic during the first week and xanthochromic in the second and third weeks of the disease but increased ICP is usually not a problem. Signs of hypothalamic dysfunction may also be noted at this time. Increasing nuchal rigidity and headache, a low-grade fever, and abnormalities of sweating may be recorded. Initially, anhidrosis first appears on the body with increased temperature sensation of the trunk and extremities and excessive sweating on the face and forehead. Later, total anhidrosis may develop. Hypersensitivity to epinephrine also develops and this is manifested by abnormal reaction of 1% epinephrine placed in the conjunctival sac.

The apoplectic onset commonly appears in patients in higher clinical grades. In these patients, clinical decompensation may occur over an interval of minutes or hours and is easily confused with rebleeding episodes. In this group, motor and sensory findings predominate while the levels of consciousness may be maintained. ICP may be high initially but does not increase markedly with the onset of clinical worsening, which helps to distinguish it from rebleeding. In both the apoplectic and gradual forms, the small penetrating arteries may be responsible for the neurological deficits that appear.

Scintigraphy and SPECT scanning at this time may show ischemic areas in the subcortical white matter and brain stem. CT infarcts develop in almost all patients who have significant amounts of blood in the subarachnoid space.[22]

Rebleeding and Disorders of Coagulation

The presence of a hematoma seems to favor rebleeding and aneurysms greater than 9 mm in any dimension rebleed more often. There does not seem to be a clear relationship between rebleeding and low clinical grade.[48]

Rebleeding in patients treated by nonoperative methods varies according to the many factors previously listed and by virtue of aneurysm location. About 10% rebleed in the first week, 12% in the second week, 7% in the third week, and 8% in the fourth week. Rebleeding levels off to about 1% to 2% per week except for AComA aneurysms, which have a late rebleeding tendency.[24] Overall, 70% of the hemorrhages have occurred by the end of 4 weeks. The most frequent time to expect this unfortunate complication is in the beginning of the second week after the first hemorrhage. There may be a peak in frequency on the same or next day of the original episode also. Rebleeding occurs when the wound in the artery is weakest, when thrombolysis occurs at the end of the first week, and before gliosis has developed.

Most rebleeding is clustered in the first few months after the initial ictus.[23] However, even late bleeding occurs.[49] McKissock[50] followed patients whose aneurysms had ruptured at least 6 months previously who were still alive. This represented approximately 64% of the original group of patients who were in the study. Ninety-seven percent of these patients were alive at 1 year, 92% at 2 years, and 82% at the end of 9 years. However, overall survival for the group was 62% at 1 year, 59% at 2 years, and 53% at 9 years when the total 364 patients were considered. Many of these were victims of recent hemorrhage.

Recently, a number of reports have appeared that seem to implicate the coagulation system in rebleeding. Both local and disseminated coagulation disorders are described. The status of the coagulation systems seems to vary in relation to the time after the onset of the intracranial hemorrhage. In patients with recent SAH coagulation, studies are often near normal. As the severity of the hemorrhage increases, there is a tendency toward both local and systemic hypercoagulability. Fibrinolytic activity also becomes elevated. The coagulogram is prognostically important for estimating rebleeding tendency. In the study reported by Zubkov and Matsko,[16] 265 patients received no antifibrinolytic therapy, 20% rebled during the first month, 8 patients had more than one bleeding episode during this interval, and there was a tendency toward late rebleeding. Seventy percent who rebled were in the high-risk group and died. In patients who rebled, there was local coagulopathy as demonstrated by variance between arterial and jugular venous fibrinolytic activity.

Clinical Grading

Attempting to balance the risks between rebleeding and cerebral vasospasm seems to require a contradictory response. In the acute stage of hemorrhage when cerebral vasospasm is reactive, surgical intervention may entail risks exceeding the natural history of the disease. Much effort has been expended in defining an interval in which operative treatment can be carried out most safely to prevent rebleeding. As SAH and its relationship to intracranial aneurysm became widely recognized, patients arrived in referral centers much earlier and in a much better condition than they had been seen in previous times. This gave surgeons the opportunity to repair aneurysms earlier after SAH. It was soon realized, however, that operative interventions in these acute cases, at least in some patients, carried extremely high risks. Thus, risk assessment became important.

Up to the present time, nearly 50 different grading systems have been offered to and used by surgeons to characterize the conditions of the acute hemorrhagic period. These grading systems separate patients, based on clinical and radiographic markers, into 2 to 12 distinct groups. Most employ some aspects of the neurological examination for grading. Among the most widely known and accepted systems are the Hunt and Hess[51] scale, the Botterell et al.[52] classification, the scales of Suzuki and Hori,[53] Yasui et al.,[54] and the grading system of the World Federation of Neurosurgical Societies.[12] Few of these grading systems take into account the underlying pathophysiological conditions of the acute stage, which greatly affects the outcome. In allocating a patient to a particular grade following SAH, many factors come into play. Few grading systems allow cross-reference, and generally they do not take into account the important variables other than consciousness. It is not our intention to further confuse clinical grading but to simplify it. The combined cases from the Polenov Institute and the University of Mississippi Medical Center (Zubkov, Smith, and Tarassoli) are grouped into four simple grades based on whether hemorrhages occurred and on overall severity of the important manifestations and pathologic processes of the event. The categories are unruptured, mild, moderate, or severe grades. Factors are added that have been shown to be most significant in determining final outcome. The grading system can be carried out simply at the bedside in a few moments and a clinical grade assigned.

Grade 0 – Patients with unruptured aneurysms
Grade 1 – Patients with ruptured aneurysms and minor signs (compensated)
Grade 2 – Patients with ruptured aneurysms and moderate signs (subcompensated)
Grade 3 – patients with ruptured aneurysms and severe signs (decompensated)

This simplified classification was derived from a computerized data base in which over 200 factors, symptoms, and signs were entered. Only 21 of these were found to be significant to the final outcome. Among these 21, some were much more important than others, and these were weighted accordingly. The following *signs* and *symptoms* were determined to be more significant:

1. General condition and health.
2. Consciousness.
3. Meningeal signs.

4. Korsakoff's syndrome.
5. Posturing.
6. Pupillary abnormalities.
7. Gaze paresis.
8. Hemispheric dysfunctions including motor paresis or speech disorders.
9. Papilledema
10. Respiratory rate and rhythm.

The following *factors* were also found to be highly relevant in assessing the outcome:

1. Age.
2. Number of subarachnoid hemorrhages.
3. Interval of unconsciousness following hemorrhage.
4. Abnormal motor movements at the onset of hemorrhage.
5. Elevated systemic arterial pressure.
6. Systemic disease.

From diagnostic studies, the following *findings* were also found to be highly significant factors in relation to outcome:

TABLE 4.1. Symptoms, factors, and findings making up grading system

Factors, symptoms, syndromes	Mild	Moderate	Severe
Factors			
1. Age	<40	40–60	>60
2. Somatic pathology	Acute pathology of the lung and heart (mild)	Acute pathology of the lung and heart (moderate)	Acute pathology of the lung and heart (severe)
3. Number of prior SAH	None	One	Two and more
Symptoms and Syndrome			
4. Primary disorders of consciousness	<5 min	<30 min	>30 min
5. Seizure and decerebrate rigidity at itcus	None	Seizure	Decerebrate rigidity
6. Disorders of consciousness	Lethargy	Stupor	Coma
7. Meningeal symptoms	Photophobia, painful eye movements, especially in extreme directions Nuchal rigidity (1–2 crossfingers) Kernig's signs up to 160°	Nuchal rigidity 3–4 fingers Kernig's signs up to 130°–140°	Nuchal rigidity 5 fingers Kernig's sign up to 130°
8. Hemispheric symptoms	Asymmetry of reflexes, mild mono- or hemiparesis Mild sensory or motor aphasia Slight amnesia	Moderate hemiparesis Moderate aphasia Korsakoff syndrome	Hemiplegia Global aphasia
9. Brain stem symptoms	Decreased corneal reflexes	Impaired upward gaze	Respiratory dysfunction Tonic clonic seizures Bilateral mydriasis
10. Vegetative – visceral symptoms	Low-grade fever Tachycardia (up to 80) BP 130/80 Tachypnea (up to 24)	Fever up to 38°C Tachycardia up to 100/min BP 160–180/110 Tachypnea (up to 26–30) Moderate disturbances of peripheral circulation; pale skin or hypexamin; moderate acrocyanosis	Fever up to 39°–40°C Tachycardia up to 120/min BP >200 or <100 Tachypnea Respiration >30/min Dysfunction of respiration rhythm Marble skin, discoloration or acrocyanosis
11. EEG	Hypothalamic dysfunction structures: diencephalic syndrome in EEG Sometimes desynchronization with sharpened alpha rhythm	Severe mesenchephalic syndrome in EEG Desynchronization of alpha rhythm Desynchronization of delta rhythm	Mesenchephalic and medullary dysfunction Slow waves with significant reduction of amplitude Photostimulation reaction absent
12. Angiography	No vasospasm or mild vasospasm No signs of ventricular dilatation	Moderate vasospasm Moderate ventricular dilatation	Severe vasospasm: >50% reduction in vessel diameter Severe ventricular dilatation
13. CT, MRI	SAH, small clots in basal cisterns on the side of aneurysm	SAH, blood clots on both sides of B. cisterns and/or Ventricular dilatation and/or Small intracranial hematoma	SAH, blood clots in ventricles and/or Ventricular dilation and/or Large intracranial hematoma

1. Location and size of the aneurysm.
2. The presence of vasospasm.
3. The amount of intracranial blood.
4. Ventricular size.
5. EEG alterations (dyssymmetry and evidence of brain stem injury).

To use these symptoms, signs, factors, and diagnostic findings effectively, each factor is weighed independently. Any symptom, sign, or diagnostic variable is assigned to one of three levels (Table 4.1)

One factor, symptom, or diagnostic test associated with higher risk automatically places the patient in a more advanced grade. The classification is a dynamic one and is continually updated, based on the patient's response on daily examination. The highest grade on any examination during the hemorrhagic period determines the grade to which he is finally assigned. This allows the surgeons to compare the results of surgery and of nonoperative treatment based on pathological events during the hemorrhagic period, which do not always correlate with clinical parameters such as consciousness alone.

Using the above system, combined mortality for grade 0 is 2%. For grade 1, with mild manifestations of SAH, management mortality was 11%. Mortality for grade 2 patients was 54% and, for those with severe signs, management mortality was 90%. In patients with intraparenchymal hematomas (less than 50 ml), 48% arrive acutely in grade 1, 50% were in grade 2, and 2% were in grade 3. In patients with larger intraparenchymal hematomas (greater than 100 ml), only 11% are found to be in grade 1, 56% in grade 2, and 33% in grade 3.[24]

This simple system of grading, applicable both at the bedside and in the angiographic suite, correlates well with outcome.

The Phases of the Hemorrhagic Period

Following rupture of an intracranial aneurysm, three phases may be recognized, and, in each, a different pathologic process intervenes. The first, or ictal phase, consists of the first 3 days after hemorrhage. Pathologic events are secondary to rupture of the aneurysm and greatly depend upon the rate of bleeding, the direction of the dissection within the brain, and the amount of blood extravasated. Intracranial hypertension, ischemic deficits, vasogenic edema, and destruction of cerebral tissue all complicate phase 1. Patients in a high grade suffer mortality due to brain herniation.

Patients who survive the ictal stage may progress to a second period, the reactive phase. During this phase, the most likely complications are vasospasm and intracranial hypertension. The reactive phase lasts from 3 days to 3 weeks, depending on the patient's clinical grade.

Phase 3, the outcome phase, lasts from 3 weeks to 3 months or longer, and during this time final outcome may be prognosticated. By this stage, the effects of reactive vasospasm have run their course, ischemic lesions may be evaluated, and chronic hydrocephalus managed.

Conclusions

The hemorrhagic period may be characterized by at least three distinct phases: the ictal, the reactive, and the outcome phase. A pattern of pathological events and complications intervene in each of these phases, manifesting different degrees of expression. Intracranial hypertension, hydrocephalus, vasospasm, and coagulation disorders make up the bulk of the problems encountered during the varying phases. Final outcome is linked closely to the most severe event that complicates each phase.

References

1. Bannerman RM, Ingoll GB, Graf CJ. The familial occurrence of intracranial aneurysms. *Neurology.* 1970;20:283–292.
2. McCormick WF, Acosta-Rua GJ. The size of intracranial saccular aneurysms: an autopsy study. *J Neurosurg.* 1970; 33:422–427.
3. Fogelholm R. Subarachnoid hemorrhage in Middle-Finland: incidence, early prognosis and indication for neurosurgical treatment. *Stroke.* 1981;12:296–302.
4. Pakarinen S. Incidence, aetiology and prognosis of primary subarachnoid hemorrhage: a study based on 589 cases diagnosed in a defined urban population during a defined period. *Acta Neurol Scand.* 1967;43(suppl 29):1–128.
5. Phillips LM II, Whisnant JP, O'Fallon WM, Sundt TM Jr. The unchanging pattern of subarachnoid hemorrhage in a community. *Neurology.* 1980;30:1034–1040.
6. Sands IJ. Aneurysms of cerebral vessels. *Arch Neurol Psychiat.* 1929;21:37.
7. Dandy WE. Intracranial aneurysms of the internal carotid artery cured by operation. *Ann Surg.* 1938;107:654–659.
8. Suzuki J. *Cerebral Aneurysms.* Tokyo, Japan: Neuron; 1979.
9. Wiebers DO, Whisnant JP, O'Fallon WM. The natural history of unruptured intracranial aneurysms. *N Engl J Med.* 1981;304:696–698.
10. Kassell NF, Torner JC. Size of intracranial aneurysms. *Neurosurgery.* 1983;12:291–297.
11. Wiebers DO, Whisnant JP, Sundt TM Jr, O'Fallon, WM. The significance of unruptured intracranial saccular aneurysms. *J Neurosurg.* 1987;66:23–29.
12. Drake CG. Report of World Federation of Neurological Surgeons Committee on a universal subarachnoid hemorrhage grading scale. *J Neurosurg.* 1988;68:985–986.
13. Wirth FP. Surgical treatment of incidental intracranial aneurysms. *Clin Neurosurg.* 1986;33:125–135.

14. Kessler CH, Vogt U. Neurologische Diagnose und Therapie der Subarachnoidalblutung. *Ther Gegerw.* 1981; 120:137–151.
15. Suzuki J, Onuma T, Ioshimoto T. Results of early operations on cerebral aneurysms. *Surg Neurol.* 1979;11:407–412.
16. Zubkov YN, Matsko DE. Some clinical and anatomical characteristics of large and giant aneurysms of the brain [in Russian]. *Zh Nevropatol Psikhiatr.* 1980;80:1809–1813. [English Abstract].
17. Fisher CM. Clinical syndromes in cerebral thrombosis, hypertensive hemorrhage and ruptured saccular aneurysms. *Clin Neurosurg.* 1975;22:117–147.
18. Ball MJ. Pathogenesis of the "sentinel headache" preceding berry aneurysm rupture. *Can Med Assoc J.* 1975;112: 78–79.
19. Okawara A. Warning signs prior to rupture of an intracranial aneurysm. *J Neurosurg.* 1973;38:575–580.
20. Graf CJ, Nibbelink DW. Cooperative study of intracranial aneurysms and subarachnoid hemorrhage: report on a randomized treatment study. III. Intracranial surgery. *Stroke.* 1974;5:559–601.
21. Waga S, Ohtsubo K, Handa H. Warning signs in intracranial aneurysms. *Surg Neurol.* 1975;3:15–20.
22. Fisher CM, Kistler JP, Davis JM. Relation of cerebral vasospasm to subarachnoid hemorrhage visualized by computerized tomographic scanning. *Neurosurgery.* 1980;6: 1–9.
23. Sahs AL, Perret GE, Lockley HB, Nishioka H, eds. *Intracranial Aneurysms and Subarachnoid Hemorrhage. A Cooperative Study.* Philadelphia, PA: Lippincott; 1969.
24. Zubkov YN. *Treatment of Patients with Intracranial Arterial Aneurysms in the Hemorrhagic Period.* Moscow, Russia: 1990. Thesis.
25. Doshi R, Neil-Dwyer G. Hypothalamic and miocordial lesion after subarachnoid haemorrhage. *J Neurol Neurosurg Psychiatry.* 1977;40:821–826.
26. Alexeev VV, Balabolkin MT, Zubkov Y. Endocrine balance in patients with brain aneurysm rupture after operation. *Med Ref J (Rus).* 1985;9:316.
27. Harden TK, Klein RL, Smith RR, Thureson-Klein AK, Lowry MW. Serum dopamine beta-hydroxylase activity following subarachnoid hemorrhage in man. *Med Biol.* 1975;53:100–106.
28. Julow J. Prevention of subarachnoid fibrosis after subarachnoid hemorrhage with urokinase. Scanning electron microscopic study in the dog. *Acta Neurochir.* 1979;52:63–62.
29. Wenig C, Huber G, Enade H. Hydrocephalus after subarachnoid bleeding. *Eur Neurol.* 1979;18:1–7.
30. Hayashi M, Kobayashi M, Kawano T, Yamomoto S, Maeda T. Cerebral blood flow and ICP patterns in patients with communicating hydrocephalus after aneurysm rupture. *J Neurosurg.* 1984;61:30–36.
31. Vassilouthis J, Richardson AF. Ventricular dilation and communicating hydrocephalus following spontaneous subarachnoid hemorrhage. *J Neurosurg.* 1979;51:341–351.
32. Ecker A, Riemenschneider PA. Arteriographic demonstration of spasm of the intracranial arteries with special reference to saccular arterial aneurysms. *J Neurosurg.* 1951;8:660–667.
33. Echlin F. Experimental vasospasm, acute and chronic, due to blood in the subarachnoid space. *J Neurosurg.* 1971;35: 646–656.
34. Crompton MR. The pathogenesis of cerebral infarction following the rupture of cerebral berry aneurysms. *Brain.* 1964;87:491–510.
35. Konovalov AN. Surgical treatment of intracranial brain aneurysms. *Medicine* (Moscow, Russia). 1973;327.
36. Wilkins RH, Alexander JA, Odom GL. Intracranial arterial spasm: a clinical analysis. *J Neurosurg.* 1968;29:121–134.
37. Clower BR, Smith RR, Haining JL, Lockard JL. Constrictive endarteropathy following experimental subarachnoid hemorrhage. *Stroke.* 1981;12:501–512.
38. Ausman JI, Diaz FG, Malik GM, Fielding AS, Son CS. Current management of cerebral aneurysms: is it based on fact or myths? *Surg Neurol.* 1985;24:625–635.
39. Finn SS, Stephensen SA, Miller CA, Drobnich L, Hunt WE. Observations on the perioperative management of aneurysmal subarachnoid hemorrhage. *J Neurosurg.* 1986; 65:48–62.
40. Smith RR, Clower R, Grotendorst GM, Yabuno N, Cruse JM. Arterial wall changes in early human vasospasm. *Neurosurgery.* 1985;16:171–176.
41. Smith RR, Clower BR, Peeler DF, Yoshioka J. The angiopathy of subarachnoid hemorrhage: angiographic and morphologic correlates. *Stroke.* 1983;14:240–245.
42. Sasaki T, Wakai S, Asano T, Watanabe T, Kirino T, Sano K. The effect of a lipid hydroperoxide of arachidonic acid on the canine basilar artery. An experimental study on cerebral vasospasm. *J Neurosurg.* 1981;54:357–365.
43. Iwasa K, Smith RR, Bernanke DH. Non-muscle vascular constriction after subarachnoid hemorrhage: role of growth factors derived from platelets. *Stroke.* 1992;23:155.
44. Hamer J, Gotte B. Incidence and neurological significance of postoperative cerebral vasospasm. A study of 80 consecutive cases with clipped sacular aneurysm. *Neurochirurgia.* 1981;24:128–130.
45. Simeone FA, Trepper PJ, Brown DJ. Cerebral blood flow evaluation of prolonged experimental vasospasm. *J Neurosurg.* 1972;37:302–311.
46. Fahmy MA, Smith RR. Identification of presymptomatic cerebral vasospasm by transcranial Doppler sonography. (17th International Joint Conference on Stroke and Cerebral Circulation). *Stroke.* 1992;23:156.
47. Kassell NF, Sasaki T, Clohan ART, Nazar G. Cerebral vasospasm following aneurysmal subarachnoid hemorrhage. *Stroke.* 1985;16:502–572.
48. Richardson A, Jane J, Yashon D. Prognostic factors in the untreated course of posterior communicating aneurysms. *Arch Neurol.* 1966;14:172–176.
49. Richardson AE, Jane JA, Payne PM. Assessment of the natural history of anterior communicating aneurysms. *J Neurosurg.* 1964;21:266–274.
50. McKissock W, Paine KWE, Walsh LS. The value of hypothermia in the surgical treatment of ruptured intracranial aneurysms. *J Neurosurg.* 1960;17:700–707.

51. Hunt WE, Hess RM. Surgical risk as related to time of intervention in the repair of intracranial aneurysms. *J Neurosurg*. 1968;28:14–19.
52. Botterell EH, Lougheed WM, Scott JW, Vandewater SL. Hypothermia, and interruption of carotid, or carotid and vertebral circulation, in the surgical management of intracranial aneurysms. *J Neurosurg*. 1956;13:1–42.
53. Suzuki J, Hori S. Prediction of reattacks following rupture of intracranial aneurysms. *Neurol Med Chir*. 1978;15(part I):35–39.
54. Yasui N, Kawanura S, Ohta H, Suzuki A, Kemiyama H, Sayama I. Prognostic factors of ruptured intracranial aneurysms: new clinical grading. In: Auer LM, Kassell N, eds. *Timing of Aneurysm Surgery*. Hawthorne, NY: Walter DeGruyter Inc; 1985:15–23.

5
Perioperative Care

The management of a patient with a saccular aneurysm is complex and involves many variables. The experience and enthusiasm of the surgical team and the facilities available are part of the decision. The definitive treatment of any intracranial aneurysm is surgical, but there are times when this therapy must be deferred. Proper management of the patient assigned a low clinical grade is not entirely settled, but many patients are operated on early, within the first few days of ictus. In patients in higher grades, early operation may be difficult to justify. Many patients who are not fully responsive initially improve after a conservative treatment program, and operative deaths decrease as conscious level rises. The purpose of a nonoperative therapy program is to assist the patient gently through this difficult phase into one in which surgery can be applied most effectively and safely.

The nonoperative treatment of a patient with a cerebral aneurysm has a short history. In 1948, Wechsler[1] reported that conservative treatment was paramount to no treatment at all. In recent years, regulated bed rest and other therapies have been added to the medical armamentarium. Few treatments have survived without modification.

Simple bed rest has long been the standard for managing a patient with an intracranial aneurysm. Since 10% of the rebleedings occur during the third week following the initial hemorrhage, the bed rest program should not be terminated before this time. Beyond the fourth week, rebleeding rates diminished to about 1% per month. Additional supportive measures are the following:

1. Hospitalization.
2. Subdued lighting.
3. Elevation of head, no more than 30°.
4. The patient is allowed to turn but not sit up.
5. Bowel habits regulated with stool softeners.
6. Bedside commode after the first week.
7. Maintenance of airway and oxygenation.
8. Seizure prophylaxis, diphenylhydantoin, 100 mg three times daily, modified by blood level monitoring.
9. Adequate fluid, 1500 to 2000 mL per 24 hours.
10. One thousand or more calories of nutrition per day.
11. Diazepam, phenobarbital with chloral hydrate for sedation or for restlessness.
12. Condom drainage for men, catheter drainage for women, only for incontinence.
13. Analgesic with codeine or meperidine as necessary.
14. Vital signs monitored periodically as needed but no more often.
15. Control of nausea, vomiting, and singultus.
16. Steroids or other edema agents.
17. Antiembolic stockings. Passive motion of the lower extremities several times daily.

The mortality rates for patients placed on this program are lowest in grade 1 and higher in more ill patients. Medical condition also effects mortality and morbidity. Those in poor condition with more than one complication carry the higher risk, over 80%. Some of these risks, such as thromboembolic disease, may be directly attributable to bed rest. Deep vein thrombosis occurs in perhaps 60% of those confined to bed rest. Pulmonary embolism is also a major factor.

Slosberg[2,3] introduced the profound hypotension regimen. Prompt reduction in arterial blood pressure by both mechanical and chemical means was recommended as soon as the diagnosis of aneurysmal subarachnoid hemorrhage (SAH) was made. Complications of this treatment have included decubitus ulceration, hypostasis pneumonia, aspiration pneumonia, cardiac arrhythmia, GI bleeding, and urinary tract infections. The worst of these, however, has been the aggravation of ischemic deficits. This form of treatment, as outlined, has largely been abandoned because of worsening of ischemic deficits. Moderate hypotension, induced by drugs alone or in combination with other types of therapy, has gained some support. In patients at risk of rebleeding, blood pressure should be controlled. However, moderate elevation of arterial pressure may be a compensatory mechanism to increase cerebral perfusion when intracranial pressure (ICP) is rising or vasospasm is increasing. If the systemic arterial pressure exceeds 180/100, treatment with quickly reversible agents may be indicated in the patient with an intact aneurysm. Apresoline is a parenteral agent that is relatively short-acting and may be administered carefully in low dosage, noting any change in neurological status as pressure is reduced. Sodium nitroprusside works rapidly parenterally but requires more intensive monitoring. ICP is also usually elevated after SAH. This is seen most often in patients with diffuse infarcts, with ventricular enlargement, or with significant amounts of intracranial hematoma. In those who deteriorate in clinical grade, over 90% succumb to their disease if ICPs are significantly elevated. Increased ICP should be treated if it exceeds 300 mm H_2O, but intracranial pressures (ICPs) below 200 mm H_2O are indicative of a good outcome. Initially, a mannitol (20–25%) solution should be administered. One gram per kilogram of body weight can be infused over a 30- to 40-min interval followed by 0.25 g/kg infusion over a 3- to 4-hour period. Hyperventilation may be used to reduce intracranial mass but Pco_2 levels of about 28 mm Hg probably work the limit of usefulness. This requires myoneural paralysis with barbiturate to accomplish and this regimen obliterates helpful neurologic signs. Barbiturates decrease metabolism also. Furosemide, 10 mg, can be used in conjunction with mannitol, but close observation of electrolytes is imperative. Ventricular drainage is useful and incremental amounts of cerebrospinal fluid (CSF) may be removed to control ICP.

Increased secretion of the antidiuretic hormone often occurs after SAH. This is usually manifested in a patient with recent SAH by somnolence and hyponatremia. A cerebral salt wasting syndrome probably also occurs after SAH and this must be differentiated from syndrome of inappropriate antidiuretic hormone (SIADH). In true SIADH, blood volume is elevated, and restriction of fluid intake must be the first priority in therapy. In salt wasting, there is a loss of sodium and water in the urine, and both must be replaced.

An unusually severe form of pulmonary edema may develop spontaneously after SAH, even in young patients. This often occurs in patients with aneurysms near the hypothalamic area and usually after the rupture of an aneurysm of the anterior communicating artery (AComA) complex. The cause has not been determined, but, presumably, the severe increase in sympathetic tone peripherally forces blood into the less resistant pulmonary circulation. EKG abnormalities include arrhythmia and ischemic changes. β-Adrenergic blockers administered early may prevent cardiac damage due to sympathetic overactivity. Some patients also require pulmonary support; ventilatory support and endotracheal intubation should be instituted if the patient is strident. If arterial blood gas measurements indicate hypoxia or hypercarbia, intubation may also be warranted. The head of the bed should be elevated slightly and mild sedatives administered. In reducing blood volume with diuretics, care should be taken to maintain adequate cerebral perfusion, especially in the presence of elevated intracranial pressure (ICP).

Treatment of Associated Disorders

Great strides have been made in the microsurgical treatment of cerebral aneurysms. Yet, overall management mortality and morbidity remain high due to disorders related to the hemorrhage. Any further gains made in the management of this disorder must come from early recognition of the many pathophysiological processes that arise after SAH and the development of treatment paradigms for these. Currently, three common complications overpower all others:

1. The effects of the immediate hemorrhage.
2. Delayed ischemic deficits.
3. Rebleeding.

The relationship between constriction of cerebral vessels and ischemic lesion of the brain is complex. Many factors impact upon this relationship, including the individual anomalies of cerebral circulation, systemic blood pressure, ICP, and probably other homeostatic mechanisms such as pulmonary circulation and function. It is known that when cerebral blood flow (CBF) reaches a critical level of approximately 20/100 g/min, infarction of tissue occurs. However, the diameter/volume flow equation is not a linear one. Volume flow, being related to cross sectional area of the vessel, is affected to a much greater extent by small changes in vessel diameter. Austin and Gaskell[4] have shown that a reduction in diameter of the middle cerebral artery (MCA) to approximately 50% of the normal reaches this critical CBF level.

Since cerebral vasospasm was first recognized almost half a century ago, many medical measures aimed at its relief have failed. Vasodilators, β-adrenergic blockers, antibiotics, local anesthetics, and many others have proven ineffective.

More recently, the calcium channel blockers have been shown to be ineffective in relieving cerebral vasospasm. The positive effects of this treatment, if there are any, may relate to dilatation of the collateral vascular bed, which could also be theoretically detrimental. There may be some improvement in outcome, however.

Over the short term, relief in some patients at least has been obtained with hypervolemic therapy. This relief has been attributed to improved rheological factors. The gains have been made at considerable cost, however. Aneurysmal rebleeding, pulmonary edema, and congestive heart failure are the major complications encountered in this group of extremely ill patients.

Intensive monitoring of central venous pressure (CVP) and systemic arterial pressure using arterial lines is required. A Swan–Ganz catheter may be used to measure pulmonary wedge pressure and cardiac output in place of the CVP line. EKG, arterial blood gases, electrolytes, and osmolarity must be monitored and controlled rigorously. Complications such as congestive heart failure and pulmonary edema can occur suddenly.

Since elevated ICP may further reduce cerebral perfusion pressure, ICP must be controlled by withdrawing CSF from a line placed in the ventricular system or by the use of hyperosmolar agents administered intravenously. Initially, hypervolemia is created by the infusion of albumin or plasminate. Thereafter, fluids and colloids may be added to create diuresis. The fluid volume intake should slightly exceed urinary output. Vasopressin may be given every 3 to 4 hours to increase peripheral blood volume. If arterial pressure does not rise, dopamine may be added to bring the systolic blood pressure to above 160 mm Hg. Digitalization may be required for the patient who has difficulty maintaining Po_2 saturation. Blood pressure elevations above 200 mm Hg systolic should be avoided since autoregulation breakthrough occurs and, for those with intact aneurysms, this form of the therapy must be limited because of induced aneurysmal rebleeding.

Many forms of the above scheme have been employed. Less vigorous methods suffice in some patients to ameliorate minor vasospasm symptoms. The simple loading of volume with plasminate or albumin, allowing blood pressure to rise spontaneously, may suffice. This treatment may be of limited use, however, if vasoconstriction continues to progress and volume blood flow cannot be maintained in the 20 ml/100 g of tissue requirements. Balloon angioplasty may be required.

Intracranial Hypertension and Hydrocephalus

The choice of treatment for intracranial hypertension depends greatly upon the cause. If ICP is increased from an intracranial hematoma, then clot evacuation may be the required treatment. The aneurysms responsible should be clipped concurrently because the rebleeding rate in patients whose hematoma has been evacuated without aneurysm clipping is extremely high. The treatment of intracranial hypertension due to brain edema is much more complex. In the acute hemorrhagic period, shunting operations, even in the case of ventricular enlargement, are not often effective. High protein and blood products together produce high levels of shunt dysfunction. External drainage, however, may be temporarily effective, but, when used over prolonged intervals, the risk of intracranial infection rises with ventriculostomy.

In patients who are in low clinical grade, medical therapy should be sufficient to control ICP. Furosemide 4 to 80 mg or mannitol in doses of 0.5 to 1 g/kg of body weight may be used to control ICP to 200 mm H_2O. These agents may be repeated every 8 to 12 hours. In patients with severe signs of increased ICP, therapy must first be aimed at the major cause. Hematomas should be evacuated or, if due to hydrocephalus, ventriculostomy is indicated. In comatose patients, both treatments may be futile.

Performing ventriculostomy in the patient with a recent SAH may be difficult and costly. The frontal horn should be selected for puncture and ventricular pressure maintained at a constant level between 150 and 200 mm H_2O. The right lateral frontal horn is preferred unless the ventricles are displaced by hematoma. For the patient decompensating rapidly, a line should be placed into both frontal horns, reducing the possibility of a major shift due to the hematoma. First, it should be determined that there is no obstruction within the ventricular system because unilateral ventriculostomy actually contributes to herniation syndromes. Approximately 16% of all patients arriving after acute onset of SAH require ventriculostomy. In those in intermediate grade, 68% require ventriculostomy, and in decompensated patients (grade 3), about one-third require this procedure. Early drainage is useful in the first few hours after a SAH, but, later, as brain swelling develops, this method loses its effectiveness. Some surgeons prefer to continue ventricular drainage throughout the perioperative and operative phases.

In alert patients, in whom ICP is not elevated, the ventriculostomy should be discontinued after 24 hours to avert infection. In lethargic and stuporous patients, the ventriculostomy should be continued. This not only allows diagnostic evaluation of ICP but also treatment by incremental removal of small amounts of ventricular fluid. If the ventriculostomy is required for longer than 1 week or if there is evidence of infection, it should be terminated or moved to another location.

Shunting is warranted occasionally in the chronic phase of hydrocephalus. In patients deteriorating rapidly due to herniation, simultaneous ventriculostomy and lumbar infusion of saline have been used with dramatic success.[5] The method needs further study.

Balloon Angioplasty

Zubkov and co-workers[6,7] first reported a balloon catheter technique for dilatation of constricted cerebral arteries after SAH. Subsequently, over 100 consecutive patients have been treated, and others have applied this technique successfully. The mechanism of action of balloon angioplasty on the spastic cerebral artery has not been clearly defined. Yamamoto and co-workers[8] showed that cerebral vasospasm may actually represent a reorganization and constriction of the collagen fibers in the vessel wall by a cell referred to as a myofibroblast (Fig 5.1). Balloon angioplasty redistributes the collagen, disrupting the binding sites from the myofibroblast, and stretches the connective tissue matrix in the vessel wall (Fig 5.2). Thus, it may be that the chronic form of sustained vasospasm that occurs 1 week after SAH results from a reorganization of the connective tissue matrices by cells proliferating in the vessel wall.

Several techniques may be employed to dilate cerebral vessels in vasospasm. In one of these, a small handmade latex balloon is prepared. The latex balloon is thin so that it can conform to the vessel in which it must be placed.

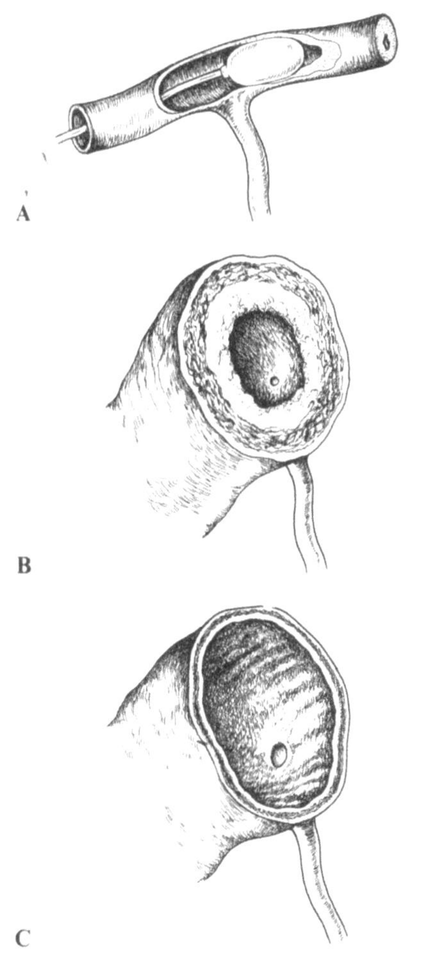

FIGURE 5.1. A scheme of cerebral angioplasty. (A) The balloon dilating the stenotic segment of the artery. (B) The ostium of the short penetrating branch before angioplasty. (C) Thinning of the arterial wall, dilatation of the lumen, and opening of the ostium after dilatation.

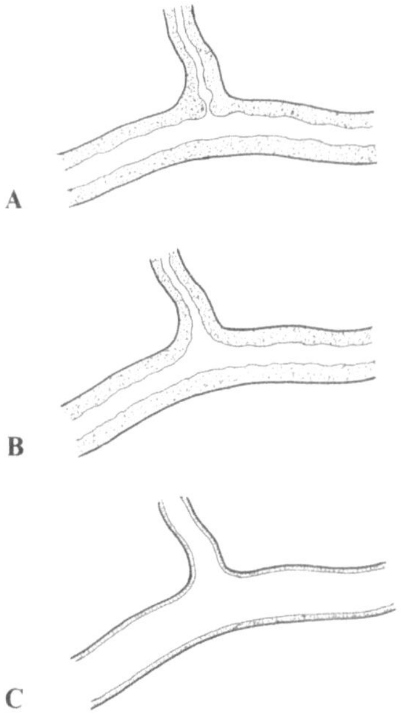

FIGURE 5.2. (A) An angiopathic artery is demonstrated schematically. The ostium has been closed by myofibroblastic reaction. (B) The short, penetrating artery is proliferated at the ostium and throughout its course. (C) An artery following angioplasty in which the ostia of the vessel was closed but the penetrating branch was not proliferated and opens after dilatation.

This is important because vessel rupture and aneurysm rupture have been the most serious complications of the method. The balloon is also specially trained to dilate first at a point distal from its tip. As the balloon is inflated, this creates a wedge that progressively opens the constrictive vessel. This technique is described in Chapter 7. The balloon is placed into the carotid artery where flow directs it through the carotid siphon into the supraclinoid portion of the carotid artery. It may also be placed in the vertebral artery (VA) via an axillary puncture. The balloon is advanced to the point of constriction and then inflated briefly. Brief inflation is emphasized in the patient with cerebral vasospasm because only short periods of occlusion may be tolerated. Contrast material is used for the inflation, and road mapping techniques are helpful. As the balloon is advanced along the cerebral arterial tree, successive dilatation is carried out until there is good anatomical vessel opening and blood flow is consequently restored.

The projection of the balloon is normally along the supraclinoid portion of the internal carotid artery (ICA) and into the M_1 branch of the middle cerebral artery (MCA). If the anterior cerebral artery (ACA) requires dilatation, the balloon may be directed into the A_1 portion by manipulation and compressive techniques. Alternately, a helper balloon may be necessary. One balloon is placed into the MCA trunk and inflated briefly, while the other balloon is directed by virtue of augmented flow into the anterior cerebral A_1 segment. Other types of balloons may be used for the treatment of vasospasm. The Stealth catheter was developed originally by Target Therapeutics for the treatment of arterial stenosis. It has a fixed volume, but a unique mechanism permits the introduction of a guidewire through it. This balloon has the advantage of a nonglobular shape and is therefore less likely to rupture a normal artery. It may be inflated to a pressure of three atmospheres without arterial damage. Higashida and co-workers[9] employ a custom-made silicone balloon manufactured for them by Interventional Therapeutic Corporation (ITC) of San Francisco, California. They use a coaxial delivery system in which a 2-0 French catheter passes through a seven French delivery system for anterior circulation spasm. The balloon measures 0.85 to 1.5 mm before inflation and is trained to inflate nearest to the attachment site first, forming a wedge. The balloon is advanced, making successive dilatations. Any skipped areas are handled on withdrawal. In their cases, four of 13 showed dramatic clinical improvement following angioplasty. One developed hemorrhagic infarction and died 24 hours afterward. Hyogo and colleagues[10] reported one case of hyperperfusion as measured with ^{123}I-IMP single photon emission computed tomograpy (SPECT) after balloon angioplasty; one patient subsequently improved clinically.

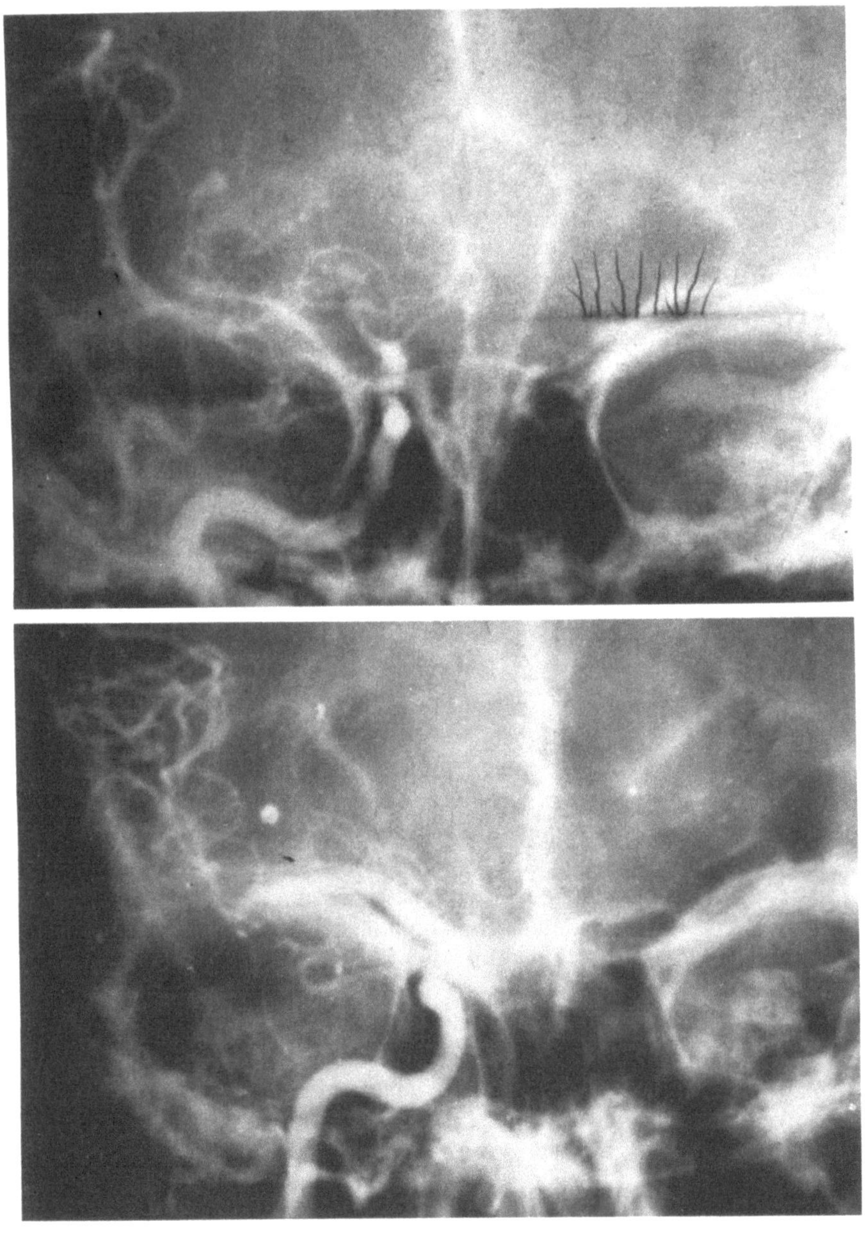

A

B

FIGURE 5.3. (A) Middle cerebral artery before angioplasty. (B) Middle cerebral artery following angioplasty.

Other modifications in balloons are possible. Takahashi et al.[11] used the silicone balloon manufactured by Dow Corning in Japan to dilate the cerebral arterial tree. They also incorporated a wire in the balloon technique to negotiate tortuous vessels in which flow was restricted. Mayberg and co-workers[12] used both the Target polyethylene balloon and the ITC microballoon. These authors reported improvement in the majority of patients in whom the arterial tree was dilated. They also used a wire in the balloon technique to negotiate tortuous vessels in which flow was restricted.

Konishi and co-workers[13] recommended inflation for an interval of 10 s and always at a different site to avoid injury. These authors advised against overinflation because of the vessel rupture problem and suggested that the MCA velocity must be maintained at 100 cm/s. In the University of Mississippi experience, velocities fall to near 0 cm/s in the MCA as the balloon is inflated in the main trunk of the MCA. Prolonged inflation, especially in the patient with symptomatic vasospasm, should be carried out with caution.

Brothers and Holgate[5] used a 0.85 × 4.1 mm silicone balloon developed by ITC Corporation that was permanently attached to a 2-0 French polyethylene nontapered catheter. The balloon is pushed to the proximal intracranial segment that is tight and then inflated as road mapping is used for a landmark. The angioplasty balloon is advanced into the first narrowed segment encountered. The balloon is inflated for 8 to 10 s and this is repeated until the vessel is dilated to a nearly normal diameter. Brothers and Holgate[5] modified this balloon by placing a small wide guidewire into it. Pushing the guidewire further deforms the balloon into a slight curve. A 25-gauge needle can be used to puncture the balloon through which the guidewire must pass. It behaves like a balloon with a moderate leak so that contrast material can still be used for angiography at the same time.

There are limitations in application of balloon angioplasty to the treatment of vasospasm. These limitations are imposed by access to the constricted areas, timing, and complications. Vessels that emanate from the main trunk of the ICA may leave at an obtuse angle and these are easily catheterized. However, those that exit at an acute angle from the ICA are more difficult to catheterize. The anterior cerebral complex and the posterior communicating artery (PComA) offer special challenges to balloon dilatation. Because flow is necessary for balloon passage in the most distal arterial tree, when flow is severely restricted, so is balloon angioplasty.

Timing of the angioplasty is important. Only about 60% of those with vasospasm progress to clinical ischemia. Because the procedure has definite risks, whether the other 40% of the population who would not advance to ischemic signs should be exposed to this risk must be questioned. Zubkov and colleagues[7] noted the fewest complications and most benefit among those who were in

A

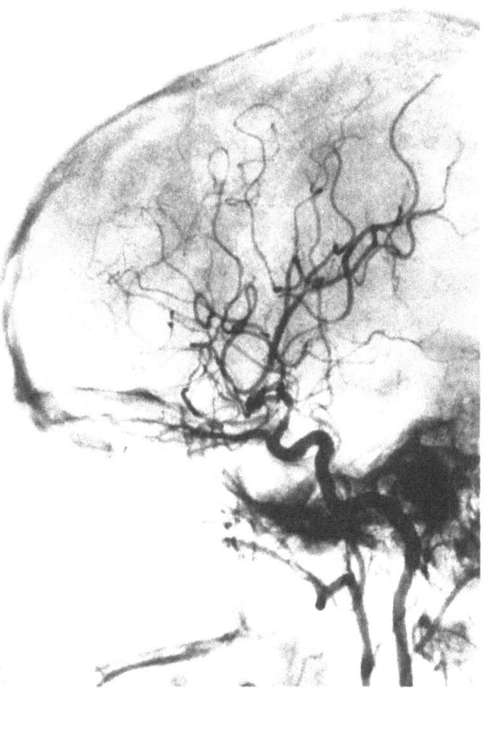

B

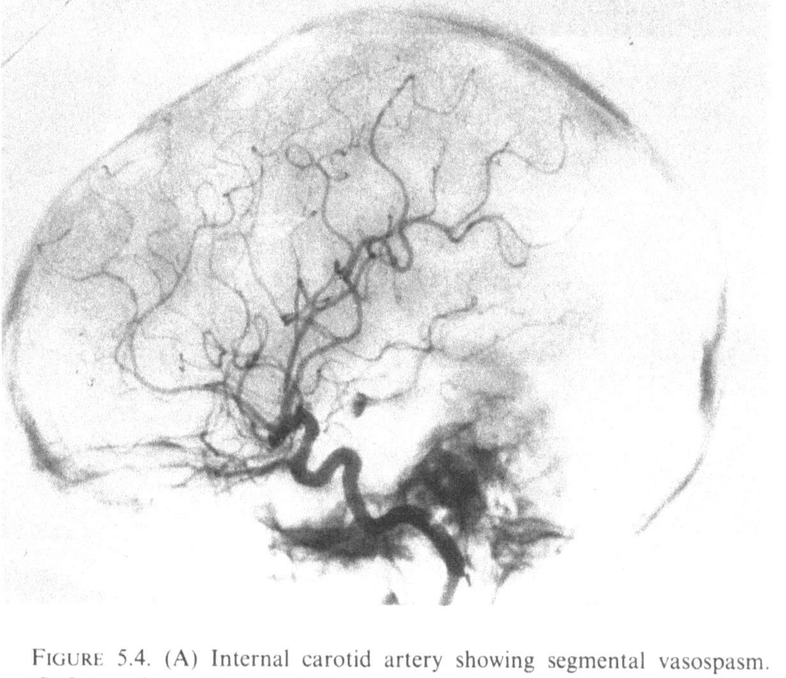

FIGURE 5.4. (A) Internal carotid artery showing segmental vasospasm. (B) Internal carotid artery following segmental dilatation.

good condition initially. Those who are obtunded had no response to angioplasty. In those who were in higher clinical grade, only 40% showed any improvement, leading to the proposal that balloon angioplasty should be used for asymptomatic angiographic vasospasm. When dilatation is performed when there was only mild clouding of consciousness, the clinical symptoms quickly ameliorate and hemicortical deficits improve. Hemiparesis in the group undergoing early dilatation recovered faster and more completely.

No attempts are usually made to pass the catheter into the distal branches since vasospasm is primarily a disease affecting vessels along the base. Angioplasty may be used in patients with intact aneurysms although arterial rupture occurred in one of Zubkov's cases. Balloon angioplasty for vasospasm followed balloon occlusion of the aneurysm. Conversion of infarct into hematoma does not often occur.

The configuration of the balloon is important. In no case should the dilatation of the vessel be extended beyond its normal diameter.

There were four major complications in this series (4.5%). In one case, the dilating balloon prematurely detached within an area of stenosis and resulted in worsening of hemiparesis despite the open surgical removal of the fragment. In another case, an aneurysm

A

B

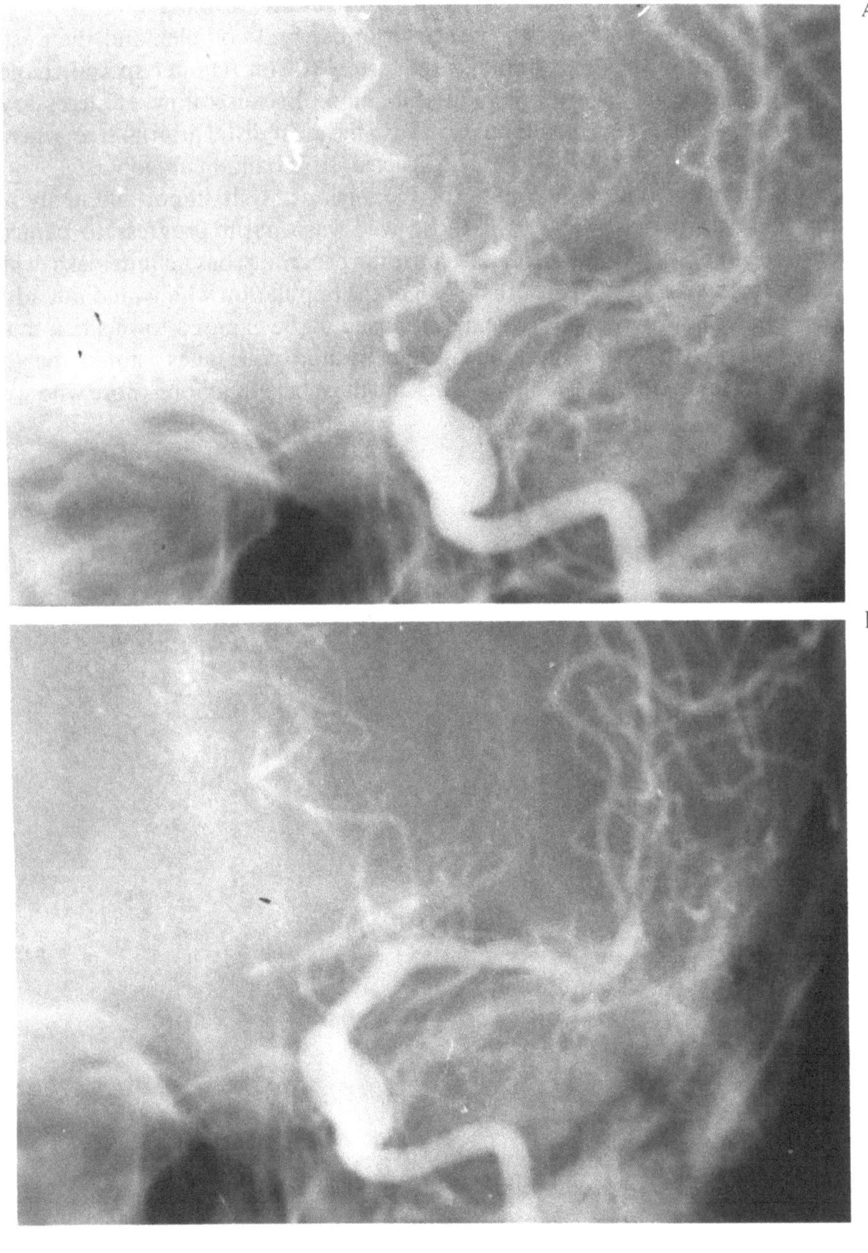

FIGURE 5.5. (A) Diffuse vasospasm in the internal carotid and middle cerebral artery. (B) The internal carotid artery and middle cerebral artery following vasodilatation using latex balloons.

FIGURE 5.6. (A) Diffuse vasospasm involving the supraclinoid portion of the internal carotid artery, middle cerebral artery, and anterior cerebral artery. (B) Following dilatation of these arteries using a latex balloon.

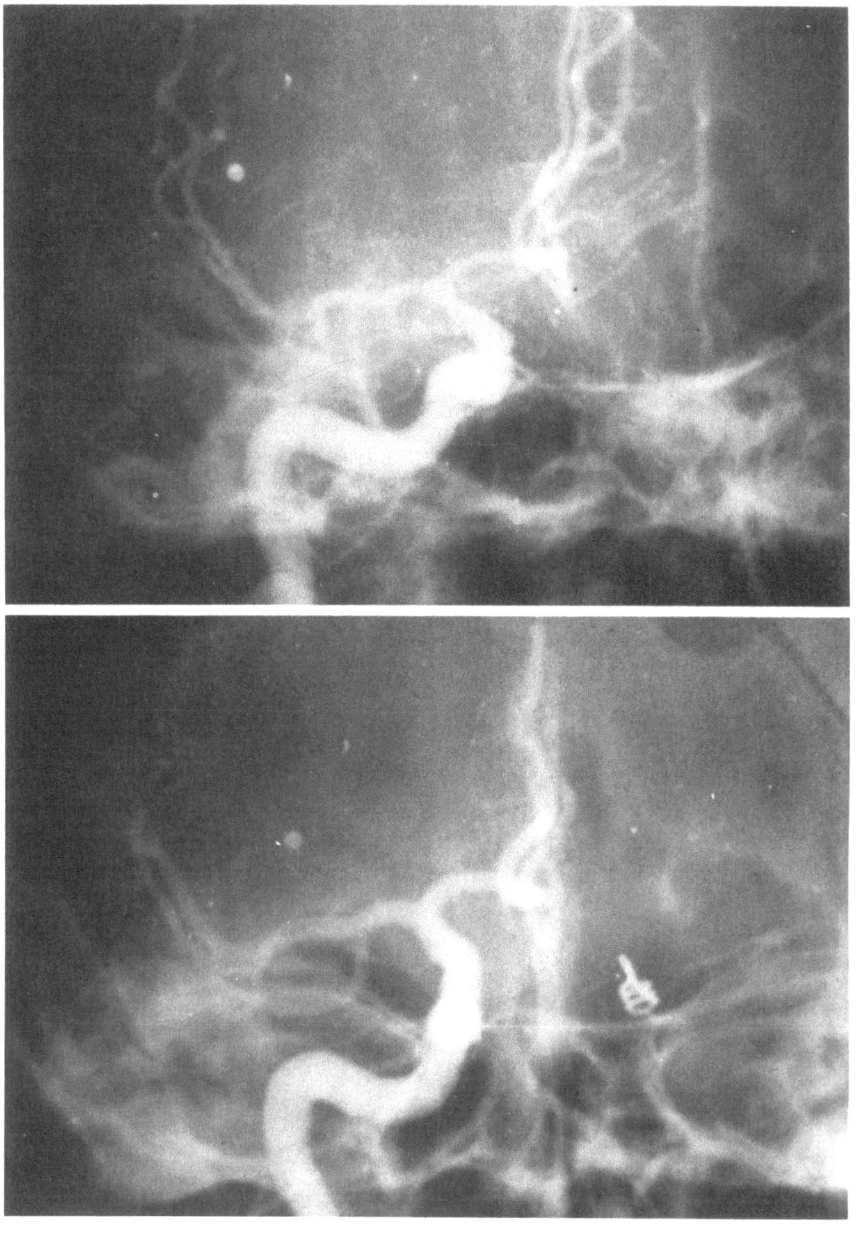

A

B

contralateral to the territory undergoing angioplasty ruptured. There was one instance of arterial rupture: in one patient, an attempt was made to occlude permanently an aneurysm with a balloon during angioplasty and this aneurysm subsequently ruptured resulting in death.

The effect of angioplasty has been assessed on outcome of surgically treated patients. Sixty patients underwent angioplasty for their vasospasm whereas 129 patients did not. The treated group also tended to be in a much more severe condition. Seventy five of the treated group had a satisfactory outcome in comparison to only 54.4% of the untreated group. Mortality was also significantly lower in the angioplastied group. Figures 5.3–5.8 show the results of angioplasty for varying vasospastic arteries.

Rebleeding

ε-Aminocaproic acid (EACA) acts by competitive inhibition of the activator converting plasminogen into plasmin. Plasmin is normally absent but it is probably the most active factor in clot dissolution. EACA crosses the CSF barrier poorly, and thus does not affect the subarachnoid clot to any great extent.

Recognizing that rebleeding from aneurysms coin-

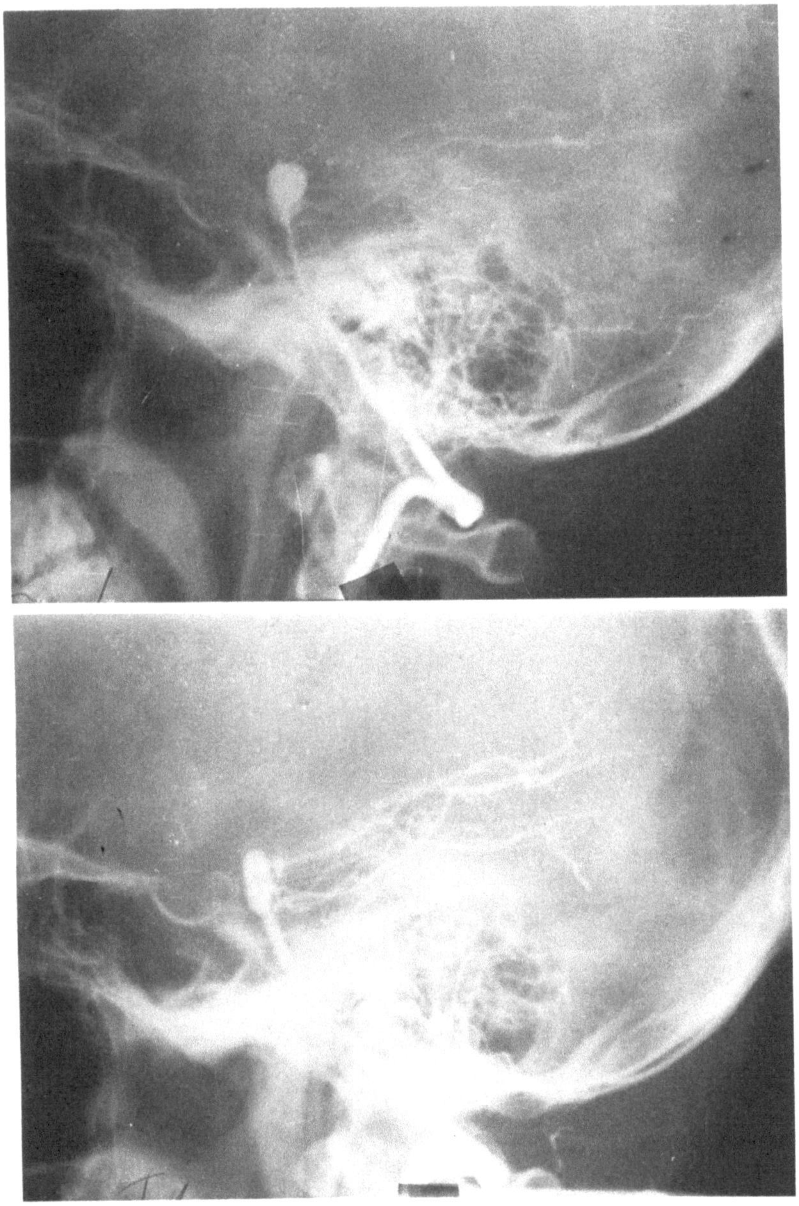

A

B

FIGURE 5.7. (A) Aneurysm of the basilar artery apex and moderate symptomatic vasospasm involving the basilar artery trunk. (B) After balloon angioplasty of the basilar artery, a balloon was placed in the aneurysm cavity, separating it from the circulation. The posterior cerebral artery fills well following angioplasty, although it was not primarily dilated. This results from dilatation of the ostium.

cided with dissolution of the clot, Mullan and Dawley[14] administered EACA to 35 patients. Only two rebled again, and there were no serious complications. This pioneer work led to a multicenter trial in which EACA was used. There were fewer rebleedings during the treatment interval in patients studied cooperatively.[15]

During the first several days of treatment, 36 to 48 g/24 h are usually administered orally or intravenously. The dose can be reduced subsequently to about 24 g/24 h. Treatment should be followed closely with clot-lysis time determinations. The effectiveness of antifibrinolytic agents in preventing premature bleeding is now accepted but the idea that this form of therapy promulgates cerebral vasospasm has, to a great extent, limited its use.

Since lysis retardation is the mechanism of action, antifibrinolytic therapy may simply prolong the interval in which recurrent bleeding is to be expected. Ideally, if this therapy is used, it should be combined with operative clipping. Complications include postoperative deep vein thrombosis. However, these complications are also known to occur more frequently in patients on bed rest and in the older population in general. Arteriopathic complications have also been described. In the University of Mississippi series, there were two instances of arterial occlusion. One femoral artery became occluded following an angiogram and a radial artery occluded after indwelling intraarterial catheter monitoring of arterial pressure. Hydrocephalus, as feared, has not been a frequent complication of antifibrinolytic therapy. Most

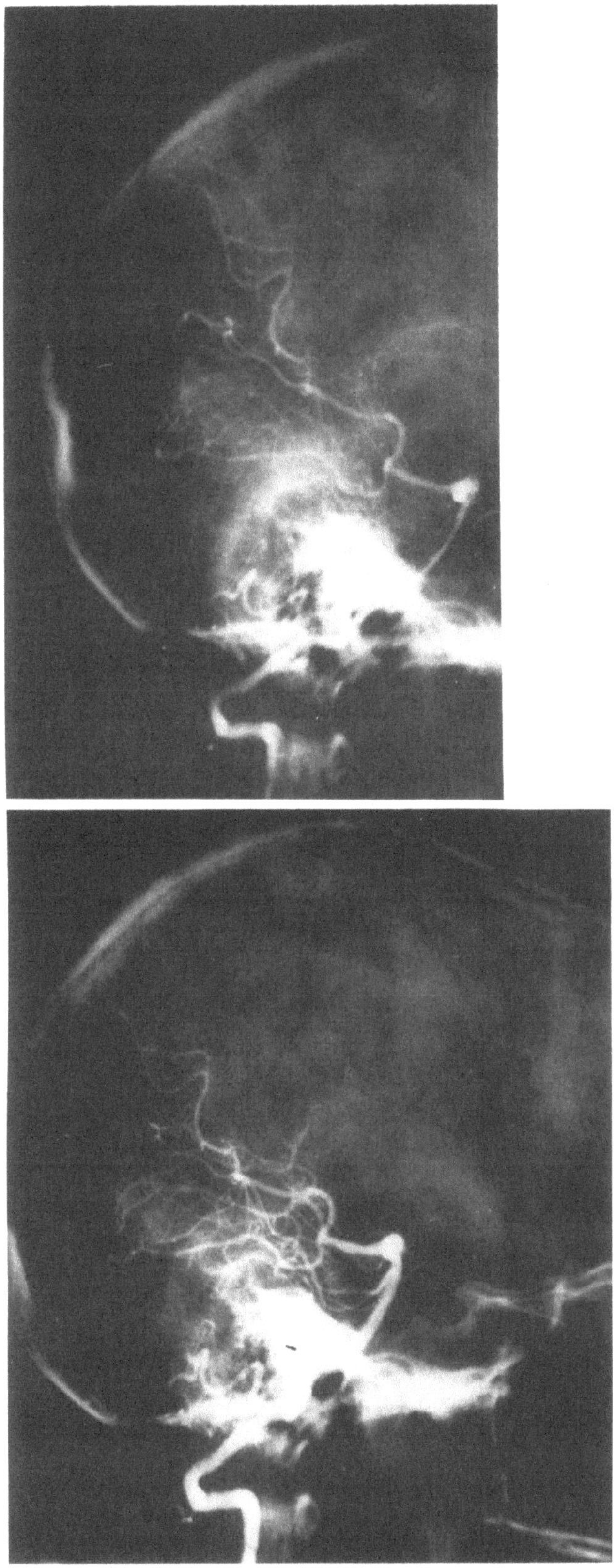

A

B

FIGURE 5.8. (A) Severe vasospasm involving the basilar artery associated with a ruptured aneurysm of P_1 branch. (B) Following basilar artery and PCA dilatation with a latex balloon.

TABLE 5.1. Therapy type and complications

Patients	Therapy	Rebleed	Ischemia	Thrombus
102	None	22.5%	15.7%	3.9%
34	EACA	17.6%	20.6%	5.9%
103	EACA + Heparin	6.8%	11.7%	0.0%

recently, the use of antifibrinolytic agents has been questioned because of the effect of these agents on vasospasm.[16] Fodstad and co-workers[17,18] found vasospasm to be activated by antifibrinolytic agents.

The causes of rebleeding were studied extensively at the Polenov Neurosurgical Institute in St. Petersburg.[19] The factors most important were related to local coagulation defects, as measured by arteriovenous differences in fibrin breakdown products and the coagulogram.[20] There was also a tendency toward generalized hypercoagulation with local fibrin deficiency. Heparin reversed the coagulation deficiencies associated with EACA therapy and prevented ischemic and thromboembolic complications.[22] Table 5.1 shows the results and complications in different treatment groups.

The drugs are administered slowly twice daily in a 5% solution containing 7500 units of heparin. If signs of diffuse intravascular coagulation develop, additional heparin is administered intramuscularly in doses of 2500 to 5000 units. The coagulogram must be used to regulate therapy and determine the need for its continuation.

Among 103 patients treated with combined heparin and antifibrinolytic regimen, rebleeding occurred in only 6.8% and five patients died. Most were in high clinical grades and the majority of the rebleedings occurred in those with aneurysms of the AComA region. In a prospective trial, the incidence of rebleeding in patients who did not receive antifibrinolytic therapy was 27.5%. The addition of heparin to the regimen reduced rebleeding and ischemia, and prevented thromboembolic complications.[20] Overall, the mortality from rebleeding in patients whose aneurysm ruptured in the hospital was 70%.

The Timing of Aneurysm Surgery

In the present era, many aneurysm surgeons are returning to an early direct operation for the patient with a recently ruptured intracranial aneurysm. The increased awareness that a large number of patients are being lost due to rebleeding during the waiting period that was advised by surgeons in the 1950s and 1960s, in part, fostered the revision. The routine use of hypotension and antifibrinolytic agents, while effective, still allows a distressingly large number of patients to rebleed. Also, there is a potential, if not real, threat that ischemic complications are exacerbated by these agents. A number of theoretical advantages apply for early surgery, including the prevention of rebleeding and the possible management of vasospasm. The fear that the aneurysm will rupture during hypertension and hypervolemic hyperperfusion can be lessened by early clipping. Additionally, in the patient whose vessels constrict, balloon angioplasty can be carried out without the threat that the balloon will rupture the aneurysm or that increased perfusion pressure will rupture it. Securing the aneurysm obviates the need for prolonged bed rest, and thus reduces the threat of deep vein thrombosis and pulmonary embolism. The patient is thus relieved of the stress of potential sudden death, and the length of hospitalization may also be reduced. Late operation brings a patient who is generally in better neurological and medical condition, with autoregulation preserved, slacked brain and improved edema. Good results are more frequently obtained when the patient is operated 2 weeks beyond initial ictus. However, this discounts the patients who may be lost to cerebral vasospasm. Although this hypothesis has not been put to randomized clinical trials, it is widely believed among senior neurosurgeons that surgery significantly aggravates cerebral vasospasm. In a cooperative study, Kassell and co-workers[21] analyzed the results of over 3500 patients. All factors were considered, but there seemed to be a window of opportunity for early surgery in good risk patients. Obviously, such factors as brain swelling, the presence of a hematoma, or the size of the hemorrhage in the cisterns as measured on the preoperative computed tomography (CT) scans are all helpful in identifying the patient most likely to develop ischemic complications during the early part of the second post-hemorrhage week; these operations should be deferred. Surgery planned for the 7- to 10-day interval seems to have the highest incidence of ischemic complications. Those patients whose postoperative CT scans showed thick subarachnoid clots remaining after operation are those most likely to suffer postoperative vasospasm.

Conclusions

The decision to perform a craniotomy for clipping of an aneurysm or to carry out an endovascular procedure is serious. The mortality and morbidity associated with either operation are still distressingly high, especially in the patient in poor clinical grade. However, not all the morbidity relates to the operation itself but to the devastating complications that intervene in the reactive phase of vasospasm, beginning in the second week. Careful preoperative evaluation allows the surgeon to be prepared for the eventualities of this serious step. Only by effectively managing the complications of the reactive period can the patient be brought to the operating room in the condition that will promote the lowest morbidity and mortality rates.

Following SAH, the first challenge is to make a prompt and accurate diagnosis. Only recognition and treatment of underlying pathological events will significantly lower the overall morbidity and mortality of this disease. The goals of therapy should be to reduce complications that occur immediately – rebleeding, vasospasm, and hydrocephalus. Intracranial hypertension should also be managed aggressively so that surgery can be applied in a safer interval. Patients thus go to the operating room in a better condition and emerge with lower morbidity and mortality.

References

1. Wechsler IS. Discussion of Dr. Wallace B. Hamby's article: spontaneous subarachnoid hemorrhage of aneurysmal origin. *JAMA* 1948;136:522–528.
2. Slosberg PS. Treatment of ruptured aneurysms with induced hypotension. In: Fields WS, Sahs AL, eds. *Intracranial Aneurysms and Subarachnoid Hemorrhage*. Springfield, IL: Charles C. Thomas; 1965:221–236.
3. Slosberg PS. Treatment of ruptured intracranial aneurysms by induced hypotension. *Mt Sinai J Med* (*NY*). 1973;40: 82–90.
4. Austin G, Gaskell R. Quantitative middle cerebral artery flow in normal and vasospastic arteries. *Neurol Res*. 1992; 14(2 Suppl):192–196.
5. Brothers MF, Holgate RC. Intracranial angioplasty for treatment of vasospasm after subarachnoid hemorrhage: technique and modifications to improve branch access. AJNR. 1990;11:239–247.
6. Zubkov YN, Nikitozov BM, Shustin VA. First experience of dilatation of spastic vessels in the acute period of aneurysm rupture. *Vopr Neurosurg*. 1983;5:17–23.
7. Zubkov YN, Nikiforov BM, Shustin VA. Balloon catheter technique for dilation of constricted cerebral arteries after aneurysmal SAH. *Acta Neurochir* (*Wien*). 1989;70:57–79.
8. Yamamoto Y, Smith RR, Bernanke DH. Mechanism of action of balloon angioplasty in cerebral vasospasm. *Neurosurgery*. 1992;30:1–6.
9. Higashida RT, Halbach VV, Cahan LD, Brant-Zawadzki M, Barnwell S, Dowd C, Hieshima GB. Transluminal angioplasty for treatment of intracranial arterial vasospasm. *J Neurosurg*. 1989;71:648–653.
10. Hyogo T, Nakagawara J, Sasaki T, Wada K, Takeda R, Nakamura J, Suematsu K. Hyperperfusion on 123-I-IMP SPECT after balloon angioplasty for cerebral vasospasm: case report. In: Sano K, Takakura K, Kassell NF, Sasaki T, eds. *Cerebral Vasospasm – Proceedings of the IVth International Conference on Cerebral Vasospasm, Tokyo*. Tokyo: University of Tokyo Press; 1990:443–444.
11. Takahashi A, Yoshimoto T, Mizoi K, Sugawara T, Fijii Y. Transluminal balloon angioplasty for vasospasm after subarachnoid hemorrhage. In: Sano K, Takakura K, Kassell NF, Sasaki T, eds. *Cerebral Vasospasm – Proceedings of the IVth International Conference on Cerebral Vasospasm*. Tokyo. Tokyo: University of Tokyo Press; 1990:429–432.
12. Mayberg M, Eskredge, Newell, Winn HR. Angioplasty for

symptomatic vasospasm. In: Sano K, Takakura K, Kassell NF, Sasaki T, eds. *Cerebral Vasospasm – Proceedings of the IVth International Conference on Cerebral Vasospasm.* Tokyo. Tokyo: University of Tokyo Press; 1990:433–436.
13. Konishi Y, Tokitsu M, Sato E, Maemura E, Hara M, Takeuchik. Percutaneous transluminal angioplasty (PTA) for vasospasm after subarachnoid hemorrhage. In: Sano K, Takakura K, Kassell NF, Sasaki T, eds. *Cerebral Vasospasm – Proceedings of the IVth International Conference on Cerebral Vasospasm.* Tokyo, 1990. Tokyo: University of Tokyo Press; 1990:440–442.
14. Mullan S, Dawley J. Antifibrinolytic therapy for intracranial aneurysms. *J Neurosurg.* 1968;28:21–23.
15. Nibbelink DW, Sahs AL. Antifibrinolytic therapy and drug-induced hypotension in treatment of ruptured intracranial aneurysm. *Trans Am Neurol Assoc.* 1972;97:145–148.
16. Smith RR, Upchurch JJ. Monitoring antifibrinolytic therapy in subarachnoid hemorrhage. *J Neurosurg.* 1973;38: 339–344.
17. Fodstad H, Thulin CA. Use of tranexamic acid (AMCA) in the preoperative management of patients with ruptured intracranial aneurysms. Unpublished data presented to Sixth International Congress of Neurological Surgery. 1977; Sao Paulo, Brazil.
18. Fodstad H, Liliequist B, Schannong M, Thulin CA. Tranexamic acid in the preoperative management of ruptured intracranial aneurysms. *Surg Neurol.* 1978;10:9–15.
19. Fradkova GV, Zubkov YN. Hemocoagulation in patients with arterial aneurysms in the hemorrhagic period [in Russian]. In: *Actual Questions Neurology, Psychiatry and Neurosurgery.* Russia: 1980;221–222.
20. Zubkov YN, Aranovich BD, Fradkova GV. Antifibrinolytic therapy in patients with cerebral vessels aneurysms [in Russian]. In: *The Annals of Saratov Medical Institute.* Russia: Saratov; 1983:52–59.
21. Kassell NF, Torner JC, Jane JA. The International cooperative study on the timing of aneurysm surgery. In: Auer LM, Kassell NF, eds. *Timing of Aneurysm Surgery.* Hawthorne, NY: De Gruyter; 1985;277–278.
22. Zubkov YN. *Treatment of Patients with Intracranial Arterial Aneurysms in the Hemorrhagic Period.* Moscow; 1990. *Thesis.*

6
Principles and Ergonomics of Direct Aneurysm Surgery

Introduction

With the operating microscope, in the 1960s came a powerful, unobstructed light source and magnified anatomy. Shortly following this development, delicate and fine dissectors, forceps and scissors became available. Aneurysm clips were gradually modified to accommodate and make best use of this new technology. Direct microsurgical clipping by craniotomy has become the most commonly applied procedure for managing an intracranial aneurysm and is currently available to virtually every aneurysm surgeon. Because of the many variations in aneurysm size, shape, and location, and peculiarities in anatomy of accompanying vessels, each operation must remain highly individualized. This chapter describes those procedures that must be used to achieve a successful outcome in a patient harboring an intracranial aneurysm and the auxiliary therapy required to accomplish this to its best advantage.

Ergonomics

For the right-handed surgeon, the first assistant stands on the right side. The anesthesiologist should be positioned to manage any airway problems that might develop. The television monitors are positioned so that the scrub nurse, anticipating the surgeon's needs, can visualize the operation at all times. Assistant surgeons should be prepared for both irrigation and suction, perhaps simultaneously. The irrigating bipolar coagulating forceps can provide continuous irrigation to prevent adherence of the instrument to the tissue being coagulated without unnecessarily encumbering the operative field. Special alloys are resistant to charring and sticking. The speaking bipolar cautery is preferred because its audible signal indicates the settings for coagulation and assures the surgeon that the bipolar has not been disconnected. The forceps pedal should be taped to the floor beneath the assistant surgeon's foot. The surgeon then has free access with the right foot for manipulating the foot pedals of the operating microscope.

Positioning

The patient's head should be placed at the far end of the operating table, facing the anesthesiologist if a temporal or parietal craniotomy is to be done. If the anterior cranial fossa must be explored, the anesthesiologist may be positioned laterally, usually on the side most convenient for access both to anesthesia supplies and to the scrub table. For approaches to the midline posterior cranial fossa, a true prone position is usually most appropriate with the anesthesiologist positioned at the patient's head. The body should be propped comfortably into a position in which it will lie in harmony with the head position. Venous drainage of the head must not be compromised and about 10° of reversed Trendelenburg compensates for any head lowering that may be required.

For posterior approaches, the head must also be flexed. For aneurysms involving the vertebral arteries at the posterior inferior cerebellar artery (PICA) junction, the microscope and patient must be placed so that the microscope can be angled toward the patient's orbit for visualizing the PICA aneurysm, beneath the cerebellar tonsil, in the prone or park bench position (Figs. 6.1 and 6.2).

For subtemporal approaches, the true lateral position is preferred. Thus, the head should be slightly flexed laterally, away from the side of approach. Hence, the temporal lobe is allowed to fall away from the middle fossa petrous bone and tentorial edge for exposure (Fig. 6.3).

Spinal drainage should be instituted prior to final positioning. Using a Touhy needle, the subarachnoid space should be entered at the L_4–L_5 interspace. As soon as cerebrospinal fluid (CSF) is obtained, the stylet should be replaced immediately so as not to collapse the dural sac. A fine catheter should be placed quickly into the Touhy needle and directed toward the cephalad position in the lumbar canal. The Touhy needle is then slipped off

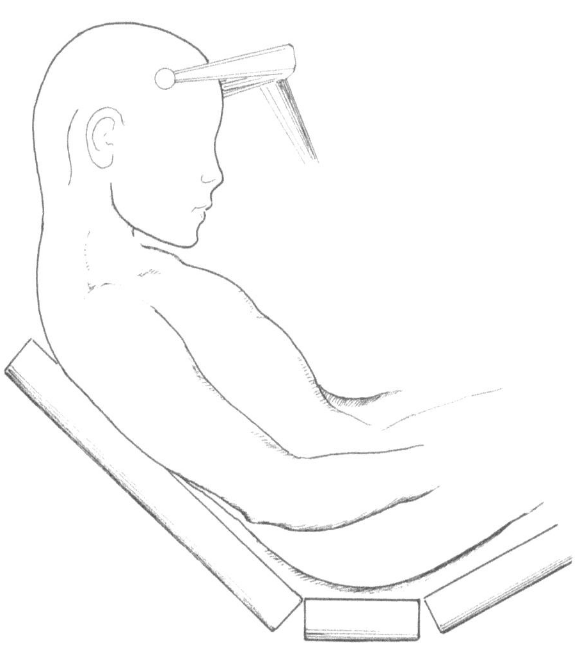

FIGURE 6.1. The sitting position for a suboccipital approach. This approach is suitable for PICA aneurysms.

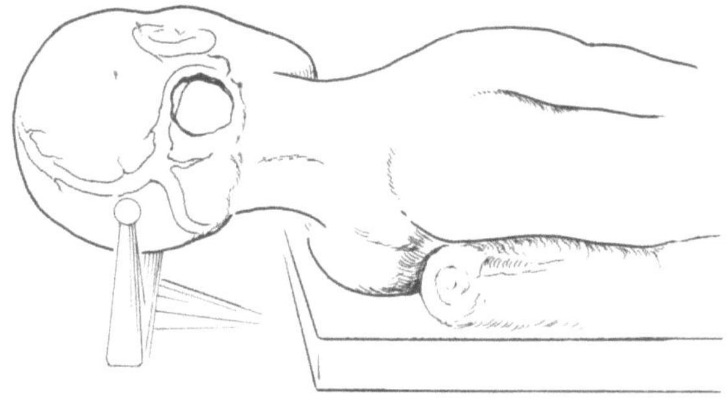

FIGURE 6.2. Suboccipital approach from the elevated supine position. The ipsilateral shoulder has been elevated with a soft roll exposing the mastoid process and midline for entry.

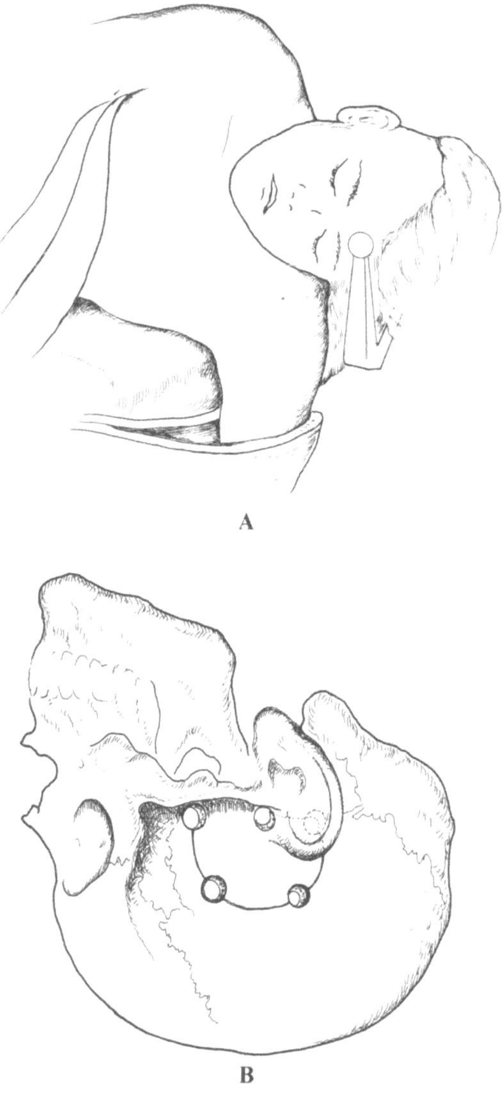

FIGURE 6.3. (A) The head position for a subtemporal approach. A true lateral position with the head slightly laterally extended permits retraction of the temporal lobe and subtemporal exposure. (B) Bone flap for a subtemporal approach for aneurysms of the basilar artery. The openings have been made in the cranium to permit removal of a free-bone flap and rongeuring to the cranial base.

the catheter, which is subsequently connected to a drainage tube and a two-way stopcock. Finally, the drainage tube is connected to a sterile bag for collection of CSF. No fluid should be removed until the dura has been opened.

Magnification and Instrumentation

Either a ceiling- or floor-mounted microscope can be used effectively. The Contraves floor stand provides float-like maneuverability, including semiautomatic counterbalancing. The motorized switch may be controlled for positioning range that would accommodate almost any neurosurgical procedure. The illumination is provided with either a halogen lamp or fiber optics. The instrument has six degrees of freedom with movement (three transitional and three rotational). The microscope and stand weigh 272 kg and movement by operating personnel may be difficult. The ceiling-mounted scope, however, does not provide the degree of freedom that may be achievable with the floor-mounted microscope. For demonstrations and teaching, the Ikegami 301 3 CCD camera provides a good-quality image at a reasonable cost. This instrument provides freeze-framing capabilities in a lightweight compact camera that is installed easily. It provides 600 TVL horizontal resolution. The camera has full 160° motorized rotation and can thus accommodate the head in almost any position in contrast

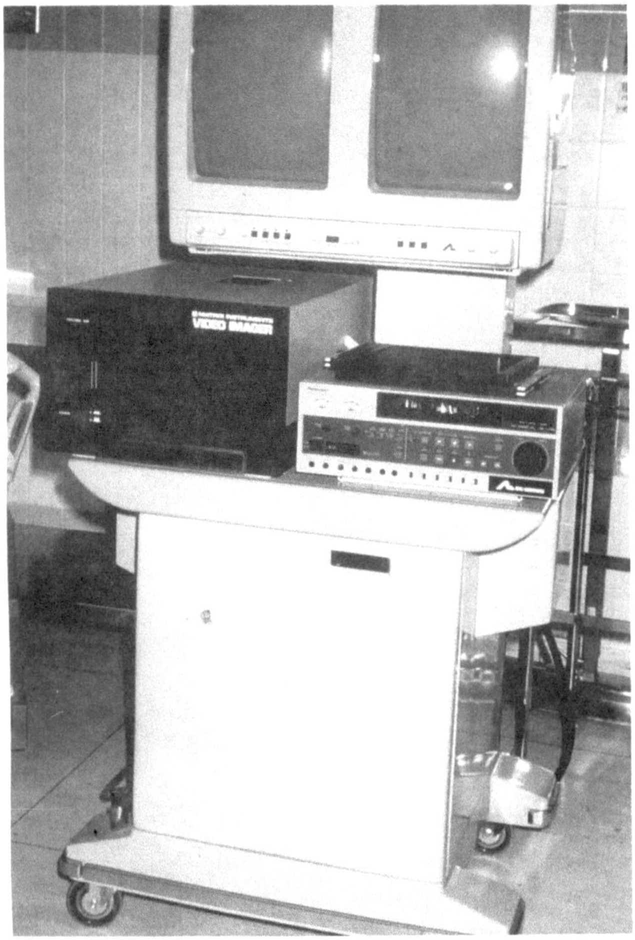

FIGURE 6.4. The OEC Diasonics neurovascular module.

to a wall-mounted unit. It operates on a 115 V, 20 A current and thus requires no special wiring.

For intraoperative angiography, a portable and mobile system such as the OEC Diasonics series 9000 C-arm is recommended (Fig. 6.4). The expanded surgical package adds the advantage of mass image storage of up to 60 images and significant image improvement by advanced digital processing. Images can be recalled later and digitally enhanced prior to hard copying. The surgical package also has digital subtraction angiography (DSA) and road-mapping capabilities. The system is simple and user friendly. The neurovascular module features a disk storage system with up to 20 s or 600 images of real-time data that can be stored for review later on a personal computer. A frame-by-frame study of minute branches of the global circulation of the intracranial vessels can also be carried out.

A radiolucent skull clamp is required if intraoperative angiography is to be employed. The Mayfield radiolucent skull clamp is made from a carbon composite fiber and is easily applied and positioned. It attaches by three-point disposable pin fixations and is compatible with the Mayfield base unit. It rotates 360° to allow positioning during angiography. The interpretation of images in unconventional planes can be extremely frustrating and thus the ability to place the patient's head in the normal lateral or anteroposterior (AP) view is essential.

For retractors, self-retaining retractors are generally accepted as being necessary for microneurosurgical procedures. Many have been manufactured. The Sugita system may be used for difficult aneurysms. This fixed head ring permits the attachment of adjustable retractors to gently hold the brain or important vascular anatomy. Attached trays hold instruments or patties. The Leyla bar provides flexibility and user ease. It provides stable fixation and multiple arms as well as hand rests. Flexible arms are available in different lengths and can be smoothly adjusted to fit any situation. It accepts both flat and rounded brain retractors and Sugita retractor blades with equal ease.

Some retractors attach to the bone margin by virtue of their single clamp. These retractors hold two blades of any size compactly against the craniotomy to permit free hand movement. Small chain links permit positioning, but the blades may still be moved slightly, even when fixed.

Microsurgical instruments generally are held with three fingers of the dominant hand. Instruments should be rounded, lightweight, and require motor power to close but have spring-action opening. They must be made from noncorrosive materials and maintain an edge after repeated handling. Titanium is light in weight but stainless steel has more balance and comfort, while still maintaining sharpness (Figs. 6.5–6.7).

There should be at least two separate wall suctions, one adjusted for high-volume evacuation and the other adjusted for fine suction. The end piece should also have adjustments available for regulating the amount of suc-

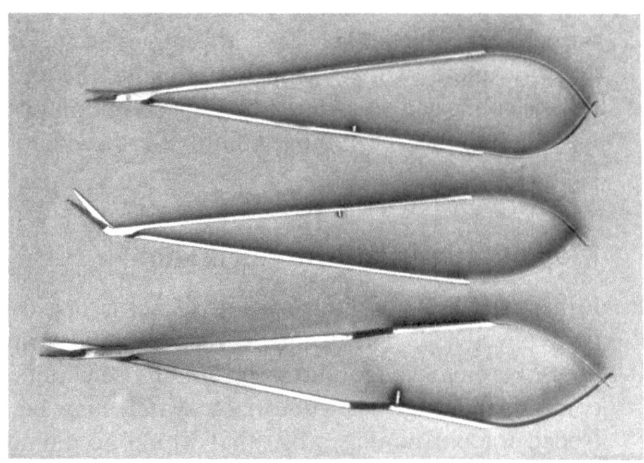

FIGURE 6.5. Stainless microsurgical scissors useful in isolating the neck of an aneurysm from the arachnoidal covering.

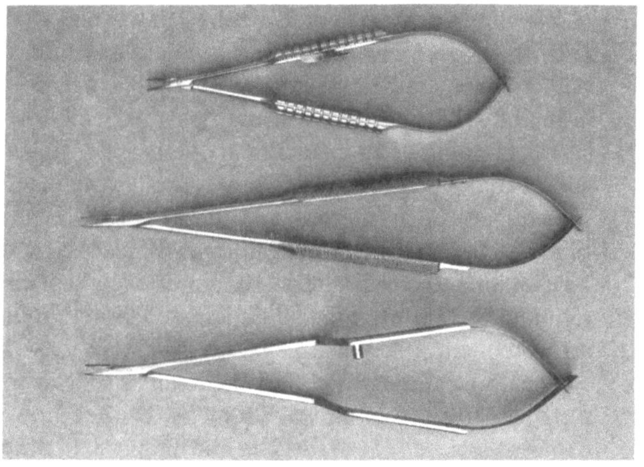

FIGURE 6.6. Different types of stainless steel needle holders that may be used for aneurysm repair.

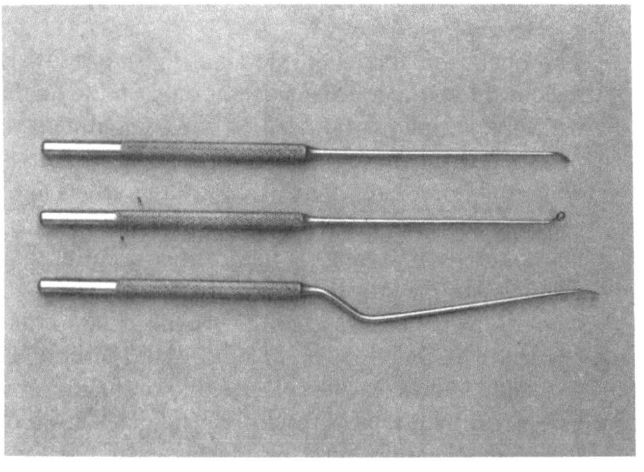

FIGURE 6.7. Microdissectors useful for isolating the neck of an aneurysm for clipping.

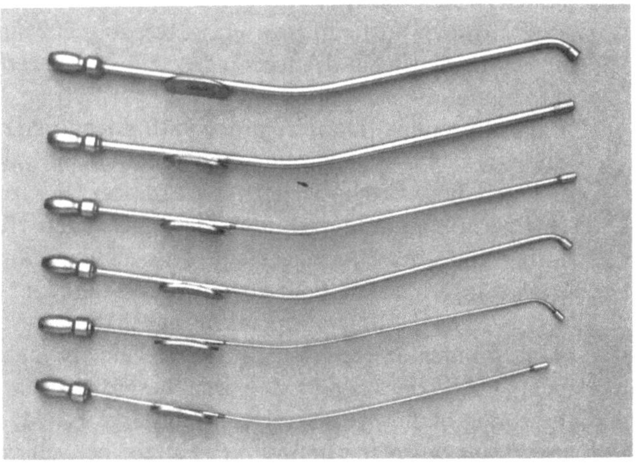

FIGURE 6.8. Microsuction devices that can be easily controlled with the thumb for dissecting and isolating aneurysms.

tion (Fig. 6.8). For coagulation, an irrigating bipolar cautery is used. The constant irrigation partly reduces adherence of the coagulum to the vessel or aneurysm surface. The audible reference is also useful because it assures the surgeon that the cautery is indeed working and at proper settings.

Anesthesia

Anesthesia for the patient with a recently ruptured intracranial aneurysm is perhaps one of the most challenging of all areas of anesthesiology. It requires close collaboration between the surgeon and the anesthesiologist to identify all the possible variations and complications that are most likely to arise in any given patient and to reduce these complications. Several points warranting consideration follow.

1. Most intracranial aneurysms lie deep within the intracranial cavity, covered by tight and edematous brain, and they lie adjacent to vital brain stem structures.
2. An intracranial aneurysm arises because of vascular disease and any aneurysm is subject to rupture with massive hemorrhage in an area where bleeding cannot be controlled easily without injuring adjacent structures.
3. Intracranial pressure (ICP) is invariably elevated during the acute period, and arterial pressure fluctuates widely. Any wide perturbations in either arterial pressure or ICP may produce premature aneurysm rupture. This may occur at any time from the moment the patient enters the operating suite until the time that the aneurysm is exposed. The manipulations necessary to place a clip on an intracranial aneurysm may involve injury to vital brain stem structures, and therefore the anesthesiologist must be cognizant of and able to manage marked reactions in all vital parameters.
4. Even after the operation is complete, the recovery period is fraught with danger due to marked changes in ICP, arterial pressure, and respiratory function. The anesthesiologist must be aware of all of the complications that may arise during this perioperative phase in order to modify his approach. Many opportunities arise for the patient with a recently ruptured intracranial aneurysm to deteriorate due to abnormal brain function. Ischemia and hypoxia may result from many variables, including cerebral vasospasm, increased ICP, altered pulmonary physiology associated with subarachnoid hemorrhage (SAH), or even concurrent cardiac involvement. The effects on the brain stem are important in determining the outcome. Ischemia, herniation, and hypoxia all have an effect on this structure, which ultimately regulates hemostasis throughout the organism. A host of abnormal cardio-

pulmonary conditions may preexist SAH, and these have a profound influence on survival and the complications seen. Among these, preexisting arterial hypertension probably affects survival the most. Aneurysms arising in patients with bacterial endocarditis, polycystic kidney disease, coarctation, and cancer can in themselves cause fatality, even without the underlying morbid condition.

The bedridden patient with a recently ruptured intracranial aneurysm is highly susceptible to complications such as pulmonary emboli and pulmonary infarction. Prior bed rest places the patient at special risk for the development of pulmonary embolization and pulmonary infarction. For instance, the aneurysm arising in the region of the anterior communicating artery (AComA) causes a form of pulmonary edema that has proven extremely resistant to treatment and sometimes causes fatality in itself. Because of the many respiratory complications that can arise, a closely coordinated effort between surgeon and anesthesiologist is paramount in deciding when extubation is appropriate and safe, when tracheostomy is preferred, and when artificial ventilation is necessary.

In selecting an anesthetic method in the acute period, the anesthesiologist should take extreme care, and all pertinent monitoring methods must be used in these extremely ill patients. Induction must be performed with minimal hemodynamic disturbances. Any perturbation may lead to aneurysm rupture. The anesthesiologist should know when the surgeon uses temporary clips. During this interval, the major arterial supply to major eloquent brain may be through collateral channels, and thus blood pressure and arterial oxygen must be made available to the organ. Generally speaking, blood pressure should be maintained at a stable preoperative rate. The anesthesiologist must recognize that good brain relaxation is needed to expose lesions along the base without undue retraction. To achieve this, edema must be reduced to a minimum by every available method. Spinal drainage must be maintained in good working order, and the hydrating agents must be administered in a timely and effective dose. The anesthesiologist should be aware that the patient with recent SAH often has altered autoregulation and that arterial pressures that would normally be acceptable may produce ischemic lesions in the patient with recent SAH. Therefore, both arterial blood gases and arterial pressure must be scrupulously monitored and maintained. Along with monitoring the many systemic variables, such as heart rate and arterial blood pressure, pulmonary function must be monitored as well. In addition, however, the monitoring of intracranial circulation and brain function becomes important in the intraoperative and perioperative period. The measurement and monitoring of cerebral blood flow (CBF) may be carried out using the transcranial Doppler (TCD), with Xe flow or with intraoperative angiography. All of these may be necessary to establish that intracranial flow is anatomically and physiologically proper.

The clipping of an intracranial aneurysm may involve substantial blood loss, occurring over an extremely short interval. An open internal carotid artery (ICA) can lose blood at the rate of 100–200 ml/min. Replacement must be available to cover at least 10 min of uncontrolled loss (3 units, i.e. 500 ml). Smaller anticipated losses should be answered with less available blood.

The above discussion offers no detail as to how to put a patient to sleep or to wake him up. It does, however, express the needs of the surgeon and emphasizes the close collaboration, that must occur during an operation for a patient with an acute intracranial aneurysmal SAH.

Monitoring

The operation for an intracranial aneurysm is always serious and outcome depends not only on the quality of operative technique but also on the commitment to the perioperative care required to return the patient to his work and home environment. Many alterations in physiology occur after SAH, including abnormalities of the heart, kidney, and lung. Complications occur both in the brain and in the intracranial compartment. The management of the patient who has undergone a craniotomy for aneurysm is therefore complex. Besides arterial blood gases, blood flow, cardiac output, and the many variables associated with the operation, ischemic deficits and systemic complications must be considered.

Many physiologic variables may be measured in the postoperative clipping phase but only a few are clinically important to the outcome. Systemic arterial pressure is a determinant of both systemic and brain perfusion. In the patient with ischemia, the blood pressure predictably rises. However, arterial pressures exceeding 200 mm Hg may have detrimental effects, especially when cerebral autoregulation is impaired.

An intracranial Doppler probe with directional capabilities is useful in determining the direction and velocity of blood flow (Eden Medical Electronics) (Fig. 6.9A). This permits minute-to-minute assessment of perfusion during and after clip placement. This method can also provide information about flow in vessels that cannot be visualized at the time of operation but that are susceptible to accidental occlusion by a clip. Velocity measurements of the opposite P_1 give reliable information as to the status of this vessel for clipping large basilar apex aneurysms when the opposite P_1 cannot be well visualized. An immediate embolus-like signal with fall in P_1 velocity indicates inclusion of P_1 in the clip blade (Fig. 6.9B).

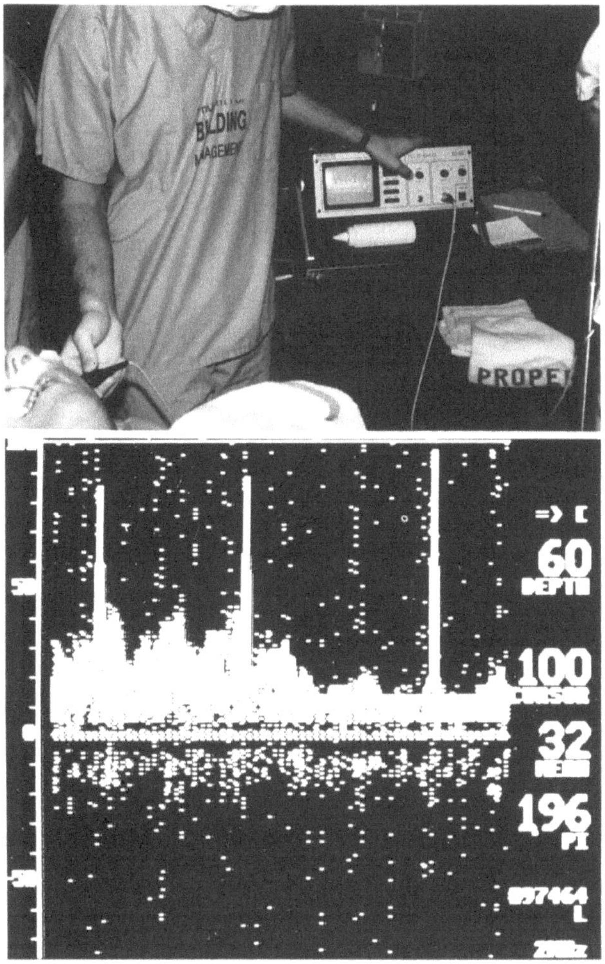

A

B

FIGURE 6.9. (A) Portable transcranial Doppler instrument for intraoperative use. (B) Transcranial Doppler recording of velocity in the left posterior cerebral artery. A right pterional craniotomy had been performed for clipping of a basilar apex aneurysm. The recording indicates three interference signals possibly related to emboli and sudden fall in velocity as the clip compromised the left P_1. The clip was adjusted and velocity returned to normal.

Blood flow velocity should be maintained in a normal range in patients who are not suffering from cerebral vasospasm. In the presence of ischemia, vasospasm, hyperperfusion, or hypertension, adjustments may be required. Velocity must be increased beyond normal levels to provide adequate perfusion. Velocity is inversely proportional to the cross-sectional area. Therefore, if the radius of the middle cerebral artery (MCA) is halved, flow velocity must quadruple to maintain constant volume flow and normal perfusion.

ICP must be maintained as close to a normal range as feasible. If ICP exceeds arterial pressure in the smallest arteries, then focal areas of ischemia may result. In general, ICPs exceeding 400 mm H_2O have been associated with ischemic lesions in the subcortical area supplied by these arterioles. Preferably, ICP should be maintained at 200 mm H_2O. To accomplish this, multiple methods may be required. A catheter may be placed in the ventricular system and CSF withdrawn as pressure becomes elevated. The catheter may be vented at specific pressures. Hyperventilation and mannitol may be employed. Generally, doses in the range of 50 mm/kg of body weight should be administered over a 6-hour interval, measuring osmolarity as a guideline to continued treatment.

Arterial P_{CO_2} measurements are a useful method for determining ventilatory status. Maximum benefits in brain relaxation can be achieved when the P_{CO_2} reaches 27 to 28 mm Hg, and hyperventilation beyond this limit is usually not productive. Barbiturate coma has been advocated for maintaining and managing elevated ICP due to a wide range of pathologic events.[1] However, the gains produced by either coma-producing drugs or paralyzing agents may be counterbalanced by the loss of the ability to evaluate clinical and neurologic signs.

In measuring ICP, compliance measurements are also useful. Saline can be introduced in small increments into the lumbar subarachnoid space as ICP is recorded. When the upsweep on the compliance curve is encountered, ICP will rise abruptly with only small amounts of fluid being added. The method can also be carried out using an intracranial subdural latex balloon filled with saline. As the balloon is inflated, in the patient who has already lost compliance, any small incremental increase in intracranial volume results in large increases in ICP by virtue of balloon inflation. This provides the surgeon with an index of intracranial space and intracranial volume.

Ventilation during induction and the maintenance of anesthesia may influence ICP. Since spontaneous breathing is usually suppressed by anesthetic drugs, it is usually necessary for the anesthesiologist to maintain ventilation mechanically. To decongest the tight and swollen brain, the Pa_{CO_2} should be maintained at about 30 mm Hg. Positive end exploratory pressure (PEEP) may be used to augment ventilation. This maneuver may have little effect on the patient with intact autoregulation but when impaired, the effect of PEEP is unpredictable.

Reducing Pa_{CO_2} shrinks the brain tissue by reducing blood flow and the intracranial blood volume. In fact, if the Pa_{CO_2} is halved by hyperventilation, CBF in tissue falls a commensurate amount, probably by vasoconstriction. Doubling the Pa_{CO_2} essentially doubles CBF, probably due to dilatation of small penetrating resistance vessels. When the Pa_{CO_2} is reduced to 25 mm Hg, the arterial saturation of oxygen also seems to decrease, probably through a mechanism involving the pulmonary circulation. Therefore, levels below this point raise the question of whether brain tissue would be adequately oxygenated and perfused. Certain inhalation agents, on the other hand, such as nitrous oxide, increase CBF at the expense of causing some increase in ICP. Most of the barbiturates decrease CBF and cerebral metabolism concurrently. The fluoranes, although they may cause some slight increase in ICP, also augment the flow.

Diuretics must continue to play a major role in controlling brain mass. Two classes of agents are generally available, the osmotic diuretics and the loop diuretics. The primary osmotic diuretic is mannitol. There are three phases associated with the use of all diuretic agents: (1) extraction of fluid from the cells, (2) hemoconcentration, and (3) rebound. Cottrell et al.[2] studied the intraoperative use of mannitol and found that a dose of 1 g/kg given at the start of the skin incision initially increased ICP slightly but reduced it effectively over the long term. Furosemide at skin incision also lowers ICP. Our regimen includes a 0.5 to 1.0 g of mannitol per kilogram of body weight at the start of the craniotomy and 10 mg of furosimide initially. Urinary output must be monitored continually with an indwelling Foley catheter. The mannitol should be administered quickly, so as to be completely infused as the dura is being opened.

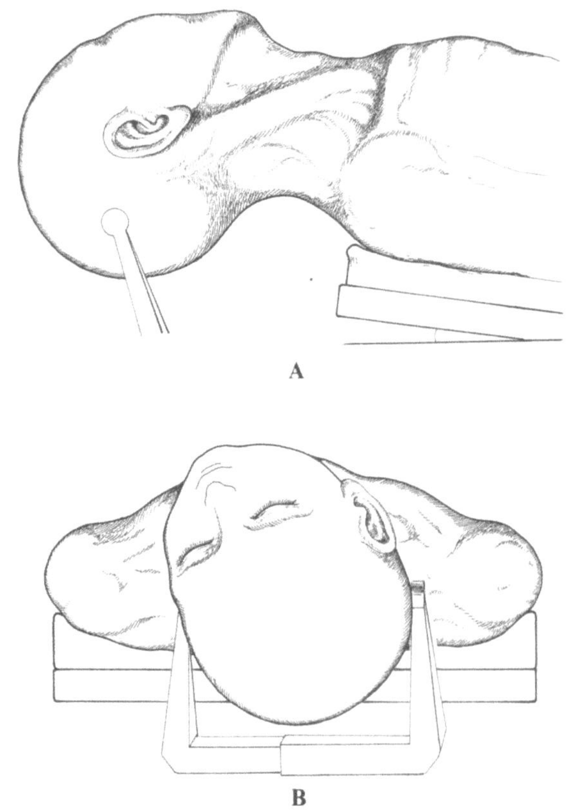

FIGURE 6.10. (A and B) The pterional approach. The head is turned at a 45° angle and slightly extended.

Pterional Approach

During recent years, the pterional approach has been used by many surgeons for managing aneurysms of both the anterior and posterior circulation. Because this is commonly used, the techniques are included here. A frontotemporal approach was introduced by Dandy[3] in 1938. Since then, the operation has been modified by many neurosurgeons. The basic features of Dandy's operation—a bone opening exposing the inferior aspect of the frontal lobe and the anterior aspect of the temporal lobe—are used by all. Although the methods used to open the scalp, the calvarian, and the dura have also varied tremendously, the basic approach, as described by Dandy, has not been altered significantly.

Position

The position of the head on the operating table depends somewhat on the position of the aneurysm and its location on the basal vessels (Fig. 6.10). For those aneurysms that project forward on the anterior circulation, a near lateral position may be preferred. If the patient's head is to be placed in a special fixation device, it should be one that will allow a certain amount of extension (10–15°) to promote exposure along the cranial base. If the head is to be held in a fixed position, the shoulder should be elevated slightly, and the feet dropped in reverse Trendelenburg style. For aneurysms occupying the basilar artery (BA) apex in which the approach is to be lateral to the carotid artery, a 45° position may be preferred. Usually, a fixed head-holding frame will be employed to maintain position. However, this must be movable because it may be necessary to change the patient's head position during the operation to facilitate angiography or carotid compression in the cervical area or to achieve better visualization along the base by increasing the amount of flexion or extension.

The Scalp Incision

The scalp incision has been modified by many neurosurgeons through the years. A curvilinear incision is probably more popular, but a linear incision may also be employed just along and slightly posterior to the hairline. The incision is carried to the superficial fascia of the temporalis muscle. Here every effort must be made to spare the temporal artery and the branch of the fifth cranial nerve supplying the temporalis muscle for motor function. Additionally, the frontalis branch of the seventh cranial nerve must be spared whenever possible. This branch is found in the fatty tissue in a separate compartment just anterior to the temporalis muscle at the pterion. An incision should be made into this fascia and the fascial compartment reflected anteriorly with the scalp flap. The incision for the scalp flap may be made in a number of positions. If the ventricles are enlarged and a ventricular puncture is anticipated, the use of Kocher's point is a good position from which to introduce a ventricular catheter into the frontal horn. This point is located 2 cm anterior to the coronal suture and 2 cm lateral to the sagittal suture. The incision can be placed to this point and then curved so as to remain in the hairline but in the line with the pupil of the eye. It begins 1 cm anterior to the tragus and 1 cm inferior to the zygomatic arch. The incision is carried superiorly and slightly curved from this point.

If ventricular puncture is not required and temporal exposure not needed, then the incision may be a linear one extending from the temporal area, slightly across the midline. The temporal muscle extends over the temporal and frontal bone in the area that must be removed. The temporal muscle must usually be disconnected from the frontal bone and reflected posteriorly. If the temporal muscle is reflected inferiorly or anteriorly with the bone flap, then it will interfere with the anterior approach, which must be carried out between the frontal and temporal lobes. Therefore, the temporal muscle is divided anteriorly and superiorly and is reflected posteriorly and held with fish hooks. This requires the removal of a free bone flap.

For a pterional approach, the methods used dictate the number of burr holes that will be required. For aneurysms involving the AComA or ICA, only small bone flaps are required. For aneurysms evacuated in the sylvian fissure or perhaps those that involve the basilar apex, the bone flap must be placed somewhat posteriorly to permit retraction and exposure. Ordinarily, one opening is placed in the frontal bone at the pterion. The second opening is placed inferiorly as far as possible along the inferior margins of the squamosal suture. Between these two openings, the greater wing of the sphenoid bone comes to the surface. It is not possible to pass the foot plate of the Midas Rex cutting instrument or, for that matter, a Gigli saw guide across this point easily. Therefore, this will be the point at which the bone flap will be broken. Usually, from these two openings, a connection is made with the foot plate of the Midas Rex instrument making the bone flap as large as necessary to permit exposure and retraction of the brain. The bone flap is broken free by using periosteal elevators at the greater wing of the sphenoid (Fig. 6.11).

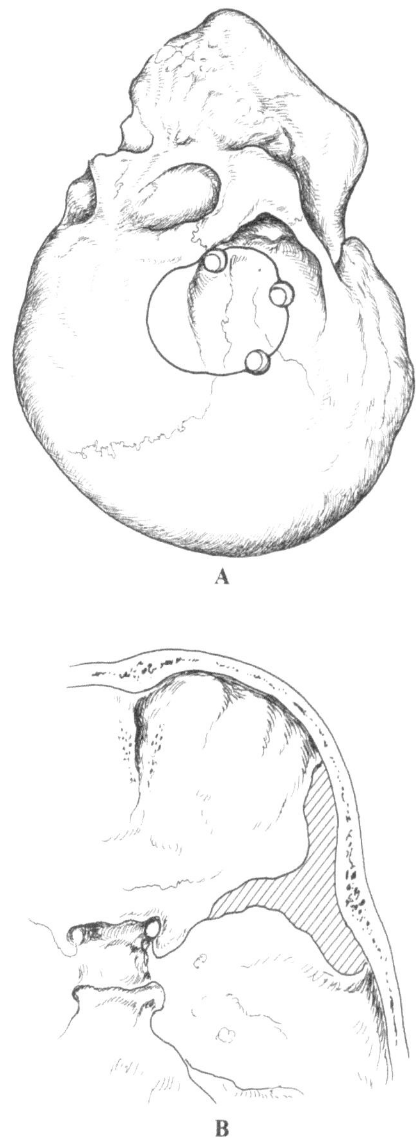

FIGURE 6.11. (A) Pterional craniotomy. Burr holes are usually placed at the inferior margin of the squamosal suture, at the pterion and others as needed. (B) This approach requires removal of the outer portions of the sphenoid bone to adequately visualize the cranial base between the frontal and temporal lobes.

The middle meningeal artery may interdigitate throughout this bone and may require coagulation before the bone flap can be removed free. The greater sphenoid bone covers portions of the frontal and temporal lobe, and this must be drilled away until a clear fissure can be demonstrated between the frontal and temporal lobes. This requires drilling approximately one-third of the external portion of the sphenoid bone to a point where the inner surface becomes pointed and projects into the dura of the sylvian fissure. This portion may be removed with rongeurs. The dura should be opened by tacking triangular flaps to the frontal and temporal musculature, exposing the frontal and temporal lobes as well as the anterior 3 cm of the sylvian fissure. The remaining dura is left in place unless it is necessary to open it to expose distal lying aneurysms. The surrounding brain is contained and protected from injury.

If a spinal drain is in place, it should be opened first. The next step is to open the chiasmatic cistern. The first retractor is placed along the inferior surface of the frontal lobe and directed toward the optic nerve. The olfactory nerve will be seen just anterior to the optic nerve entry into the optic foramen. After the olfactory nerve has been identified, the retractor is shifted somewhat posteriorly until the optic nerve has been visualized. The arachnoid covering the nerve and chiasmatic cistern appear slightly blue in color and should be opened using fine forceps and microscissors. Bipolar coagulation also breaks arachnoidal adhesions. This releases CSF from the chiasmatic cistern. A cotton pledglet or Miracel® strip should be placed under the retractor and gentle suction applied until the chiasmatic cistern has been emptied of CSF. This will permit further adjustment of the retractor.

At this point, a second retractor should be introduced along the anterior aspect of the temporal lobe. Gentle retraction is applied until the veins connecting the temporal tip to the sphenoparietal sinus have been identified. These should be coagulated and divided to facilitate displacement of the temporal lobe slightly posteriorly and inferiorly, opening the sylvian fissure further. Just inferior and posterior to the optic nerve, the arachnoidal cistern containing the ICA can be identified. The membrane should be coagulated and divided, opening the cistern to expose the ICA. The arachnoid should be opened as much as necessary along the anterior and lateral surfaces of the carotid artery. For aneurysms located anteriorly on the supraclinoid portion, this opening may be shortened. For those aneurysms occupying the basilar apex, the incision will be lengthy and the sylvianotomy extended.

The extent of the sylvianotomy depends on many factors but much is determined by the tightness of the brain (Fig. 6.12). The thickened and triangular-shaped arachnoidal covering may be opened deep into the basal part of the fissure with exposure of the main trunk of the MCA and its major branchings. This depends greatly on how much exposure is needed. In a patient with a slack brain, a single retractor may be placed in the notch separating temporal and frontal lobes and adequate exposure obtained for clipping of an anterior circulation aneurysm. When the brain is tight, a considerable sylvianotomy may be needed in order to gain exposure of the aneurysms of the posterior circulation, especially if they project high along the basilar apex.

For aneurysms that arise on M_1 or M_2, a carotid cistern opening is not required. The sylvian fissure may be opened laterally, exposing the M_2 and M_1 branches directly in the fissure. Further descriptions of the pterional approach as it relates to aneurysms in special locations will be described in detail in the appropriate chapters.

Retraction of the Brain

Many different types of self-retaining retractors are available to promote exposure of the basal arteries and aneurysm. Of these, the Yasargil and Sugita retractor systems have achieved popularity. A Leyla bar may be used to affix the Yasargil retractor system. For the Sugita system, a special ring may be used or fixed to the frame of the instrument directly. Usually, one or perhaps two retractors are necessary. One retractor is usually placed on the frontal lobe and the second at the crotch between the frontal and temporal lobes in the sylvian fissure. The Sugita retractors are especially useful for deep approaches such as for a pterional visualization of the BA apex aneurysm. The Sugita retractor has a wide base but tapers quickly to a finer configuration at the tip. A fine layer of cotton, latex, Miracel®, or plastic should be placed between the retractor and the brain.

In the acute SAH case, brain retraction may be particularly difficult and retractor damage may occur. While it is not settled whether intermittent traction versus steady continuous traction gives the best results, it is reasonable to believe that removal of the compressive forces every few minutes may allow perfusing of brain tissue otherwise rendered ischemic by the retractor blade. If possible, every vein must be preserved. If the retractor seems to compress especially those vital veins, the retractor should be removed every 10 to 15 min and circulation in the vein reestablished. This prevents thrombosis of the cerebral vein.

Managing the Veins

The veins of the brain may be subdivided into superficial and deep systems. The superficial veins usually arise in the brain substance and cross the subarachnoid and subdural spaces to drain into the sinuses. The veins that usually arise on the tentorial aspect of the brain empty into the transverse and the superior petrosal sinuses. The anastomotic veins connect the superficial and deep systems.

There is little scientific information concerning the effects of occluding superficial cerebral veins. However, anecdotal reports from the descriptive work of surgeons indicate that complications were thought to have arisen from sacrifice of various deep and even some superficial veins. A sound working principle is to avoid the sacrifice of any vein unless the risk of leaving it intact is greater. Certain veins should not be divided.

The veins that bridge the sylvian fissure and enter the sphenoparietal sinus at the temporal pole must occasionally be sacrificed if they limit downward and lateral retraction of the temporal lobe. The middle cerebral vein runs along the sylvian fissure and lateral sulcus, is sometimes quite large, and drains deeply through veins connected to the sphenoparietal sinus or cavernous sinus. This vein should be preserved and usually retracted toward the temporal side of the opening. We have observed temporal lobe swelling due to venous occlusion. Kaplan[4] describes facial palsy and focal epilepsy, begin-

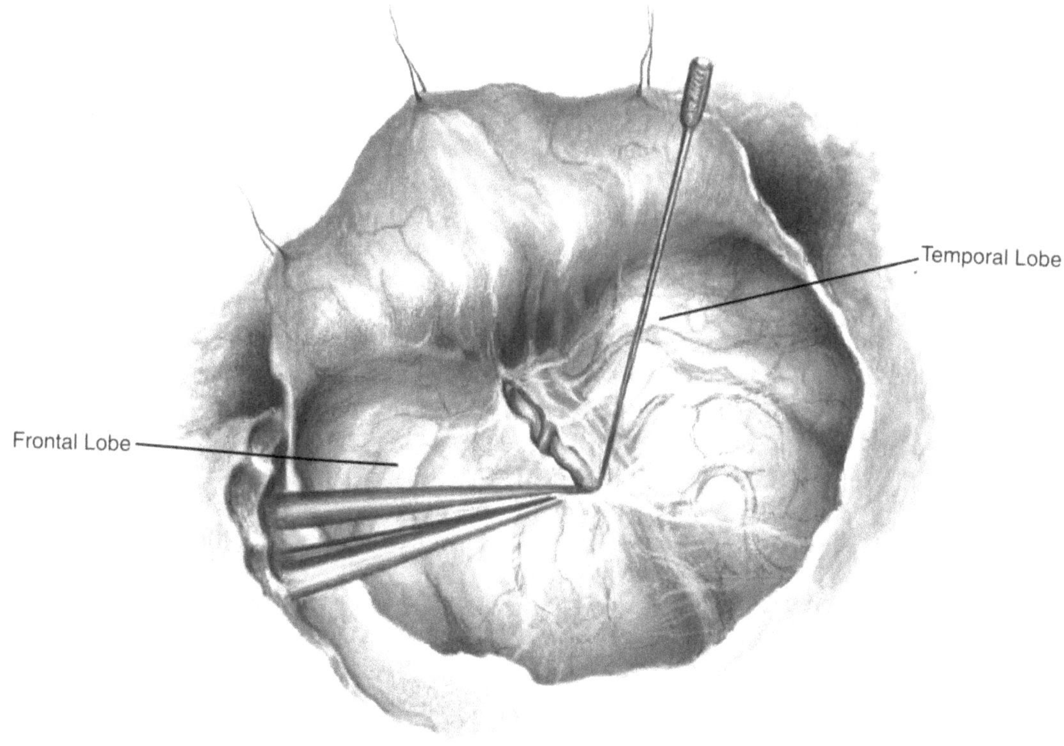

A

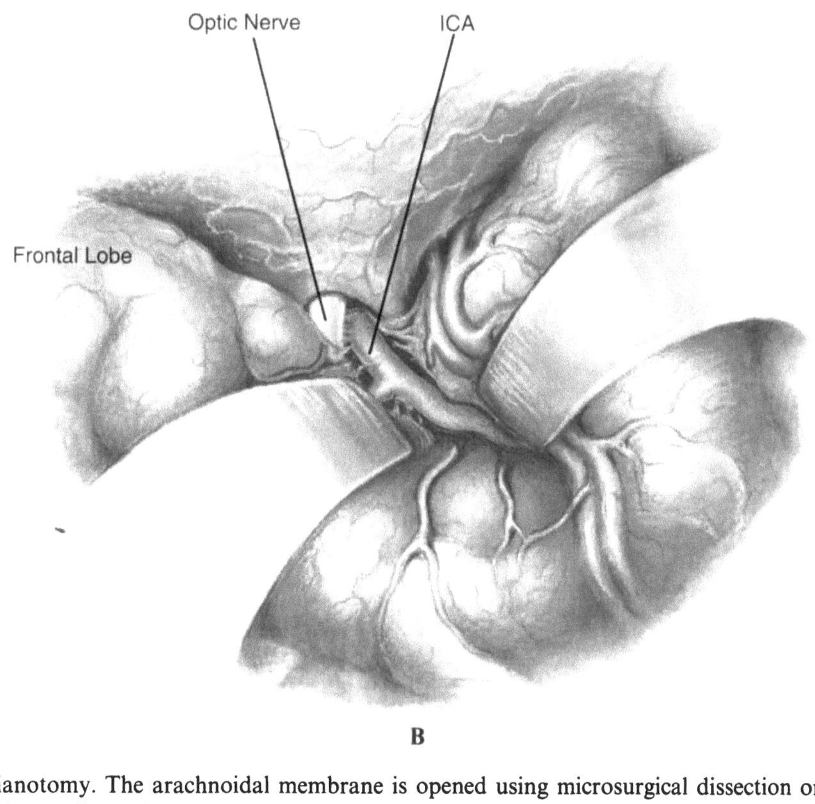

B

FIGURE 6.12. (A) Sylvianotomy. The arachnoidal membrane is opened using microsurgical dissection on the frontal side of the middle cerebral vein. The small crossing vessels must be coagulated and divided. (B) The dissection is carried deep, retracting the veins temporally to expose the internal carotid artery (ICA) and middle cerebral artery. The extent of the sylvianotomy is variable, depending on the location of the aneurysm.

ning in the throat and face following occlusion of this vein. Aphasia may also accompany occlusion of this vein. The rolandic vein, or Trolard's vein, need not be sacrificed because of its posterior position. Occlusion may result in contralateral hemimotor and sensory disturbances, usually temporary. This vessel arises in the posterior extremity of the lateral fissure and courses in the central gyrus. Headaches, dizziness, and weakness in the contralateral forearm have been described in association with thrombosis. The lateral occipital veins drain the occipital lobe and pass beneath the temporal and occipital lobe to enter the transverse sinus. Ligation of these veins may produce aphasia or hemianopsia.

The vein of Labbé arises as a continuation of the superficial sylvian vein. However, it receives many tributaries from both the parietal and temporal cortices and passes across the posterior temporal lobe diagonally to join the transverse sinus. Many cortical veins may accompany the anastomotic vein of Labbé. The inferior anastomotic vein of Labbé must be preserved because sensory, motor, and speech disorders follow sacrifice in some cases, and these cannot be predicted beforehand. Thrombosis of this vein may result in hemiparesis, especially involving the upper extremity and aphasia when on the left hemisphere. Occlusion of these veins may also lead to increased venous pressure and temporal lobe hematomas.

Temporary Clipping

Recently, fine and delicate temporary clips with variable closing pressures have become available. Closing pressure as well as intraarterial blood pressure, size of the vessel, and other factors are probably important in recognizing the amount of damage done by temporary clipping.[5] Sugita et al.[6] advises that the differentiation between temporary and permanent clipping is a blade pressure of 80 g. However, Gertz et al.[7] using a Heifitz clip, showed that pressures of even 30 g could cause recognizable defects when the scanning electron microscope was used to evaluate the endothelial surface. Other pathological changes, including the proliferation and migration of smooth muscle cells into the subintimal areas, also occur after temporary vascular clipping. In Symon et al.'s[8] view, temporary clipping is safe, but still it should be used as an elective rather than as a prophylactic procedure.

Separation of the Neck of the Aneurysm from the Parent Vessel

During microdissection of an aneurysm, total exposure of the fundus is usually unnecessary. The dissection should proceed around the neck of the aneurysm where the clip will finally rest. If an important vessel arises from the fundus, then complete dissection must be carried out. Careful study of the angiogram, both before surgery and intraoperatively, will assist the surgeon in identifying major vessels and their origin. If the angiogram has been selective, large and important vessels will usually not escape detection. However, aneurysms of the M_1–M_2 junction and of the BA apex may be accompanied by perforators of such small size that they do not appear on the angiogram, and they must be identified anatomically by the surgeon at dissection. When the dome of the aneurysm is to be dissected free, the use of temporary clips may be advantageous. Reducing the pressure in the aneurysm allows manipulation of the aneurysm sac, reducing the chance that it will rupture. The use of temporary clips also assists in the control of bleeding, should it occur, and allows intraoperative bleeding to be manageable with minimal compression and retraction. Two microsurgical instruments should be used to separate the neck or dome of an aneurysm from an artery to which it seems attached. One is used to retract the aneurysm or artery, and the other to strip away adhesions between the two. A wide selection of instruments, however, must be available. Some, such as the small spatula-like microdissecting tool, allows gentle separation with traction. A small pick (or a small instrument with a right-angle terminal point) may be used to retract the artery. Occasionally, sharp dissection is necessary with microscissors or sharper dissectors. The origin of the aneurysm from the parent vessel must be shown so that the clip can be applied parallel to the parent vessel to preserve its normal flow channel. Clips placed too far distally on the aneurysmal sac will leave a rest that may form secondary aneurysms at a later time.

Clipping

Many types of clips are now supplied for occluding the neck of an aneurysm, and a wide selection of clips should be available. Each clip has a specific clip applicator, and these must also be available as well as familiar to the assistant. Some applicators allow placement of clip at an arbitrary angle, and some have straight directed tips. Others may be manipulated so that the applicator tip can be adjusted to the angle needed or so that the aneurysm clip itself can be rotated on the applicator to achieve the angle necessary for clipping.

For fusiform aneurysms, a wide variety of fenestrated clips are required. In these, the arterial channel will be formed through the fenestration and the blades of the clip placed upon the wall of the vessel containing the most outpouching. There are several general rules and principles that should be adhered to during aneurysm clipping.

1. The aneurysm clip should be applied parallel to the axis of the vessel from which it arises.
2. The clip should be applied along the shortest dimension of the aneurysm neck. Clips applied in the long direction may not be sufficient to completely occlude the neck but, more importantly, they may distort the flow in the parent artery due to traction on its wall.
3. The size of the clip selected is important. The clip should slide onto the aneurysm neck without protruding more than a millimeter or so on the opposite side. Always inspect the blades of the clip after applying. The blades of the clip should be as narrow as possible in order to avoid compromising flow in the primary arterial channel.
4. If the neck of the aneurysm cannot be clipped close to the parent artery because of perforating or important channels that exit there, the residual neck must be invested or wrapped with muscle to protect it from future growth and rupture.
5. The presence of an atheroma, near the orifice of the aneurysm or along the parent artery, may call for modification of the clipping technique. The presence of an atheroma in the vessel usually mandates temporary clipping. Care should be taken not to dislodge the atheroma in an aneurysm neck back into the parent artery, causing thrombosis or embolization.
6. Manipulation around an aneurysm may precipitate mechanical vasospasm. Mechanical and manipulatively induced vasospasm may be relieved by the application of a 2% solution of papaverine HCl through a small needle to the adventitial surface of the artery.
7. Clots surrounding the aneurysm and parent vessel should be removed to prevent vasospasm later.
8. Thrombosed aneurysms require special care. The application of a clip to a hard thrombus may be unsuccessful due to migration of the clip, whether toward the dome or toward the parent vessel. To achieve successful clip, a temporary clip may be placed on the parent artery, the aneurysm opened, and the thrombus removed before final application of the clip.
9. Atheroma in a vessel may interfere with clipping. If the clip migrates either toward the dome or toward the parent artery or if there is crushing and extrusion of the atheroma, the use of temporary clips on the parent artery is preferred. The aneurysm should be opened, and endaneurysmectomy performed. The surgeon should be comfortable with microsurgical suturing in order to repair vessels so endarterectomized.
10. The method of application of the clip is important. The clip blades should first be opened fully and snapped into locking position. In approaching the aneurysm, the blades should be released to approximate the size of the neck of the aneurysm. In passing the blades around the neck of the aneurysm, a gentle side-to-side motion or a slight opening and closing movement prevents the clip blades from stabbing and puncturing the dome of the aneurysm that may be protruding into the blades from the posterior surface.

Difficult Aneurysms

Some aneurysms must be approached when circumstances are suboptimal. Occasionally, with restricted or limited access, the dome of an aneurysm may be encountered before the parent artery can be visualized and isolated. The fundus must be mobilized and manipulated in order to expose the neck and the parent artery from which this lesion arises. Several methods may be used to achieve this end. Intraoperative hypotension may be used when the patient's clinical condition permits. Mean arterial blood pressure may be reduced to 40 to 50 mm Hg in a healthy young individual for prolonged periods, probably an hour or longer. This does not apply to the patient who has cerebral vasospasm, impaired renal function, severe arteriosclerotic vessels, or other compromising vascular lesions. However, brief periods are tolerated in almost all patients. By reducing systemic arterial pressure, the fundus of the aneurysm can be mobilized easily, compressed by microretractors, and visualization around the dome achieved. This may permit the placement of temporary clips. The placement of temporary clips must take into account short arteries that penetrate the brain substance. Certain penetrating arteries carry high risk for deep infarction when prolonged temporary clipping is required. A poor second choice for visualizing the environment of a giant aneurysm that must be approached from the fundus is the use of a mirror. This may be heated slightly in the microscope lamp to prevent fogging. Reversal of anatomy may be confusing under these circumstances but this technique can often be used to assure that an opposite P_1 has not been included in a clip or that Percheron's arteries have been spared. A third possibility for effecting visualization is by operative or needle decompression. The aneurysm clip is advanced on either side of the dome as far as it can be visualized safely. The clip is positioned and, making certain that the fundus is well occluded and selecting a site where connective tissue appears to be preserved, a 27-gauge needle is inserted into the fundus. The needle should never be inserted into the thin membrane-like covering where the hemorrhage occurred because this may produce bleeding that is difficult to tamponade. As decompression is accomplished, the clip is advanced along the fundus each time achieving better visualization. The commitment to open the aneurysm and evacuate its contents (either with a needle or by suction) does limit some of the options available for correction since bleeding will certainly occur if the clips must be removed for any reason.

Some aneurysms are unclippable by virtue of their contents. Aneurysms that arise in an atheromatous bifurcation may have enough hardening in the wall that standard clips will not close and, even so, could provoke occlusion of feeding arteries by the atheromatous material. Such lesions must not be handled with ligature because, invariably, this forces the atheroma back into the nutrient artery lumen. When clip blades fail to close securely, an atheroma-free area in the nutrient artery, both proximal and distal to the aneurysm orifice must be occluded with temporary clips. If possible, short arteries are always excluded from the temporary clip. Then the aneurysm is opened, usually along its longest axis, terminating the incision several millimeters distal to the intersection of the aneurysm and the nutrient artery. Then, using microdissection, the aneurysm may be entered and evacuated of its contents by endaneurysmectomy. The atheroma is then slightly stretched, pulled into the aneurysm and divided. A clip is then applied to encompass the recently freed portion of the aneurysm neck and the temporary clips are removed (Fig. 6.13).

Some aneurysms, notably the variety described as fusiform aneurysms, cannot be clipped. Only rarely are these aneurysms responsible for SAH, but they may be a source of emboli. The hallmark of fusiform aneurysms is that they contain thrombi in their walls. Therefore, placing clips upon these lesions is extremely dangerous. Forming a new lumen by the exclusion of a portion of the wall with fenestrated clips is rarely feasible, unless the aneurysm does not contain clots. Management therefore may be extremely difficult. If it is a long lesion and the parent artery cannot be sacrificed, then a bypass using an external carotid branch may be considered. If the length is short, the lesion may be excised and an end-to-end anastomosis of the proximal and distal segments carried out. The limits for safe occlusion times for many intracranial vessels have not been established. Many variables must be considered, including the angiographic collateral channels that are present. There is little published information concerning safe occlusion times for the major intracranial arteries in man. The A_2 branch at the frontopolar artery may be occluded for 45 min without infarction in some patients. In primates, occlusion of the main trunk of the MCA proximal to the lenticulostriate arteries results in small infarcts in only 15 min unless the animal is heparinized. Clipping distal to the short arteries is tolerated for longer periods. In our cases, temporary clipping for as short as 12 min has produced infarction while other patients have tolerated 40 min without deficits.

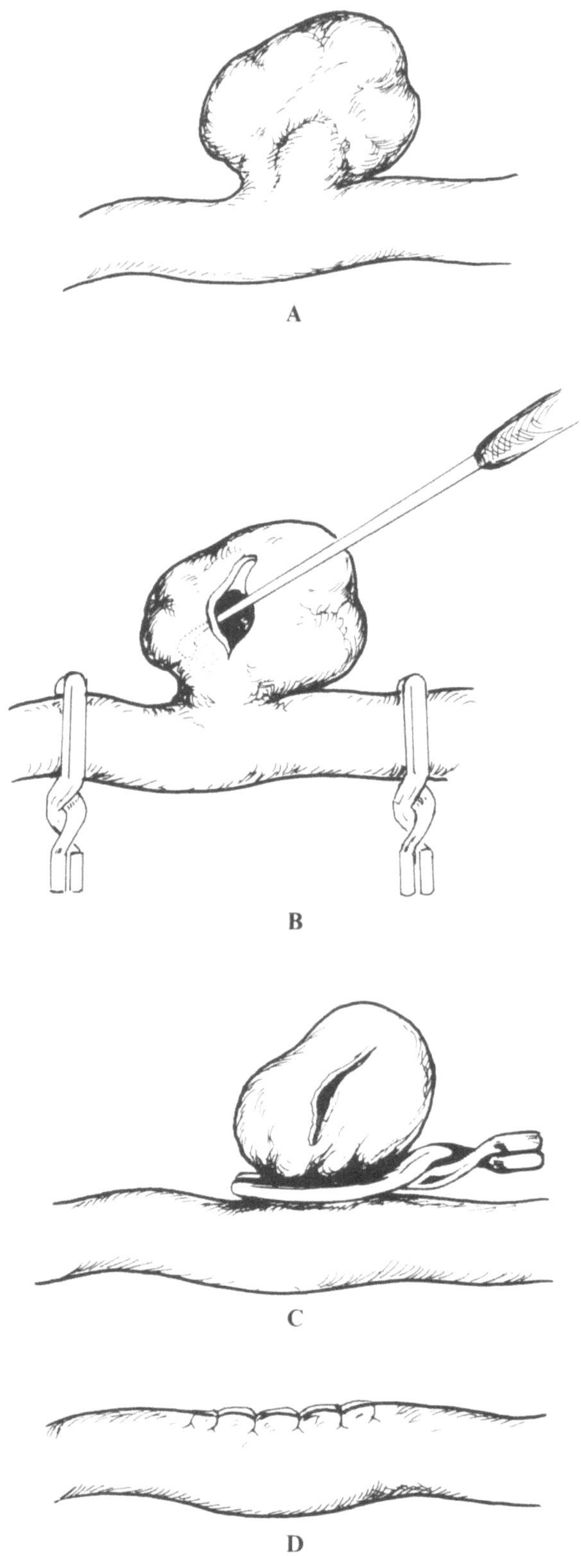

FIGURE 6.13. (A) Complex aneurysm containing atheroma preventing clipping. (B) After placing temporary clips on proximal and distal feeders, the aneurysm is opened and the atheroma dissected free. (C) A clip has been placed on the neck after endaneurysmectomy. (D) The aneurysm has been excised and microvascular suture performed.

Intraoperative Aneurysm Rupture

This is a complication most feared by the aneurysm surgeon, although if properly anticipated, much of the risk and most of the stress with this complication can be eliminated. Premature rupture must still be regarded as a complication of dissection. It occurs in 18% to 61% of all aneurysm cases.[9] Most of the hemorrhages occur during dissection of the fundus near the previous hemorrhage site. For this reason, preliminary dissection must begin along the parent artery from which the aneurysm arises so that temporary clips may be used if necessary. Batjer and Samson[10] have reviewed their operative experiences with premature rupture. They have seen spontaneous hemorrhage during induction of anesthesia and even perhaps at dural opening. However, these complications fortunately occur rarely, and when they do, there is only one alternative—to place a clip upon the bleeding aneurysm. This requires rapid exposure, high suction, and hypotension in order to gain control. This is perhaps one instance where microsurgical techniques must be abandoned in favor of expediency. When all else fails, the suction should be used as a dissecting instrument and the arachnoid quickly removed from the proximal artery from which the aneurysm arises. This fearful complication arises usually from a carotid artery aneurysm, and, if it does involve the BA, other complications can be anticipated. When only a small rent or laceration has occurred, the bleeding may be controlled with the use of a small suction placed against the wound with small cotton pledget. The pressure may be reduced if temporary clips have not been applied. When bleeding can be controlled, the preferred careful microsurgical dissection about the neck should be carried out. Any perforating arteries that are attached to or surround the aneurysm should be dissected away carefully. This may be accomplished bluntly using a variety of the small retractors and microdissecting instruments. Stretching the arachnoidal adhesions makes it possible to lyse it with scissors. Maximum magnification and lighting are essential. When the rupture occurs in a secondary loculation, a temporary clip may be applied at the base of this outpouching in order to gain adequate exposure of the neck. When bleeding occurs as the clip is being applied or released, if the clip seems to be in good location, closure should be continued. Sometimes, as the clip blades close, an adhesion along the fundus of the aneurysm may cause rupture, which becomes sealed with complete blade closure. If the clip blades fail to close securely and bleeding continues, another clip is advisable. Two or more clips may be used but they usually obstruct the surgeon's view. Therefore, if two clips will not suffice, then these clips must be removed and repositioned. If the first clip does not close completely, there may be thrombus or irregularity in the wall of the aneurysm or a defective clip may prevent complete sealing. A reinforcing clip might be placed along the axis of the first if this happens.

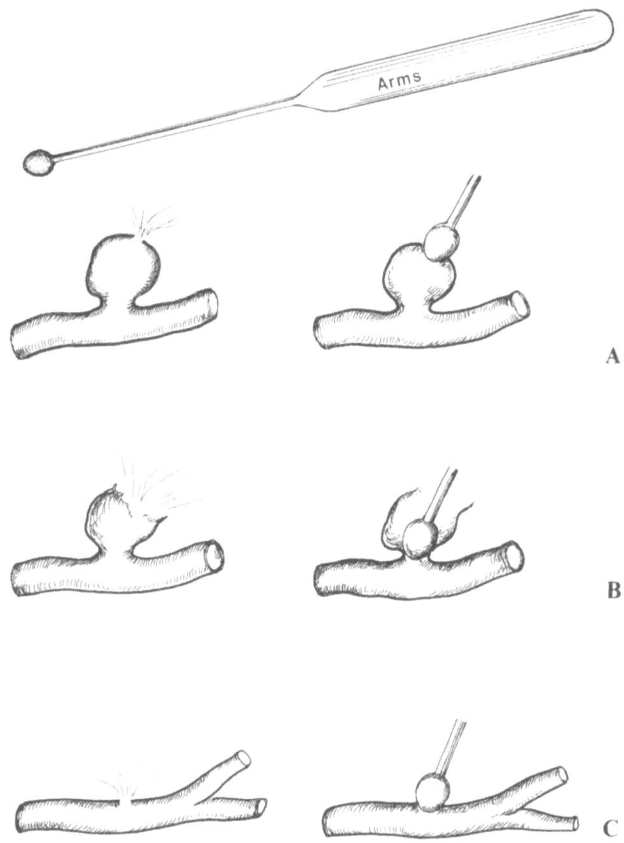

FIGURE 6.14. The use of Zubkov's ball. (A) The aneurysm has ruptured and the ball has been used to staunch flow from the aneurysm while the clip is applied to the neck. (B) The aneurysm has massively ruptured and the ball is used to occlude flow into the aneurysm at its orifice while a clip is applied. (C) The ball may be used to control flow from a rent in a vessel while primary repair is done.

Finally, Zubkov's ball may be used when massive bleeding from an unidentified area or source occurs (Fig. 6.14). Using large suction, this is directed toward the stream of blood until the major rent can be identified. The ball may be used in several ways. If the rent is small, the ball may be used to create just enough external compression to seal it. Dissection proceeds until a clip can be fastened around the neck or fundus if further dissection is necessary. If the rent is a large one, the ball is inserted into the aneurysm and gently manipulated toward the direction of the stream. The ball is then placed into the neck of the aneurysm, partly compromising flow in the parent artery also. At this time a clip is selected and placed preliminarily around the shaft of the ball. Now, while suction is still applied, the ball is removed and the clip is allowed to close.

When all else fails, Poppens' technique may be employed in which the entire aneurysm sac is engulfed into a large suction tip. This method may yet be useful in the so-called type 4 rupture as described by Pertuiset.[11] The entire fundus is contained in the suction, the large suction is advanced to the parent artery and then backed off slightly. An angled clip is usually needed and may be placed distal to the suction apparatus. If continued bleeding takes place, additional clips may be used or sutures may be needed in the parent artery if the rent enters this vessel. A piece of temporalis muscle is still useful for tamponade in the massively bleeding aneurysm. This may be held in place with clips for permanency.

In evaluating operative aneurysm mortality by postmortem angiography, Karhunen[12] concluded that bleeding from the aneurysm or adjacent arteries accounted for 25% of the deaths. Clip-induced obstruction of adjacent arteries accounted for 11% of the deaths. Kinking of adjacent arteries due to malposition of the clip could be substantiated. All complications occurred more frequently in patients with aneurysms of the BA type.

Aneurysm Excision and End-to-End Anastomosis

When important arteries enter an aneurysm and it is impossible to preserve these channels, one option for their preservation is an end-to-end anastomosis. The procedure is applicable to the branches of M_1 or M_2 and branches of the anterior cerebral artery (ACA) where length can be achieved. Especially, in older individuals, the arteries may be somewhat redundant. Prior to applying temporary clips, as much length as possible should be achieved by isolating the artery proximally and distally along its course. If there are any short penetrating branches that restrict movement of the vessels, this may mitigate against such a procedure. When applying temporary clips to the proximal and distal branches, short penetrating branches should be excluded when possible. At this time, the blood pressure should be elevated slightly, and heparin should be administered. To present an even surface for anastomosis, the arteries should be divided. If one channel is smaller than the other, it may be divided tangentially in order to provide more surface for the end-to-end anastomosis. Fine 9-0 or 10-0 sutures are employed, using a fine beveled needle. About 8 to 10 interrupted sutures are usually placed around the anastomosis after anchoring points are placed at 0°, 90°, 180°, and 270°. The endothelium on both sides should be examined and included in the suture. At various points during the procedure, a blunt 27-gauge needle may be placed in the lumen of each vessel for heparinized saline irrigation. This will ensure that the endothelium is not compromised by suture material. After the anastomosis is complete, the site is wrapped with Gelfoam sponge and the clips removed first on the distal side and then on the proximal side. If bleeding persists after 10 to 15 min, additional sutures may be necessary.

Wrapping Techniques

Wrapping techniques may be used both for large and small aneurysms. Wrapping may be used for an infundibulum or an outpouching to prevent enlargement. Once the aneurysm is formed, wrapping techniques are usually not successful because they cannot adequately contain the large growing aneurysm. They may be the only alternative, however, when multiple perforators exit the dome and the aneurysm has not ruptured. Surgical cotton, muslin, or Gortex may be used. Surgical cotton develops perhaps the best fibrous reaction, and this probably provides the best investment material.

Summary

There are many ways to clip an intracranial aneurysm. A successful neurosurgeon strives for uniformity, with gentle dissection and retraction. A surgical maxim is that all vessels must be saved if possible. No tissue must be sacrificed by prolonged temporary clipping if it can be preserved safely. Thorough knowledge of the anatomy and physiology of the vascular bed assists in surgical planning, both preoperatively and intraoperatively. Monitoring is an essential part of today's neurosurgical operation. All instruments must play in harmony. There must be no discord due to clumsy or inappropriate equipment. However, none of these can replace preparation. The surgeon should plan beforehand to handle virtually any eventuality. This will lead to a successful outcome, sometimes even under the worst of circumstances and conditions.

References

1. Traeger SM, Hemning RJ, Dobkin W, Gianotta S, Weirl MH, Weiss M. Hemodynamic effects of pentobarbital therapy for intracranial hypertension. *Crit Care Med.* 1983;11:697–701.
2. Cottrell JE, Robustelli A, Post K, Turndorf H. Furosemide and mannitol-induced changes in ICP and serum osmolarity and electrolytes. *Anesthesiology.* 1977;47:28–30.
3. Dandy WE. *Intracranial Arterial Aneurysms.* New York: Comstock; 1944, reprinted 1969.
4. Kaplan HA. Results of obliteration of specific cerebral veins and dural venous sinuses: animal and human studies. In: Kapp JP, ed. *The Cerebral Venous System and its Disorders.* Boca Raton, FL: Grune and Stratton Inc; 1984:275–282.
5. Dujovny M, Kossovsky N, Perlin A, Segal R, Diaz F, Ausman JI. Intracranial clips: an examination of the devices used for aneurysm surgery. *Neurosurgery.* 1984;14:257–267.

6. Sugita K, Hirota T, Iguchi I, Mizutami T. Comparative study of the pressure of various aneurysm clips. *J Neurosurg*. 1976;44:723–727.
7. Gertz SD, Rennels ML, Forbes MS, Kawamura J, Sunaga J, Nelson E. Endothelial cell damage by temporary arterial occlusion with surgical clips: study of the clip site by scanning and transmission electron microscopy. *J Neurosurg*. 1976;45:514–519.
8. Symon L, Momma F, Murota T. Assessment of reversible cerebral ischemia in man: intraoperative monitoring of the somatosensory evoked response. *Acta Neurochir (Wein)*. 1988;42:3–7.
9. Batjer H, Samson DS. Management of intraoperative aneurysm rupture. *Clin Neurosurg*. 1990;36:275–288.
10. Batjer HH, Samson DS. Retrograde suction decompression of giant paraclinoidal aneurysms. Technical note. *J Neurosurg*. 1990;73:305–306.
11. Pertuiset B. Intraoperative aneurysmal rupture and reduction by coagulation of the sac. In: Pia HW, Langmaid C, Zierski J, eds. *Cerebral Aneurysms—Advances in Diagnosis and Therapy*. Berlin: Springer-Verlag; 1979:398–401.
12. Karhunen PJ. Neurosurgical vascular complications associated with aneurysm clips evaluated by postmortem angiography. *Forensic Sci Int*. 1991;51:13–22.

7
General Methods for Endovascular Neurosurgery

Introduction

During the past decade, endovascular techniques for intracranial aneurysms have flourished. The original indication, giant unclippable intracranial aneurysms, has been extended to include small aneurysms and those that have recently ruptured. In addition to balloons, the introduction of coils and hardening materials has allowed extension of the technique to virtually any aneurysm of the intracranial circulation. Hardening materials can be introduced into the aneurysm within a balloon or directly into aneurysm cavities.

Each aneurysm requires a special technique, but common rules apply. Equipment in the operating room, monitoring of the procedure, preoperative and postoperative care, and preparation of catheters are common requirements that must be addressed by the endovascular therapist. This chapter will outline the general methods and the special techniques required to manage both common and unique aneurysms.

Ergonomics in the Endovascular Operating Theater

High resolution imaging equipment is the number one priority for endovascular neurosurgery. Digital methods, subtraction angiography, and road mapping are required for best results. The radiation source must be mobile in relation to the head. Good lateral, anterior–posterior, oblique, and submentovertex views are important. The power of the system is perhaps of less importance than the software used to display the image. The energy source must be checked periodically to assure a consistent and safe dose. Annually, the endovascular team should review the hazards of radiation and methods to protect themselves and the patient. The procedure may be carried out in the radiographic suite or in the operating room (OR), depending on the patient's condition and needs. In the OR, either fixed-beam or mobile sources may be used.

The OEC diasonics neurovascular module includes road mapping, real time angiography, and subtraction imaging from all views. This instrument emits 10 to 20 rad/min in the boost mode and perhaps more in some instances. Careful attention must be paid to safe usage. Doses exceeding 1500 rad may cause superficial skin reactions.

Equipment for monitoring is also required. Transcranial Doppler (TCD) sonography as well as intra-arterial lines for continuous arterial pressure monitoring should be available, and intracranial pressure (ICP) lines and monitors should be used when needed.

Instrumentation for Endovascular Surgery

Sterile instruments are needed for use in catheterizing the carotid and femoral vessels. For puncture of the cervical common carotid artery, a 5-cm-long needle with an internal diameter of at least 2 mm is needed. The needle terminates distally with an angle of 45°. The bevel is rounded somewhat so as not to present a sharp point to the wall of the artery (Fig. 7.1). If the needle tip has been filed to a sharp point, the needle may injure or damage the catheter or balloon, on passage or retrieval. Two ports are available at the proximal end of the needle. One of these is in line with the axis of the needle and the other enters 45o from the primary axis. The direct entry port is used for the introduction of balloons and guidewires. The 45° port is connected to plastic tubing for introduction of contrast material or to flush the catheter and balloons placed into the primary port. A stylet extending 2 mm beyond the blunted needle tip will be introduced through the primary port. The stylet, however, has been sharpened and is used to penetrate skin, subcutaneous tissue, deep tissue, and both walls of the carotid artery. An obturator is also available for occluding either the side port at 45° or the direct port. This inserts with a simple twist into the port. A diaphragm mechanism is also incorporated into a special adapter that can be placed in either the direct or the angled port. This special adapter permits the introduction of catheters and bal-

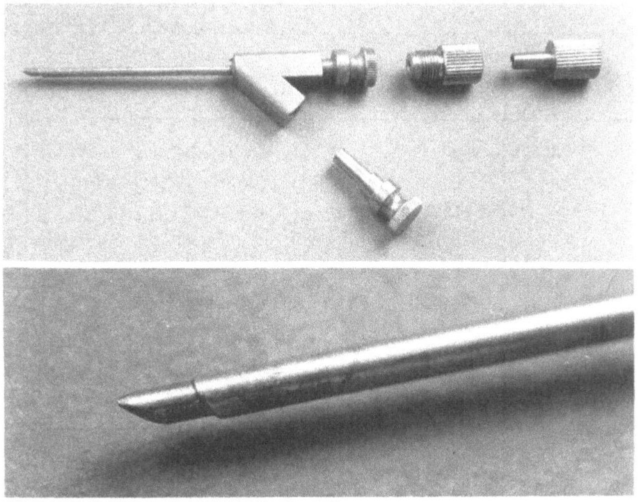
A
B

FIGURE 7.1. The needle used for carotid artery puncture.

loons and forms a tight seal to prevent the retrograde release of blood once the artery is punctured. A small syringe of 1 ml total volume with 0.1 mm gradations may be used to inflate the balloon or to place agents within the catheter.

Puncture of the common carotid artery (CCA) permits the use of short balloon catheters, which are more manageable. The metal but blunted needle end allows manipulation within the carotid artery. A more flexible plastic catheter will not permit change in direction by external manipulation.

The Seldinger approach may also be used to introduce catheters into the internal carotid artery (ICA). The sheath is somewhat more flexible, but movement within the artery is also limited.

For vertebral artery (VA) catheterization, the axillary artery is preferred because it is the most direct and shortest route to the artery. Balloon catheters of 25 to 30 cm may also be used, shorter than those required for the femoral route. The distal end of the catheter (approximately a 2 cm portion) has been previously stretched and thinned to make it more flexible. A gentle curve is placed at the end of this catheter. This is accomplished by holding the catheter under a steam kettle for approximately 20 s. After heating under the steam, the catheter is gently molded around the finger tip in order to create a gentle curve for the transition between the subclavian and the VA. The balloon catheter is introduced through this catheter after it has been directed in the VA.

Balloon Catheters

Serbinenko's[1] latex balloon catheter was first developed in 1971. Two types of balloons were used, detachable and nondetachable. Polyethylene was used for the catheter and latex for the balloon itself. For nondetachable balloons, the balloon was affixed to the catheter with a fine monofilament suture. The first detachable balloon prepared by Serbinenko was affixed to a catheter slightly flared at the tip. The orifice of the balloon contained a thickened area of latex that functioned as a valve. The balloon was then inflated with hardening material. After hardening, it was possible to detach the balloon from the flared catheter maintaining inflation of the balloon. However, this balloon does not lend itself well to liquid materials because the liquid escapes from the orifice and deflation occurs. Later, Serbinenko and Filatov[2] developed a valve system designed to prevent deflation.

Zubkov's[3] detachable balloon was developed in 1972. This balloon was made from latex, but the catheter was made from thoroplast, an agent similar to Teflon. For nondetachable balloons, he employed a fine monofilament suture to affix the balloon to the catheter in this way. Afterward, the balloon was redipped into latex to form a cohesive unit. For detachable balloons, Zubkov employed a latex thread. As the catheter was withdrawn from the balloon, the latex thread tightened, allowing the balloon to maintain inflation, even when liquid materials were employed. Later, Zubkov prepared balloons that were trained to assume a certain shape in an aneurysm when inflated and he modified the method for attachment of the balloon to the Teflon catheter. Since this time, many balloons have become available through the reports of individual surgeons or from commercial companies. The construction, design, and materials used are listed in Table 7.1.

Inflating Materials

Both liquid and polymerizing materials may be used to inflate the balloon. Contrast materials used for angiography, such as Venografin, Omnipaque, or Conray, are acceptable. Nonionic contrast materials are less toxic and are therefore preferred. Sometimes, inflation with isotonic saline is preferred. If, for instance, the balloon has been placed in a position that will produce stenosis of the parent vessel, this would not be seen on the angiogram if the balloon were inflated with contrast material. Therefore, the lumen of the parent vessel may be more adequately evaluated if the balloon is inflated with saline. The ideal properties of a polymerizing material are the following:

1. Polymerization must be accurately controlled and measured.
2. The polymerizing material must be inert in relation to the balloon material so that erosion and rupture will not occur.
3. The material must be of low viscosity so that it can be injected through fine catheters in a reasonable time frame.

TABLE 7.1. Balloon catheters used in the intracranial vessels

	Balloon type		Balloon material		Catheter material		
Author or company	Nondetach	Detach	Latex	Silicone	Polyethylene	Teflon	Silicone
Serbinenko (1970)	+	+	+		+		
Zubkov (1972)	+	+	+			+	
Debrun (1975)	+	+	+			+	
Scheglov (1975)	+	+	+		+		
Hieshima (1981)	+	+		+	+		
Kerber (1975)	+			+			+
Taki (1979)		+	+		+		
Interventional Therapeutics Corp.	+	+		+	+		
Meditach	+	+		+		+	
Target Therapeutics	+	+		+	+		
Jugenor Medical, Inc. Paris, France	+	+	+			+	

4. It must be biocompatible and approved for medical use.
5. The volume of the material must not expand or contract during polymerization from the liquid phase. The liquid and solid states must not vary in volume by more than 1% to 2%. If it shrinks, the aneurysm may fill angiographically. If it expands, the aneurysm may rupture.
6. The material should be visible radiographically.

Popular polymerizing agents include silicone, 5-hydroxy ethyl methacrylate (hema), and isobutyl-2 cyanoacrylate (IBCA). Each of these materials must be combined with its own catalyst in order to polymerize. The polymerization time is determined by the amount of catalyst in proportion to polymer. Currently, no radiographically opaque polymer is available.

The aneurysm is first filled with liquid contrast material while it is determined angiographically that the aneurysm is completely occluded. The contrast material is then withdrawn and the amount that was used to produce the desired effect is measured carefully. Only this amount of polymerizing agent will then be injected back into the balloon. During the polymerization process, angiography is used to make certain that the balloon occludes the aneurysm. If insufficient polymer is present, more may be added with its catalyst to achieve the desired effect.

Coils

During recent years, many endovascular surgeons have turned to platinum microcoils to induce thrombosis in intracranial aneurysms. Various materials (such as wool, silk, cotton, or Dacron) have also been incorporated into the microcoils to form a fibrous network or mesh to entrap the blood particles and enhance clot formation. Gianturco and co-workers[4] were the first to use coils to occlude the vasculature to a hypernephroma. The diameter of these coils was large, and the delivery system was not suitable for neurosurgical use. Originally, the coils consisted of fragments of the guidewire used for angiography catheters. At first, 5-cm lengths of 0.89-mm wire were used in the renal system. In 1979, Anderson and co-workers[5] introduced "mini" Gianturco stainless steel coils for transcatheter vascular occlusion. The mini coils are made from segments of guidewires 5 cm long by 0.46 mm in diameter. Dacron threads were included in these original stainless steel coils which were introduced through a 5-F French catheter, but these were still not appropriate for neurosurgical use.

Yang and coauthors[6,7] reported using platinum wire in patients with arteriovenous fistulas (Target Therapeutics) (12,13). They used distal tips with .014- and .013-in steerable guidewires. The length of the coils produced was 0.5 to 1.5 cm. Hilal and co-workers[8] used coils of platinum coated with synthetic fibers (Hilal Microcoils, Cook Inc). Guglielmi and co-workers[9] developed a new type of coil, the so-called detachable coil, that could be used for electrothrombosis prior to separation.

Handmade Balloon Catheters

In the former Soviet Union, the development of the balloon catheter differed considerably from those developed later in the United States. For the balloon itself, latex was used exclusively. The method used in preparation of the balloon and the catheter and the method for attaching the balloon to the catheter varied among the three major investigators—Serbinenko,[1] Zubkov,[3] and Shcheglov[10]—who were developing this field simultaneously. Serbinenko and Shcheglov used polyethylene catheters of fine caliber while Zubkov preferred a Teflon catheter. In Zubkov's view, the Teflon catheter is much more hydrophobic, less likely to attract platelet and blood thrombi, and therefore less likely to produce thromboembolic complications. The surface is smoother, facilitating detachment of the balloon without producing undue traction on a vessel. Teflon is somewhat stiffer than polyethylene and thus can be guided through the basal intracranial vessels somewhat independently of blood flow, a quality that makes it particularly suitable for the treatment of vasospasm when flow may be diminished considerably. Serbinenko and Shcheglov both flared the catheter tip, and the balloon was attached by virtue of its own sphincter mechanism, being somewhat thicker at the attachment site. The thickened area also secured the balloon to the catheter. This method, not using suture, permitted easy detachment, but the sphincter mechanism was not tight enough to retain nonviscous liquids. Silicone and other hardening agents could be used safely however. Shcheglov also employed a thrombogenic substance in the wall of his balloon to further promote occlusion of the aneurysm.[11] Zubkov first used a latex thread to secure the balloon to the catheter. This created a sphincter mechanism that, upon detachment, was capable of retaining nonviscous liquids in the balloon. Later, other catheters were developed that permitted an easier access into the neck of an aneurysm by virtue of the configuration of the tip of the catheter.

Each balloon should be prepared individually for each patient and for the particular pathology to be treated, including cerebral vasospasm (Fig. 7.2). The size of the balloon, its configuration, and its filling properties are all important in planning therapy. A special form is used to prepare each individual balloon. The size of the form generally determines the size of the balloon that will be produced at full inflation. A blunt needle with a 0.3- to 0.4-mm diameter may be used to prepare a latex balloon for the treatment of vasospasm involving the middle cerebral artery (MCA). The balloon is made longer than necessary, usually about 1 cm in length. This is accomplished by placing a rounded-point needle 1.5 cm into pure medical latex. Each batch of latex has its own particular hardening characteristics available from the supplier of the medical latex. Each batch may also vulcanize at different temperatures; therefore, only experience can produce the best balloon. After dipping into latex, the needle is withdrawn and the latex allowed to air dry along the shaft of the needle. Then the needle containing the latex coating is placed in water at 45°C for approximately 30 min. The needle and latex are removed and air-dried. After air-drying, the balloon-tipped needle is placed into an oven at 70°C for 3 to 5 min for final hardening. Afterward, the balloon is slipped off the end of the needle with talc coated finger tips.

Preparation of the Catheter

A Teflon catheter, having a 0.3- to 0.4-mm internal diameter, should be used for intracranial catheterization. For the anterior circulation, using the carotid artery as a primary route, approximately 40 cm of Teflon tubing is needed. For use in the VA using an axillary artery approach, a 60 cm Teflon tube is required. The distal

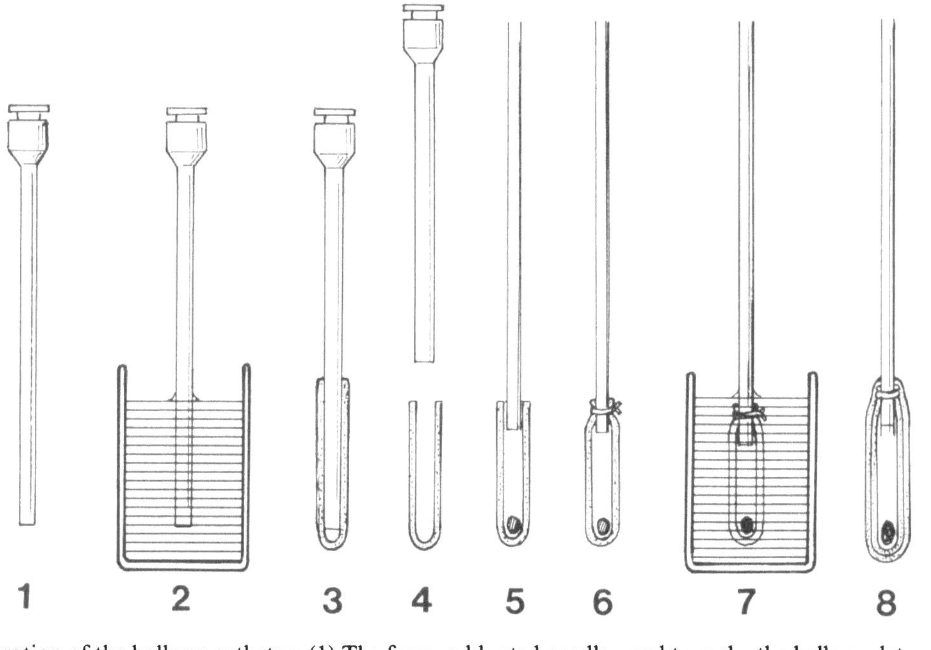

FIGURE 7.2. Preparation of the balloon cathetex; (1) The form, a blunted needle, used to make the balloon determines the ultimate size of the balloon; (2) the form has been dipped into medical grade latex and coated; (3) the latex is allowed to harden about the form; (4) the latex has been slipped off and trimmed; (5) a marker has been placed in the apex of the balloon and the balloon connected to a Teflon catheter; (6) The balloon has been affixed to the catheter using latex thread; (7) The balloon is once again dipped in latex to present a nonthrombogenic surface; (8) finished balloon ready for use.

8 cm of the catheter is extended by traction to 10 to 12 cm to make it both thinner and more flexible for negotiating the tight curves of the intracranial circulation. Any irregularities may be trimmed from the distal tip so that the terminal 6 to 8 cm of the extended segment are left attached to the catheter. With a scalpel blade, the catheter is then cut off at the end at an angle of 45°.

The tip preparation depends greatly on the type of balloons needed: detachable versus nondetachable. For a nondetachable balloon, such as those required for angioplasty, the tip of the catheter must be flared slightly. This is accomplished by the insertion of a blunt needle or stylet into the opening and rotating it at approximately 30°. This produces a very slight flare (approximately 1 mm maximum) at the tip. For vasospasm, the uninflated balloon must be 0.5 to 0.6 cm long. The remainder of the balloon is cut away and discarded.

A radiographic marker must be prepared and inserted into the balloon. This may be accomplished by making transverse cuts across the blades of a silver clip, producing a small piece of silver that measures approximately 0.3 to 0.4 mm. A 0.3-mm silver wire may also be used. Using fine forceps and magnification, the small piece of silver must be introduced into the balloon. Manipulated into the apex of the balloon, this marker will identify the most distal site that the balloon has passed.

The balloon is also connected to the catheter using magnification and manipulation. The balloon should be inserted over the catheter until it comes in contact with the apex. The balloon is then fixed to the catheter, using 8-0 nylon or Prolene suture material. The ends of the suture are then trimmed closely with microscissors and the nondetachable balloon is thus secured. Finally, the affixed balloon is dipped into the latex mixture once more. The latex is allowed to cover the balloon entirely, extending over about 0.1 mm of the catheter to affix further the balloon to the catheter. This produces a smooth nonthrombogenic surface connecting the catheter to the balloon. The diameter of the finished balloon is critical. In no case should the inflated diameter of the balloon exceed 115% of the normal vessel diameter. Purinja and Kasjanov[12] reported that some arteries rupture when expanded 115% above normal diameter. However, the latex balloon is so flexible that it assumes a sausage shape in the vessel. Balloons made from silicone assume a globular shape and may cause vessel rupture.

For detachable balloons, both the catheter tip and the balloon must be prepared differently. Again, the catheter tip should be stretched and lengthened in its terminal 8 to 10 cm. No flare is placed upon the end of the catheter.

Detachable balloons are fixed and hardened similarly to nondetachable balloons. A small piece of silver is also placed in the apex of the detachable balloon. This balloon is then slipped over a Teflon catheter with an internal diameter of 0.3 to 0.4 mm. Fixation, however, is different. The balloon is attached to the catheter with 0.3- to 0.4-mm diameter latex thread, using a locked surgeon's knot. The final tension placed upon the latex thread determines the detachment force needed for detachment. The latex thread is trimmed adjacent to the knot with microscissors. Finally, this prepared balloon is dipped into latex extending the latex coating beyond the proximal portion of the latex balloon by approximately 0.1 mm (Fig 7.3).

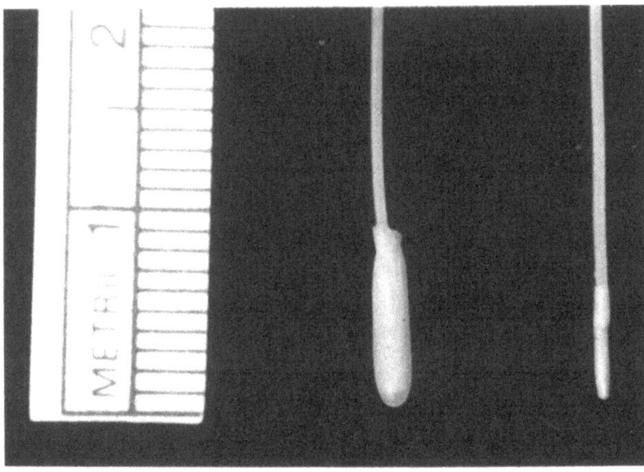

FIGURE 7.3. Handmade latex balloons. On the left, the larger balloon is for occlusion of a large aneurysm and on the right the smaller balloon was prepared for vasodilatation of the the vessel in vasospasm.

The size of the balloon is again critical to the structure that must be occluded. If the balloon is to be placed into an aneurysm, careful measurements must be made to ensure that the apex of the balloon fits snugly against the dome of the aneurysm but also projects far enough proximally to obstruct the neck of the aneurysm. Inflation must begin at the tip of the balloon and proceed backward toward the detachment site. Inflation of the balloon must not place additional pressure upon the thin aneurysm wall. The diameter of the inflated balloon must always be slightly wider than the neck of the aneurysm. The diameter of the noninflated balloon must be small enough to pass through any stenotic area in the vessel leading to the aneurysm and into the orifice of the aneurysm as well.

In making the balloon, the size of the form needed depends on the size of the aneurysm to be occluded. The larger the diameter of the aneurysm, the larger the form required. Forms measuring 0.4 to 1.0 mm create balloons in the range 0.5 to 1.0 cm when they are fully inflated. The length of the balloon is determined by the length of exposed latex on the end of the catheter.

Sterilization of Balloon Catheter and Instruments

The methods used to sterilize the balloon and catheter must not change their physical properties. Latex balloons are usually made from natural products, and hot sterilization methods may change the chemical structure of the balloon, weakening it or reducing its elastic properties. Commercially made balloons and catheters may arrive in a sterile pack. They should also be tested by inflation before they are placed in an aneurysm to assure that elastic properties have not been altered. In time, both latex and silicone materials tend to deteriorate. Therefore, they should be used as quickly as possible after preparation. Handmade balloon catheters should be sterilized immediately before use. Many types of antiseptic solutions may be used for chemical sterilization. Absolute alcohol, alcohol in chlorhexidene, or iodine-containing compounds may be used for sterilization.

All types of balloons and catheters may be sterilized in a gas autoclave and by gamma rays. Dry heat should not be employed for latex balloons because latex has a low melting point. Boiling or steaming is also inappropriate for latex microballoons because of weakening of the wall produced by heat.

Removal of Air from the Balloon

In the deflated state, the catheter and balloon contain a certain amount of dead space. This must be displaced by a small amount of contrast material. The balloon is held in an upward position between the thumb and index finger while being inflated with contrast agent. The air representing the dead space is allowed to migrate to the apex of the balloon. The tip of the catheter is advanced toward the apex of the balloon containing the air. As the balloon is deflated, air leaves first and contrast material later. After the air has entered the syringe, the balloon may be inflated with the syringe pointed downward to entrap the air in the upper portions. Any time the syringe is detached from the needle, a small drop of contrast material should be placed in the needle hub to make certain that contrast material fills the pavilion of the syringe before reconnecting. Otherwise, a small amount of air may be injected back into the balloon.

Training of the Balloon

At this point, the catheter projects nearly to the apex of the balloon. To prepare a detachable balloon, the balloon should be shifted toward the distal end of the catheter, leaving approximately 2 mm of the catheter extending into the orifice of the deflated balloon. During the process of tying the balloon onto the catheter, some grooving has been made into the catheter by the tying suture. This makes detachment somewhat forceful. If the sphincter is displaced or shifted toward the end of the catheter, this presents a smooth surface for the sphincter mechanism to slide upon. Latex suture also creates a furrow in the Teflon catheter that makes more detachment force necessary. As the untrained balloon is expanded, inflation proceeds in random configuration. The surgeon should train the balloon to inflate in proper order. For angioplasty and vasodilatation, the inflation process should begin proximally and proceed distally, expanding the vessel wall in the process. The balloon serves as a wedge creating a position for advancement into the distal arterial stream. For inflation within an aneurysm, the inflation process should begin at the apex and proceed to the orifice, ie., distal to proximal; otherwise, obstruction at the neck may cause pressure within the aneurysm. To train the balloon, the surgeon compresses the part of the balloon to be inflated last between the fingertips while test inflation is carried out several times. For a vasodilatation balloon, the surgeon compresses the apex of the balloon in the fingertips, leaving only the proximal portion exposed. He then inflates this several times to weaken the proximal portion.

Anesthesia

Local anesthesia with neuroleptics is preferable for most patients. For agitated or confused patients and those with impaired consciousness and responsiveness, general anesthesia may be preferred. When ventilatory support is needed, general anesthesia is required. The equipment and personnel needed for rapid general induction must always be available in the endovascular operating theater. Suction, anesthetic gases, and monitoring equipment should be available for emergency care.

Position of the Patient

The patient should be brought to the operating room or angiographic suite premedicated, with an established intravenous line. The patient is placed on the operating table in the supine position with the head extended by placing a 10- to 15-cm roll beneath the shoulders (Fig 7.4). After preparation of the skin of the cervical area from the chin to the clavicles, the lower portion of the torso is draped. The face is left exposed so that the patient can communicate freely and so that vision, speech, and pupillary reaction can be tested easily. Light neuroleptic anesthesia and local analgesia are obtained with fentanyl and droperidol combined with 1% lidocaine. If the procedure is performed outside the surgical suite, an operating room should be on alert and available should

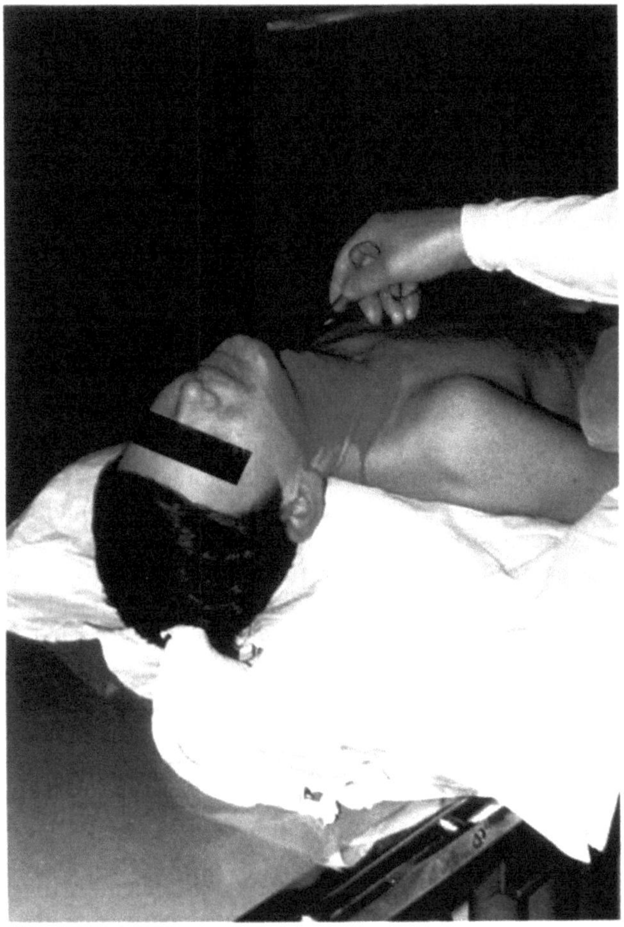

FIGURE 7.4. Position of the patient for puncture of the common carotid artery and for introducing a needle into the internal carotid artery.

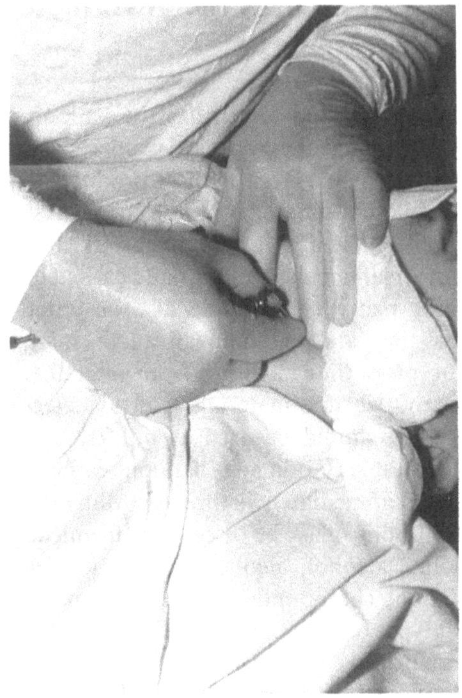

FIGURE 7.5. The preferred position for puncture of the common carotid artery.

complications occur. Possible complications that would necessitate operating room use include rupture of an artery, rupture of an aneurysm, dissection, thrombosis, or embolization.

Puncturing the Artery

The artery should be palpated between the fingertips and more or less impaled between two fingers (Fig. 7.5). Preferably, the needle should be introduced 2 cm proximal to the bifurcation of the common carotid artery because of the risk of atheroma or stenosis at the bifurcation. Both walls of the artery are punctured and the stylet removed. The needle is then withdrawn slowly until brisk backflow bleeding is seen. The thumb is placed over the orifice of the needle as it is threaded into the internal carotid artery. This reduces the possibility that balloons will be placed into the external carotid artery segment. The needle, being blunt and at 45° angle, can be compressed against the posterior wall of the carotid artery to reduce back bleeding. Tubing and two-way stopcocks are then connected to the side port for flushing and the injection of contrast material. The other port may be occluded with cotton, latex, or a special adapter. The adapter, by virtue of a central opening allows introduction of the balloon catheter.

The Seldinger method can also be used. The skin should be punctured with a No. 11 blade in order to pass the dilator over the guidewire. In this technique, the artery is punctured and the stylet withdrawn. A short guidewire is introduced into the Seldinger needle. Over the guidewire, the vessel dilator is then placed. After dilating the opening of the carotid artery, finger pressure should continue to be applied to prevent bleeding from the dilated opening. A plastic sheath is then passed over the guidewire and attempts made to direct it into the ICA. The sheath is flexible and bending, and prevents the passage of balloons. If the sheath is not absolutely straight and in the center of the arterial stream, as the balloon is withdrawn, it may be detached prematurely by kinks in the tip of the plastic sheath. It has the advantage, however, of having a closable diaphragm. This diaphragm covers the side port and prevents backbleeding at the time of introduction of the balloon catheter.

General Technique of the Endovascular Operation

Balloon Occlusion of Arterial Aneurysms

After preparing the neck with antiseptic solution, analgesia is achieved with 1% lidocaine. The artery may be partially immobilized by injecting small amounts of lidocaine on either side. The needle should rest within 1 cm of the origin of the ICA. This is achieved by direct puncture of the common carotid artery threading the blunt needle into the internal segment.

For catheterizing the VA, a Seldinger technique is preferred. The arm is extended on an armboard and the axilla is prepared. Local anesthesia is used to infiltrate the axillary skin and the tissue surrounding the axillary artery. After the pulse of the axillary artery is identified, an 18-gauge Seldinger needle is used for puncture. After the stylet has been removed, a guidewire is passed into the axillary artery and the needle sheath removed. A dilator is then used to enlarge the opening in the axillary artery. A catheter with a 2-mm internal diameter is passed over the guidewire and advanced toward the VA using direct imaging. The VA having the most direct route to the aneurysm in question should be selected. However, if one artery is dominant, the nondominant artery should be chosen because sacrifice may be required. The less serpentine artery should otherwise be selected because the curves interfere with the passage of the balloon and catheters. A catheter containing a small terminal flexure is then introduced into the VA and extended approximately 1 cm into the VA.

Good patient preparation and anesthesia are important to the success of the endovascular operation. Atraumatic puncture facilitates passage of the balloons and avoids intimal flaps and dissections. The hemodynamic status of the patient is also important. Arterial blood pressure should be normal and intracranial hemodynamics must be stable. Most balloons are directed by virtue of blood flow, and, if this is impaired, balloon passage will be retarded. An intravenous solution should be administered continuously during the endovascular procedure. This lessens the risk that contrast material will damage the kidneys and also improves blood flow and blood pressure.

At the time of injection of the carotid artery, the sympathetic ganglion may also be anesthetized to prevent prophylactically the acute vasospasm that may come with arterial manipulation. After puncture of the carotid or vertebral artery, 2000 to 3000 units of heparin sulfate are administered *slowly* intraarterially in 10 ml of physiological saline. Two to three thousand units of heparin are also added to 400 to 500 ml physiological saline for irrigation.

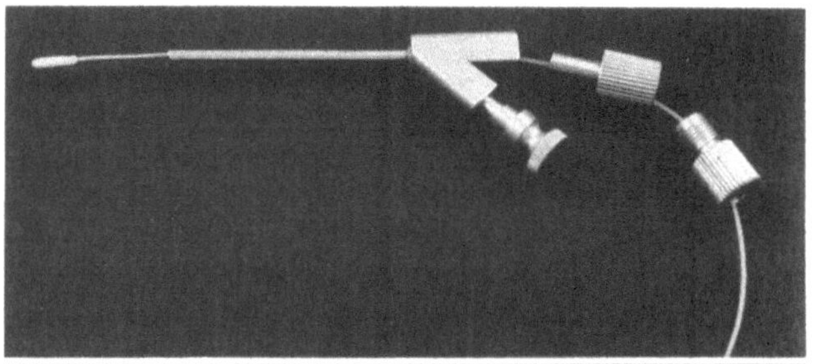
A

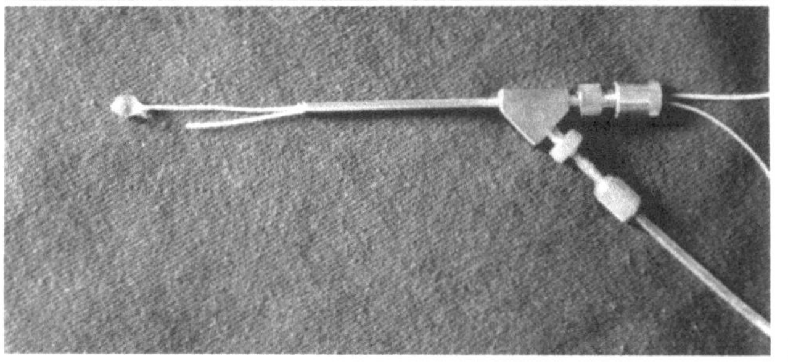
B

FIGURE 7.6. (A) A single balloon catheter has been passed through the straight port of the needle. (B) Two balloons have been introduced into the straight port. One balloon has been inflated after passage.

Prior to introduction into the intracranial circulation, the balloon must be inflated and measured. Both length and diameter must conform to the aneurysm that is to be treated. Additionally, the balloon should be tested for leakage and then trained. For an aneurysmal balloon, inflation begins first at the distal site and progresses toward the attachment site on the catheter. The latex thread holding the balloon to the catheter has created slight fissuring in the catheter. To prepare for detachment, it must be shifted toward the end and out of the groove previously made. One or two balloons may be introduced into the needle via the straight port as the side port is injected with saline. These balloons are directed toward the aneurysm by the endovascular surgeon (Fig. 7.6). The balloon is not inflated until the radiographic marker can be seen near the orifice of the aneurysm in question. Periodically, injections are made, and road mapping techniques are employed. In this way, the orifice of the aneurysm has been identified before the balloon reaches the target site. In some cases, the aneurysms may be occluded using only a single balloon. Two balloons are preferred for most aneurysms. First, the helper balloon is used to alter the flow of blood in the arterial tree. By inflating or deflating this balloon, the primary balloon may then be directed into whatever flow channel results from the occlusion by the helper balloon[11] (Fig. 7.7A). Second, the helper balloon may be used as a deflector of the primary balloon (Fig 7.7B). The helper balloon is advanced beyond the orifice of the aneurysm.

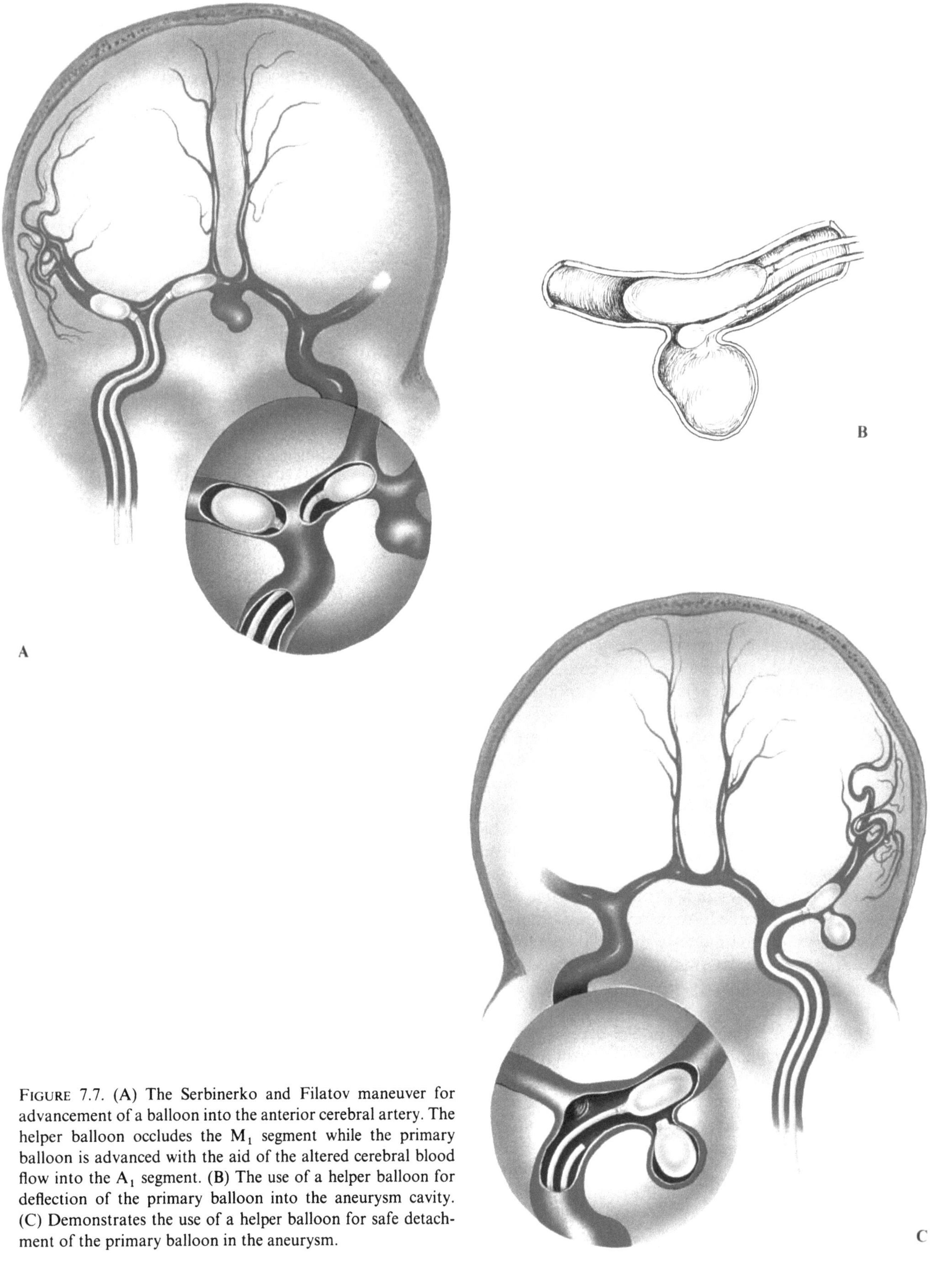

FIGURE 7.7. (A) The Serbinerko and Filatov maneuver for advancement of a balloon into the anterior cerebral artery. The helper balloon occludes the M_1 segment while the primary balloon is advanced with the aid of the altered cerebral blood flow into the A_1 segment. (B) The use of a helper balloon for deflection of the primary balloon into the aneurysm cavity. (C) Demonstrates the use of a helper balloon for safe detachment of the primary balloon in the aneurysm.

The primary balloon is then advanced until it deflects into the orifice of the aneurysm. The helper balloon is then deflated and retracted slightly. Third, the helper balloon is used to safely detach the primary balloon (Fig. 7.7C). After inflation of the primary balloon, in the aneurysm, the helper balloon is advanced into a position where it occludes the orifice of the aneurysm. The catheter from the primary balloon passes it in contact with the side wall of the parent artery. This provides safety since the very flexible latex balloon tends to deform and pull into the arterial lumen as the catheter is retracted. Last, the helper balloon is deflated after the catheter is detached from the primary balloon and both catheters and the helper balloon are removed from the artery. The helper balloon may be held in a waiting position near the orifice of the aneurysm while the primary balloon is being inflated. Should the artery or the aneurysm rupture, the helper balloon is rapidly advanced and inflated, reducing blood flow and causing tamponade. Then the patient should be taken immediately to the OR for direct surgical repair of the bleeding site via craniotomy.

Endovascular Manipulation

As the balloon catheter or catheters are advanced slowly, direct and continuous imaging is essential. Inflation of the balloon is normally not required. Inflation is contraindicated as long as the radiographic marker proceeds along the vascular channel of interest. If the balloon catheter stops its distal migration due to tortuosity, or a bifurcation of a vessel is encountered, minimal inflation may be needed to create a bolus for flow directed movement. Maximal inflation, on the other hand, produces tamponade and retards forward migration. The balloon is directed slowly toward the orifice of the aneurysm. Special maneuvers may be needed to force the balloon into the aneurysm where flow is slow. Occasionally, minimal inflation of the balloon causes turbulent flow, directing the balloon into the orifice of the aneurysm. The direction of blood flow may be altered by compression of the opposite cervical carotid artery, directing the balloon toward the aneurysm or collateral artery. This is a useful maneuver when the balloon must be directed into the A_1 branch. Occlusion of the opposite carotid artery augments flow in the ipsilateral A_1 segment, reversing flow in the opposite A_1 segment. It may also create enough flow aberration to direct the balloon into an anterior communicating artery (AComA) aneurysm. The contrast material that is used to inflate the balloon may be somewhat heavier than the blood in which it passes. Thus, when the balloon is inflated, gravity can be used to direct the movement of the balloon. The patient's head may be turned so that the aneurysm becomes the most dependent portion,

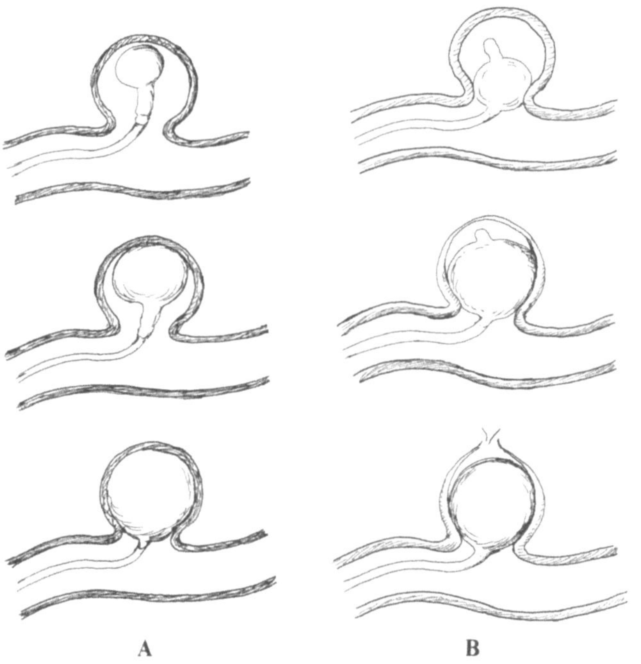

FIGURE 7.8. (A) The correct method for inflating a balloon in an aneurysm cavity. Inflation begins at the fundus and advances to the orifice (B) The incorrect method for inflating a balloon in an intracranial aneurysm, blocking the neck. Further inflation causes pressure on the wall and consequent rupture.

thus facilitating passage of the heavier balloon into the aneurysm.

After the balloon is introduced into the aneurysm cavity, temporary inflation is carried out in order to assess its position. At this time, the balloon is inflated from the fundus progressing proximally toward the orifice. This prevents the entrapment of blood within the aneurysm and the creation of abnormal stresses on the aneurysm wall (Fig 7.8). Temporary occlusion allows testing of the effect of the balloon on local circulation. Occasionally, an inflated balloon may protrude into the lumen blocking distal flow. The volume necessary to produce the desired balloon size must be calculated carefully. The usual temporary occlusion time is 20 to 30 min, and this provides ample opportunity to study intracranial flow patterns that will result after detachment. The clinical status of the patient is evaluated, keeping in mind that inflation of the balloon may precipitate vasospasm or produce ischemic signs. In addition, the TCD may be used to monitor cerebral blood flow (CBF) velocity. During test occlusion, a significant fall (50%) in velocity alerts the surgeon that balloon occlusion will probably not be tolerated.

In the next stage, permanent occlusion is carried out. The balloon is deflated by gentle suction applied to the catheter via a small syringe. The decision must be made as to what the permanent inflating or hardening agent will be. In each case, the decision is made based on the individual characteristics of the patient and the aneurysm to be treated. Aneurysms that have a large internal diameter (greater than 10 mm) should be treated with soft balloons, filled with contrast material. For smaller aneurysms, a hardening agent is usually preferred. Silicone may be used as a hardening agent prior to detachment of the catheter. With large and giant aneurysms, some shrinkage is desirable. If the hardening agent is firm, this will not occur. Soft balloons filled with contrast material permit thrombosis and fibrosis, eventually leading to shrinkage of the aneurysm. Invariably, there is some leakage through the latex membrane. Smaller aneurysms (less than 10 mm) rarely produce mass effect even locally, and therefore shrinkage is not required.

After permanent occlusion of the aneurysm, detachment is the final stage. If the balloon is filled with contrast material, it may be detached at any time. If it is to be filled with a hardening agent, it must be left in place until solid. This can often be determined by examining the residual material that remains after mixture of the compounds; when hardening takes place, it has usually taken place within the aneurysm, and the balloon may be detached at this time. The amount of agent placed in the balloon for temporary occlusion is determined by measuring the amount removed after temporary inflation. Only that amount can be reintroduced into the balloon for permanent detachment. Before the balloon is detached, aneurysm occlusion is evaluated angiographically and the status of the parent artery is examined. Occasionally, a small amount of additional hardening agent will be needed to produce total occlusion. A helper balloon is always preferred in detachment whether the aneurysm has been preliminarily filled with soft or hard materials. Occasionally, however, detachment must proceed without the aid of a helper balloon. This occurs in aneurysms with small necks in which the balloon is well seated within the dome or fundus and also when the helper balloon cannot be advanced into a small artery, such as the AComA, to assist in the detachment. If the balloon seems well seated and unlikely to migrate back into the artery, detachment proceeds.

After detachment of the balloon, the operation may be terminated. This requires gentle retraction of the catheter from which the balloon was attached, and, subsequently, the catheter and helper balloon are removed. Again, this should be done with imaging so that the helper balloon will not be detached by kinking or by contact with the needle or catheter. Afterward, the needle is removed and compression is applied to the carotid artery for at least 10 min. A small amount of Xylocaine may be infiltrated around the carotid artery prior to the withdrawal of the needle to prevent pain that might be caused by the compression.

The patient should be observed at this time for the development of ischemic and hemorrhagic complications. Anticoagulation should not be reversed, but control of blood pressure is essential. A preoperative coagulogram allows identification of potential bleeding complications. The evaluation of neurological signs of ischemia and hemorrhage are carried out at regular intervals. Postoperatively, the patient should be under the direct supervision of an internist and/or a neurosurgeon.

Occlusion of the Parent Vessel

Occasionally, the vessel on which an aneurysm arises must be sacrificed for definitive treatment. When the balloon can be passed directly into an aneurysm, thus preserving the parent artery from which it arises, the term *reconstruction* is applied. This operation is not always feasible, however, and depends upon the relationship of the parent artery to the aneurysm, the size of the aneurysm, its orifice, and its location in the arterial tree. In some cases, the parent artery upon which the aneurysm arises along with the aneurysm may be occluded. This is referred to as a *deconstructive operation* and is sometimes acceptable, even when minor deficits are anticipated, when overall risks are weighed against a possible SAH. Deconstructive operations are feasible when the vessel upon which the aneurysm arises can be sacrificed without profound neurological impairment. The determination of collateral patterns and the safety of a deconstructive operation can only be made by temporary balloon occlusion of the artery in question, combined with careful monitoring and neurological testing.

Before deconstructive operations are carried out, complete angiographic visualization of the cerebral circulation (including both intracranial VAs) is requisite. If the injection of one VA does not fill the opposite VA intracranially, the other VA must be injected. Both carotid arteries, including their cervical portions, must also be visualized.

Angiography of the opposite arterial tree must be performed during the balloon occlusion tests. In the case of carotid artery occlusion by balloon, for instance, the contralateral carotid artery should be injected to assess cross-filling in the transcerebral circulation during the time of balloon inflation. The TCD is also useful for determining safety of occlusion.

If the balloon cannot be placed opposite the orifice of the aneurysm, thereby excluding the orifice from circulation, then proximal occlusion of the parent artery must suffice. The same precautions prevail before proximal occlusion as in other deconstructive operations. Temporary occlusion must be performed with testing before balloon detachment. The balloon should not be placed opposite perforating or short arteries. These vessels often lack collaterals, and infarction often follows their obstruction. These perforating or short arteries include Heubner's artery, the PICA, the lenticulostriate artery, the anterior choroidal artery, and the penetrating arteries from the basilar and P_1 segments. Even temporary occlusion may occasionally produce small infarcts. Deconstructive operations are applicable under certain circumstances, such as when there is a fusiform aneurysm or when the aneurysm involves the cavernous portion or surgically inaccessible arteries. These lesions are prone to form intravascular thrombi and embolize. Therefore, in certain instances, proximal balloon placement is preferable to placing balloons directly into the thrombus-filled sac. Additionally, these lesions may become symptomatic because of compression, embolization, or hemorrhage.

Deconstructive operations in which major vessels must be sacrificed may not be tolerated because of distal ischemia. In this case, the operation must be abandoned in favor of some blood flow augmenting procedures, such as extracranial–intracranial bypass, as a preliminary measure. After bypass, angiography must be performed again, and balloon test occlusions must be carried out.

Angioplasty for Vasospasm Treatment

The direct port or straight port through which the balloon will be passed is closed by a twist of cotton or diaphragm. The lateral port connects with tubing for irrigating and for the administration of contrast agents. Angiography is carried out to verify the position of the needle and the status of the intracranial vessels, allowing confirmation of vasospasm and the status of the aneurysm, and assuring correct positioning.

The angioplastic balloon must be modified for entering the cerebral circulation. The balloon catheter is then fed through an adaptor that prevents backbleeding around it. The catheter is advanced in the needle and moved into the artery by flushing. The blunt 45° needle has been placed against the ICA back wall to prevent backbleeding. The needle must be turned 180° to place the needle freely in the open channel of the ICA, away from the back wall. As the catheter and balloon are advanced, saline may be injected into the side port to assist in carriage into the ICA. The catheter is gently fed into the vessel until it reaches the intracranial circulation. The balloon usually stops spontaneously as it reaches the vasospastic portion of the MCA or carotid artery. At this point, the proximal part of the balloon is gradually inflated. As this takes place, the proximal inflated balloon comes in contact with the wall of the artery, securing it. Subsequently as the distal portions of the balloon are inflated, it assumes a sausage shape and expands into the constricted portion of the vessel. This inflation only requires a few seconds to carry out, and then the balloon is quickly deflated. The balloon and catheter are then advanced along the vessel, dilating 1.0 to 1.5 cm of the vessel on each successive turn. The limits of angioplasty for the MCA are usually reached at the bifurcation. The balloon and catheter may be advanced into the M_2 branches, but these arteries, being smaller, may rupture when the balloon is fully inflated. Usually, vasospasm terminates at the distal end of the M_1 branch. This procedure, however, allows augmentation of blood flow to the important short branches that enter the basal nuclei, usually proximal to the M_2 branches.

The same balloon catheter may be used to perform angioplasty on the supraclinoid portion of the ICA and the M_1 branches. Anatomical peculiarities of the A_1 and the anterior cerebral artery (ACA) make it somewhat more difficult. The A_1 segment may originate from the ICA at an acute, an obtuse, or a straight angle. The maneuvers employing two balloon catheters helped introduce the dilating balloon into the A_1 portion. Two balloon catheters must be used to perform this maneuver. One is advanced into the M_1 segment and inflated briefly while the other is pushed into the A_1 from the ICA. Inflation of the M_1 balloon deflects flow and the balloon into the A_1 branch. Then the M_1 balloon is deflated and removed.

Angioplasty in the vertebrobasilar system is best performed with a catheter of an internal diameter of 2.0 to 2.5 mm. An axillary artery puncture allows quick entry, but longer catheters must be employed for a femoral route. The short length through the axillary approach allows easy manipulation of the catheters once they enter the intracranial vasculature with less dead space. The patient should be monitored neurologically throughout the angioplasty, and the TCD is also helpful. The TCD measures CBF and assures that compromise by catheter or balloon has not occurred. Following angioplasty, the catheter is removed from the vessel and the needle removed under direct imaging. Bleeding from the vessel is controlled by 10 to 15 min of compression.

The following general observations apply to balloon angioplasty for vasospasm.

1. Local anesthesia is preferred because it allows constant neurological evaluation during the procedure.
2. Generally, angioplasty should be performed on the most severely affected hemisphere first. This is based on both radiographic and clinical criteria.
3. A single dilatation provides permanent relief from vasoconstriction. Dilatation for more than a few seconds causes deterioration due to worsening ischemia.
4. Control of intracranial pressure (ICP) is essential to successful angioplasty.
5. The coagulation system must be normal.
6. Heparinization with 3000 to 5000 units is required during manipulation of the balloon and catheter.

Occlusion Tests

Preoperative evaluation gives information regarding how aggressive the surgical procedure can be with regard to carotid artery sacrifice, and it also identifies patients who are potential candidates for revascularization procedures, such as superficial temporal artery anastomosis to the middle cerebral artery or a direct saphenous vein bypass of the cavernous ICA.

1. *The clinical balloon occlusion test.* The balloon is passed into the artery from which the aneurysm arises. Inflation excludes both the parent artery and the aneurysm from cerebral flow. For approximately 30 min thereafter, vital signs, the electroencephalogram, and appropriate neurologic signs are monitored. If an aneurysm of the vertebrobasilar circulation is being excluded, visual fields and eye findings are of interest. If anterior circulation vessels are to be occluded, motor, speech, and consciousness are all important. If vital signs remain normal, the neurological status does not change, the EEG is not altered in amplitude or frequency, then it may be concluded that this procedure carries low risk. After 30 min, if the patient is stable and the EEG is unchanged, then the balloon may be detached from the catheter.
2. *Temporary occlusion with distal back pressure.* In this test, a special balloon is prepared in which a catheter passes through the balloon and projects into the lumen distal to it.[13] Another smaller catheter attaches to the balloon for inflation and deflation. Thus, a double-lumen catheter is passed (Fig. 7.9). The balloon is slowly inflated with contrast material in the parent artery as an angiogram is being carried out. After the vessel is occluded, the syringe is left attached and the balloon is maintained at a constant volume and pressure. The catheter passing through the balloon into the distal lumen is connected to a transducer, and intraarterial pressure is measured before and after balloon occlusion. If back pressure does not fall more than 30% below the baseline, balloon occlusion should be tolerated. A decrease of 30% to 50% in back pressure defines the intermediate zone in which there is greater risk for ischemic deficits. If pressure falls more than 50%, ischemic complications are virtually assured.
3. *Balloon occlusion with TCD testing.* Patients have been studied using the Matas compression test and TCD in our center. They were placed in either the high- or the low-risk group based on the following: Patients whose MCA velocity was reduced by less than 50% during external compression of the carotid artery and whose ACA flow reversed were placed in the low risk group; none developed neurologic deficits after permanent occlusion. High risk patients were those who had a reduction greater than 50% in the MCA velocity or whose ACA flow failed to reverse on compression. Fifteen percent of those in our small series undergoing permanent occlusion developed ischemic deficits.

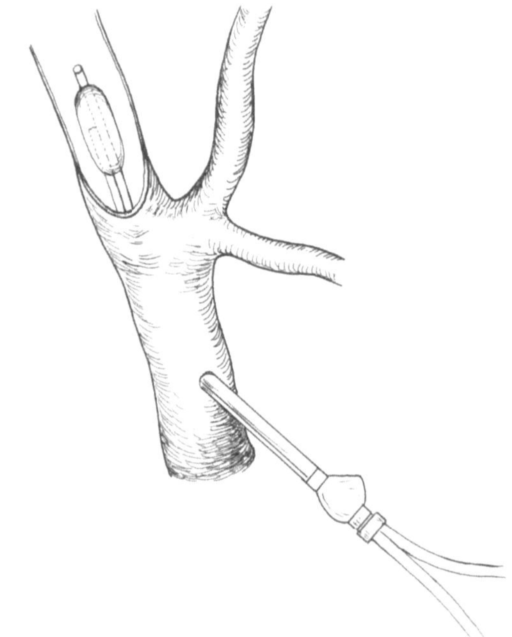

A

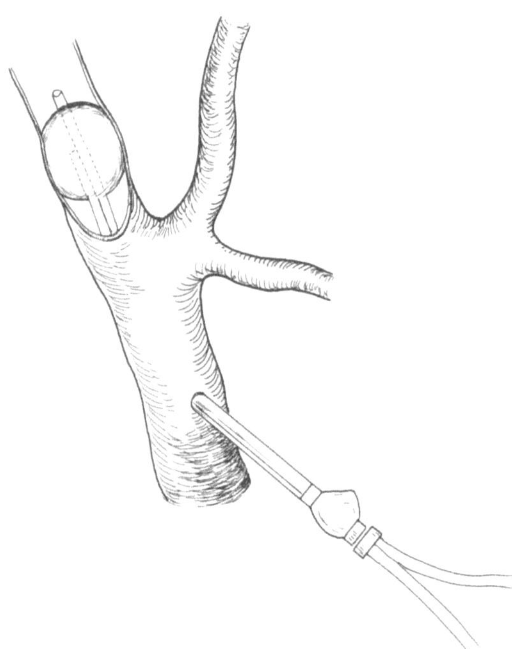

B

FIGURE 7.9. (A, B) The double lumen catheter technique for measuring distal pressure.

Some patients also underwent balloon test occlusion. In general, the results were complementary. However, 50% of the patients who underwent test occlusion had a complication. This included one dissection, pain, and several vasovagal responses.

The Matas test was generally well tolerated by patients (Fig. 7.10). Approximately 5% complained of pain at the

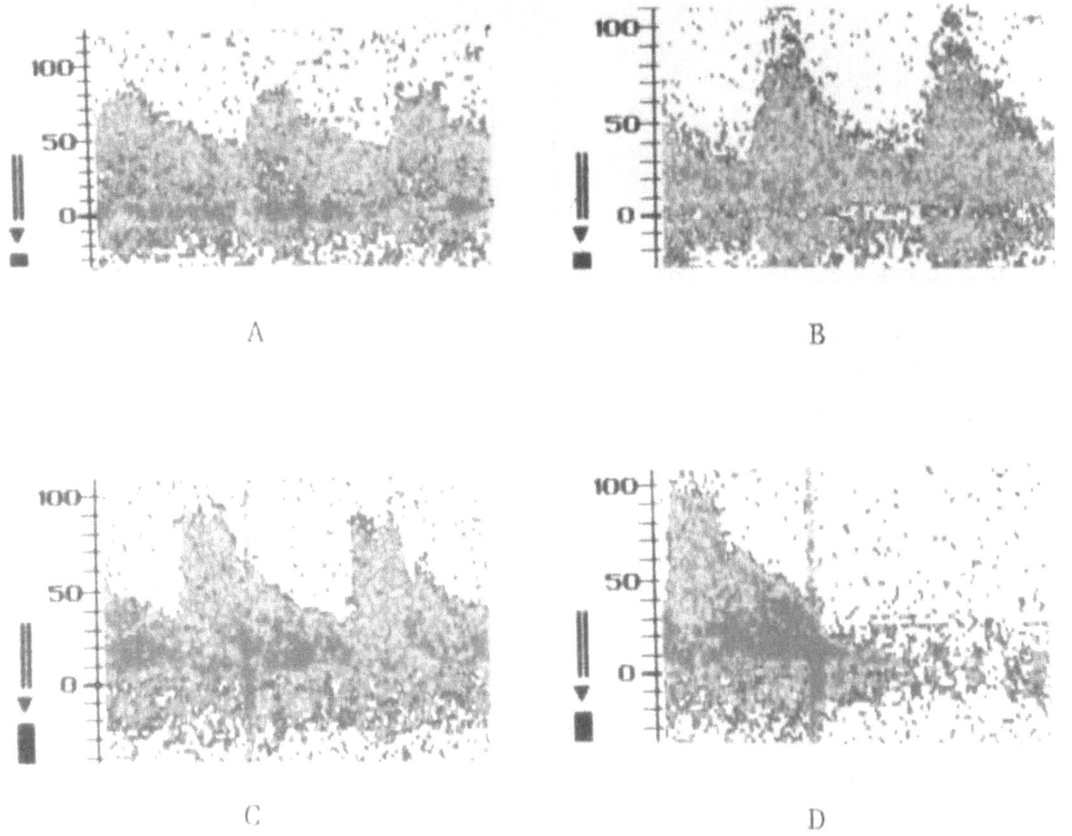

FIGURE 7.10. The Matas TCD test. (A) MCA velocity prior to carotid artery occlusion. (B) Velocity is unchanged during common carotid artery compression. (C) Flow in the aneurysm prior to compression. (D) Aneurysmal flow with compression. The aneurysm promptly thrombosed following carotid artery occlusion and the patient suffered no ischemic deficits.

site, but all were able to complete the procedure. No patient experienced any neurologic symptoms during the procedure or any systemic hemodynamic events.

The TCD may be useful as a safe noninvasive method to evaluate patients who may need carotid artery occlusion for the treatment of aneurysms with detachable balloons. It offers safe, low cost, and easily repeatable risk assessment that will allow identification of the patient most apt to develop ischemic deficits. Extracranial–intracranial (EC-IC) bypass or carotid-to-carotid shunt must be employed in these cases to preserve neurological function when the parent artery must be sacrificed to achieve complete extirpation of the lesion. Other testing methods, such as intracarotid balloons and ^{133}Xe, may also be used.

Special Difficulties of Balloon Occlusion of Aneurysms

Unusual anatomy and patterns of blood flow create special challenges for the endovascular surgeon. Inadequate equipment for imaging and for performing balloon occlusion testing leads to poor results. Inadequate training or poor technical skills can also lead to complications.

The endovascular treatment of a patient with recent SAH carries special risks and complications not usually associated with the unruptured aneurysm. The surgeon must be aware of these special problems when planning early treatment. In addition to hemorrhagic complications, the patient's general cerebrovascular reserve may be compromised due to ischemia or local coagulopathic defects. The arterial wall after acute SAH is covered with a platelet fibrin deposit, and there is a widespread degeneration in the endothelial layer. These events promote a coagulopathic reaction that may lead to thrombus formation in the vessel to be treated or around the balloon and distally. Angioplasty, like surgery, can precipitate a cascade of events leading to severe neurological deficit if the surgeon does not exercise due care. If endovascular surgery is to be undertaken in the acute phase, for instance, 1 week following a major SAH, the patient must be in good neurological condition, compensated, in grade I or grade II of the Hunt and Hess scale. There should be no evidence of cerebral vasospasm based on clinical examination, the TCD, CBF, or the angiogram done immediately before balloon therapy. The exception, of course, is the angioplastic treatment for vasospasm in which the aneurysm will be managed concurrently.

Aneurysms develop peculiar shapes (L-shaped configurations or multiple lobulations), and these create special problems for the endovascular surgeon. Peculiarly shaped balloons may be designed to facilitate closure of the orifice of the unusually shaped aneurysm. The size of the balloon must be configured carefully in order to occlude the neck and rest on the dome of the aneurysm distally. When inflated, it thus extends across the longest length of the aneurysm with the proximal end projecting almost to the parent artery orifice. The remainder of the aneurysm need not be filled with a balloon. If the orifice is sufficiently blocked or occluded, thrombus will form in the aneurysm and it will gradually shrink as balloon volume decreases.

The next major challenge that the endovascular surgeon faces relates to the size of the blood vessel and the orifice of the aneurysm to be treated. When the parent artery presents a stenotic channel, flow may be accelerated. Guidance of the catheter in the poststenotic channel may be impossible. Sometimes, stenosis is so great that the balloon catheter itself will not pass. Tortuous and serpentine arteries also sometimes present difficulties to the endovascular surgeon because catheters and balloons tend to hang up at sharp angles. If the communicating arteries are inadequate, the balloon catheter may not pass through these small channels in which blood flow is reduced. Aberrations in the circle of Willis must also be considered. If the A_1 is hypoplastic or absent, the endovascular surgeon may be unable to modify blood flow adequately by carotid compression. These obstacles may be overcome by modification of technique.

Zubkov designed a special balloon for aneurysms with tight orifices (Fig. 7.11). This balloon is inflated distal to the aneurysm orifice in such a way as to deflect the distal tip at right angles to the introduction catheter. Thus, the balloon and catheter deflects in a pattern that is perpendicular to the wall of the artery (Fig. 7.11B). The catheter is then slowly withdrawn until the distal tip of the balloon enters the neck of the aneurysm (Fig. 7.11C). This is accomplished by placing a weak segment at the inferior position. This weak segment inflates first, deflecting the distal tip perpendicularly. As a third technique, the primary balloon may be inflated minimally with contrast material just opposite the neck. The helper balloon is then advanced into a contiguous position along the arterial wall where inflation drives the primary balloon into the neck of the aneurysm where it is inflated temporarily. The helper balloon may then be deflated slightly and pulled back.

Generally, the size of the deflated balloon should be proportionate to the size that it will be in its final form. A large aneurysm with a small neck thus may not be occluded adequately with a small noninflated balloon that will pass through the orifice. The surgeon must, therefore, weigh the relative chance of being able to produce adequate occlusion of this aneurysm with a thin balloon in relation to the risk of an open and direct operation for clipping of the aneurysm neck. These alternatives must be discussed by the neurosurgeon and the patient.

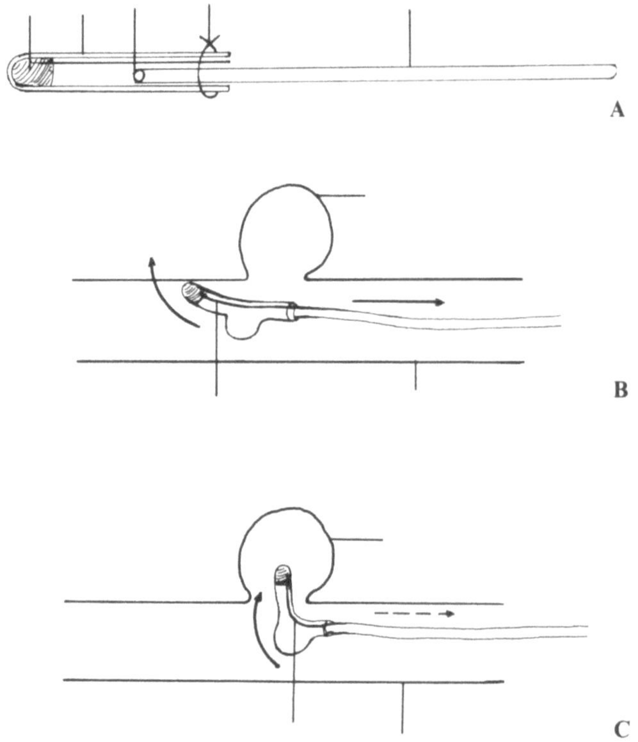

FIGURE 7.11. (A–C) Special balloon for right-angle introduction from the primary artery. The balloon is weakened on one side, which causes it to dilate at this site first, deflecting the tip into the aneurysm.

This situation occurs commonly in arteriosclerotic aneurysms or giant aneurysms arising from large arteries, such as the ICA or the basilar artery (BA) near the apex, the VA near the craniovertebral junction, or along the main trunk of the MCA. Usually, the stenosis occurs within a few millimeters of the orifice of the aneurysm to be occluded. If the stenosis is severe, alternate routes of treatment may be required. Moderate stenosis may be handled using endovascular methods. On the distal side of the stenosis, some turbulent flow is almost always encountered that may interfere with passage and proper direction of the balloon. When the stenosis is on the proximal MCA or carotid artery, it may be dilated using a hard balloon. The hard balloon has a fixed volume, is less flexible, and passes with much greater ease through stenotic areas. It may be manipulated irrespective of the blood flow pattern but requires a guidewire in order to be advanced through the stenotic area. If the plaque is extremely hard, it may not respond to balloon dilatation. In this case, stereotaxic methods may be employed to introduce a balloon into the fundus of an aneurysm.[14]

Technique

Any stereotaxic frame may be used. However, the holder must be adapted to contain a long needle with an internal diameter of 1.5 mm. The introduction of the needle is carried out using angiographic control. The needle is advanced, using the stereotaxic coordinates, toward the dome of the aneurysm. By compressing the aneurysm as seen on the angiogram, the surgeon recognizes when the dome has been encountered. The aneurysm wall is deformed by the blunt needle, and a rounded trocar point is used to puncture the aneurysm. More contrast is injected to insure that the needle is properly placed within the aneurysm cavity. Then the trocar is withdrawn and a Teflon catheter with detachable balloon is introduced into the aneurysm cavity. Under angiographic fluoroscopic control, the balloon is inflated until there is no angiographic filling of the aneurysm as the balloon occludes the neck. When the aneurysm no longer fills, the balloon is detached by the gentle traction on the Teflon catheter, using the needle for counter pressure. Two cases were handled without incident using stereotaxic methods at the Polenov Institute (Fig. 7.12).

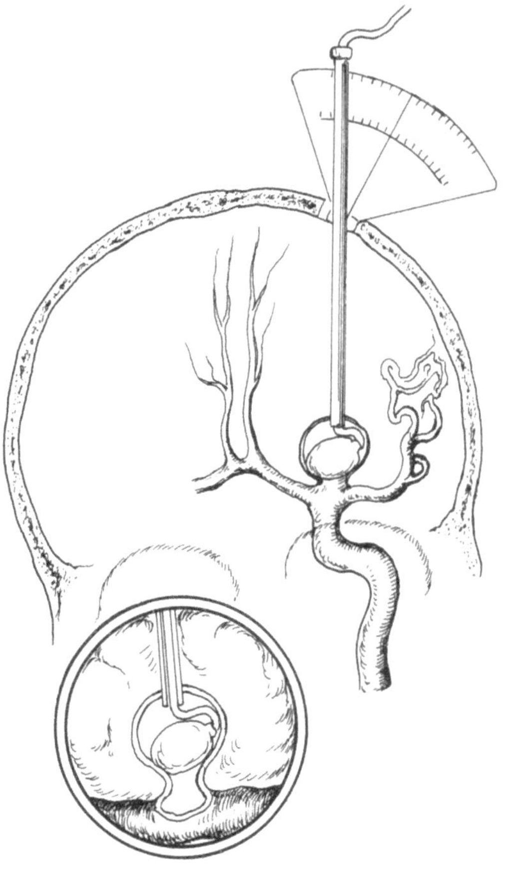

FIGURE 7.12. Stereotaxic introduction of a catheter and balloon into an intracranial aneurysm through a specially designed catheter.

Serpentine Arteries

Tortuous arteries cause difficulty in passing the balloon catheter. The balloon hangs up at sharp curves in the artery. Resistance develops when the wall of the vessel and the catheter come into contact and friction prevents their further passage. Lengthening the taper on the end of the catheter may facilitate passage of the balloon through a tortuous artery. Most catheters have only the terminal 5 cm or so tapered. The taper may be extended 8 to 10 cm from the distal tip carrying the balloon, thus adding flexibility. Minimal inflation and deflation of the balloon during passage assists in migration of the balloon to the target site. As the balloon tip is inflated, blood flow assists in carrying the catheter and balloon. In some circumstances, the endovascular surgeon must be prepared to accept defeat because of tortuosity.

In the patient with reduced cardiac output, flow may be impaired so that catheter passage becomes impossible. This also occurs in the patient with decreased CBF in such conditions as vasospasm or major vessel occlusion, hypotension, or decreased peripheral blood volume. Systemic arterial pressure (SAP) should be maintained near-normal when an intact aneurysm is present. In the patient with good communicating arteries, blood flow may be augmented unilaterally by compression of the opposite carotid artery. This facilitates passage of a balloon through sites where resistance is encountered due to tortuosity or stenosis.

Like surgery elsewhere, knowledge of the angiographic anatomy, of the physiology of the cerebral circulation, and of the particular vessel in question is also required. Familiarity with acceptable occlusion times for the various vessels is also needed. Balloon occlusion of large arterial trunks along the base might be well accepted in a patient who has good collateral and cross-filling. More distally in the arterial tree, if the balloon occludes the orifice of a major short artery such as Heubner's artery, the lenticulostriate artery, or Percheron's artery, infarction may result in only a few minutes. Considerable skills and training are required to prepare a small balloon, attach it to a catheter, and pass it into the intracranial circulation just as they are for microdissecting an aneurysm away from the MCA and applying a clip. Motor skills are developed only through experience.

If the procedure seems to be going poorly on any given day, it may be better to request the assistance of another skilled endovascular surgeon to puncture or pass a balloon into a difficult area. If a proper start is not achieved by correct needle placement, the operation may fail because of hematoma and abandonment may be necessary.

Although there are common rules for endovascular operations, much depends upon the technique and methods familiar to thc individual surgeon. If he has been trained with a latex balloon system, changing to a silicone system requires further training. Silicone, having a smooth surface, is less thrombogenic when placed in an aneurysm. The endovascular surgeon should be familiar with all balloon systems, however, in order to modify his operations to suit the patient's disease. Occasionally, one catheter or balloon system will clearly have advantages over another.

Prevention of Endovascular Complications

In patients harboring recently ruptured cerebral aneurysms, in contrast to those with AVMs and fistulas, reduced blood flow may be expected. Recognizing the threat of ischemia prepares the surgeon for managing ischemic complications associated with passage of a balloon through vessels that are already compromised. Patients who have the poorest collateral circulation and the poorest reserve are the ones most likely to develop complications. Translated to the patient with vasospasm and SAH, the patient who is becoming lethargic or febrile in the early stages of vasospasm would be at greatest risk for balloon occlusion of the aneurysm.

Clinical testing is an essential feature of balloon occlusion of aneurysms. Test occlusion must be carried out to assess the patient's tolerance for manipulation. During test occlusion, the balloon is advanced into the intracranial ICA and inflated with contrast material. If the patient tolerates 3 to 5 min of occlusion, planned treatment proceeds. If the patient does not tolerate brief balloon occlusion, then modifications in technique must be made. Volume augmentation, hypertension, or balloon angioplasty of the stenotic vessels are needed prior to balloon occlusion of the aneurysm. Intolerance or even brief periods of ischemia also requires modifying the use of the helper balloon technique because the balloon partially occludes the parent artery.

The endovascular surgeon must have some intuition concerning the wall of the cerebral vessel to be treated and the unique rheology of the circulating blood. Blood clotting may be a factor. In addition to heparinization and blood volume expansion, the use of dextran is helpful in preventing catheter complications. Five hundred milliliters of dextran 40 may be administered initially.

Patients who harbor intracranial aneurysms often have vascular disease proximally in the arterial tree. The endovascular surgeon must be familiar with the status of the vessels preoperatively so as not to dislodge plaque material by the introduction of the catheter and balloons. Collateral blood supply and the peculiarities of the circle of Willis should be known. If a balloon should project from the aneurysm and block the parent artery to a minor degree, the surgeon should know that collateralization from the opposite hemisphere or from nearby vessels would be sufficient to maintain the distal tissue. Monitoring blood flow and functional physiology is therefore essential in the endovascular operating area and may be accomplished by the EEG, volume or velocity flow measurements, all supplemented by the clinical examination. In the event of ischemic events, as measured by the above methods not clearing in minutes, the operation should be terminated immediately. If the patient develops a deficit with temporary balloon occlusion of a parent artery, the operation should be terminated and started again on another day when the patient is hemodynamically stable. Sometimes, other treatment methods must be chosen.

Complications of Vasodilatation

There are three primary complications associated with vasodilatation: ischemic complications, hemorrhagic complications, and general complications of the endovascular approach.

Ischemic complications occur due to excessive occlusion times during the procedure. Stenosis also occurs because the diameter of the noninflated balloon is equivalent to the vessel's diameter. In this situation, the balloon adds to ischemia of the vasospasm even before dilatation. Occasionally, the procedure is carried out in patients whose blood flow has been critically reduced even before dilatation. Only short periods of vasodilatation will be tolerated.

The most feared complication of angioplasty is separation of the balloon from the catheter and distal migration into the intracranial arterial tree. This occurs most often when a detachable balloon has been used for occlusion of an aneurysm. To prevent ischemic complications, the balloon and catheter should be as small as possible, firmly attached to the catheter, and the dilatations carried out rapidly. The balloon should then be rapidly deflated to augment flow. Acute local vasospasm may be precipitated by manipulation of the artery. The injection of a small amount of papaverine may relieve this kind of vasospasm. The segment of vasospastic artery to be dilated should be a short one. The segment to be dilated should include, if possible, the primary collateral channels and penetrating branches. If further dilatation is needed, a second session should be scheduled.

Should the balloon separate and migrate into the arterial tree, prompt craniotomy is required. In this case the artery containing the balloon must be exposed surgically, opened, and the embolus extracted. The artery is then closed with a few interrupted 10-0 nylon sutures.

Hemorrhagic complications occur due to rupture of the primary vessel or the aneurysm. Fortunately, in over 100 patients, this complication has occurred in only one. The complication, however, probably arises when dilatation exceeds normal diameter of the artery. In no case should the balloon diameter exceed 115% of the normal vessel diameter. Also, if there is any clear evidence of arteriosclerotic vessels, these should be spared since the hard artery tends to fracture more easily. Older patients with aneurysms have arteriosclerotic plaques that may be confused with vasospasm. Aneurysms rupture coincidental to angioplasty, due to loss of coagulation, to traction or maneuvering during the angioplasty near the aneurysm neck, or to a misplaced balloon in the neck of an aneurysm, causing increased arterial pressure or dynamic pressures within the aneurysm. During test occlusion, only a short segment of the vessel should be closed, the balloon size should be correct, and test occlusion should not be carried out near the aneurysm. The surgeon should always be prepared for an open prompt craniotomy and should try to preserve flow in the affected arterial branches should they become obstructed with a catheter, balloon, or by thrombus.

Certain complications are common to all endovascular procedures. These arise due to the difficulties during puncture. Subintimal threading of the catheter or needle may give rise to dissection syndromes and ischemic complications resulting from these. Neck hematomas may develop, requiring termination of the procedure. Occasionally, a punctured artery develops thrombus and becomes a surgical emergency. Neurological deficits may appear even during primary vessel puncture.

Conclusion

Endovascular operations, much like direct operations, are invasive and carry with them inherent risks. Because the endovascular procedure is done remotely from the end of a fine catheter, control and manipulation are also issues. Unusual complications arise because of these variables, and the endovascular surgeon should always have these in mind. The loss of a balloon into the distal arterial tree or rupture of a parent artery aneurysm may lead to serious morbidity or mortality. Preparation and prompt action by craniotomy may lessen the ultimate risk of these serious complications.

References

1. Serbinenko FA. Catheterization and occlusion of magistral brain vessels. In: *Abstract Book of the First Congress of Neurosurgeons of USSR*. Moscow, Russia: 1971;1:121–123.
2. Serbinenko FA, Filatov YM. Method of catheterization of anterior cerebral artery. In *Proceedings of the Third Congress of Neurosurgeons*. Baltic Republic, Riga; 1972:160–762.
3. Zubkov YN. Catheterization of brain vessels [in Russian]. In: *Neurosurgery*: Annals of the Polenov Neurosurgical Institute (Leningrad, Russia). 1973;5:218–227.
4. Gianturco C, Anderson JH, Wallace S. Mechanical devices for arterial occlusion. *Am J Roentgenol*. 1975;129:428–435.
5. Anderson JH, Wallace S, Gianturco C, Gerson LP. "Mini" Gianturco stainless steel coils for transcatheter vascular occlusion. *Radiology*. 1979;132:301–303.
6. Yang PJ, Halbach VV, Higashida RT, Hieshima GB. Platinum wire: a new transvascular embolic agent. *AJNR* 1988;9:547–550.
7. Yang PJ, Halbach VV, Higashida RT, Hieshima GB, Seigel RS. Platinum wire: a new transvascular embolic agent. *AJNR*. 1988;9:1030.
8. Hilal SK, Khandji A, Solomon RW, Chi L. Obliteration of intracranial aneurysms with preshaped thrombogenic coils. Presented at the 1989 Annual Meeting of the Radiological Society of North America; November 26–December 1, Chicago, Illinois; 1989.
9. Guglielmi G, Vinuela F, Dion J, Duckwiler G. Electrothrombosis of saccular aneurysms via endovascular approach. Part 2: preliminary clinical experience. *J Neurosurg*. 1991;75:8–14.
10. Shcheglov VI. Endovascular interventions in neurosurgical pathology [in Russian]. In: *Sjezd Neirokhirurgov USSR*. Moscow, Russia: 1979;558–559.
11. Romodanov AP, Shcheglov VI. Intravascular occlusion of saccular aneurysms of the cerebral arteries by means of a detachable balloon catheter. Kiev Research Institute of Neurosurgery, Kiev (USSR). *Adv Tech Stand*. 1982;9:25–49.
12. Purinja BA, Kasjanov VA. *Biomechanics of Large Balloon Vessels in Humans* [in Russian]. Riga, Russia: Zinatne, 1980:260.
13. Asaturyan GA, Dubikajtis YV, Zubkov YN, Panuntsev VS, Rikunov MA, Semenjutin VB. Modern possibilities of estimate of functional significance of brain vessels in neurosurgical clinic [in Russian]. In: *Actual Problems of Neurology and Neurosurgery*. 1981;3–7.
14. Khilko VA, Zubkov YN. Intravascular surgery of intracranial aneurysms. In: Khilko VA, Zubkov YN, eds. *Endovascular Neurosurgery*. Leningrad, Russia: Medicina; 1982:150–153.

8
Cavernous Sinus Aneurysms

Aneurysms of the cavernous portion of the internal carotid artery (ICA) make up 5% of all intracranial aneurysms. Some aneurysms, also referred to as paraclinoid and subclinoid variants, are located intradurally but are not totally confined to the cavernous sinus. Aneurysms that are confined to the cavernous sinus and rupture produce carotid cavernous sinus fistulae. If the aneurysm projects above the cavernous sinus into the subarachnoid space, subarachnoid hemorrhage (SAH) or even subdural hematomas may occur, depending on the location of the bleeding point (Fig. 8.1).

Microvascular Anatomy

In 1965, Parkinson[1] reported the first attempt of a direct surgical approach to lesions involving the cavernous sinus, reemphasizing the important anatomical landmarks of the region. The cavernous sinuses are formed by dural layers located within the lateral side of the sella turcica, surrounding the pituitary gland, and by the body of the sphenoid bone. Along the anterior border, the cavernous sinus is attached to the anterior clinoid process and extends to the subclinoid space and the superior orbital fissure. It attaches posteriorly to the posterior clinoid process and extends to the apex of the petrous bone.

The third segment of the ICA, sympathetic fibers, and abducent nerve course within the cavernous sinus, but the oculomotor nerve, trochlear nerve, and the ophthalmic and maxillary divisions of the trigeminal nerve pass within its lateral wall.

The Roof of the Cavernous Sinus

The anterior clinoid process is located in the anterior part of the roof of the cavernous sinus. Removing the anterior clinoid process creates a dural space that is called the "clinoidal space" or "carotid cave" (Figs. 8.2 and 8.3).

The dura mater covering the inferomedial surface of this space is thinner than its lateral wall, and the anterior vertical segment of the intracavernous ICA may be seen easily through it. The clinoidal space may be used to approach lesions of the anterior and superior part of the cavernous sinus. This space is separated from the optic canal by the posterior part of the "optic-strut," which is the inferior root of the lesser sphenoidal wing. Both sides of the optic strut are covered by dura mater.

The ICA leaves the roof of the cavernous sinus in an oblique direction, surrounded in the dural exit area by dural bands that attach to the ICA, making a ring around it. This "pericarotid dural ring" is thin in the anteromedial part where it may be easily separated from the ICA. The medial part of the dural ring is continuous with the dura of the diaphragma sellae. The pericarotid dural ring is thicker dorsolaterally to the ICA and connects firmly to the caroticoclinoid ligament. The caroticoclinoid ligament is a thick fibrous band that forms the posterolateral part of the pericarotid dural ring and connects the anterior and middle clinoid processes.[2]

The middle clinoid process, when it exists, is located in the area lateral to the tuberculum sella and medial to the carotid sulcus. Another dural ligament in the roof of the cavernous sinus, called the caroticooculomotor membrane, extends from the lateral part of the ICA to the posterior clinoid process.[3] The anterior part of this ligament separates the clinoidal space from the cavernous sinus and attaches to the interclinoid ligament and folds superiorly.

The oculomotor nerve penetrates the roof of the cavernous sinus in the anterolateral part of the oculomotor trigone, lateral to the ICA exit site and close to the lateral wall in the area between the anterior and posterior clinoid processes. The oculomotor trigone, situated in the most posterior part of the roof of the cavernous sinus, is formed by three dural folds or ligaments:

1. The anterior petroclinoid fold is the anterior extension of the free margin of the tentorium, extending

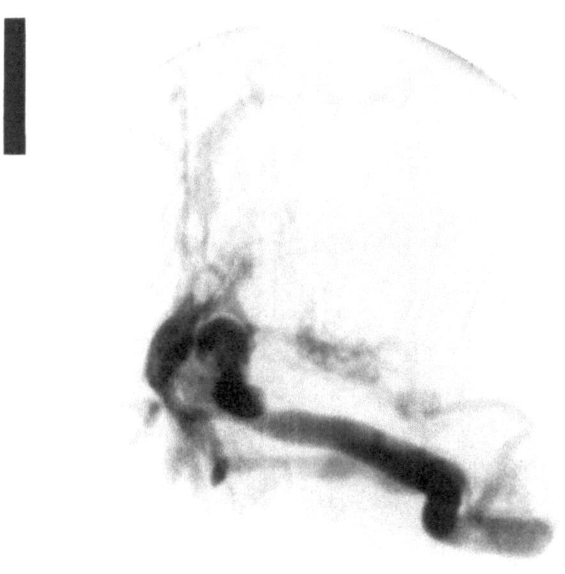

A

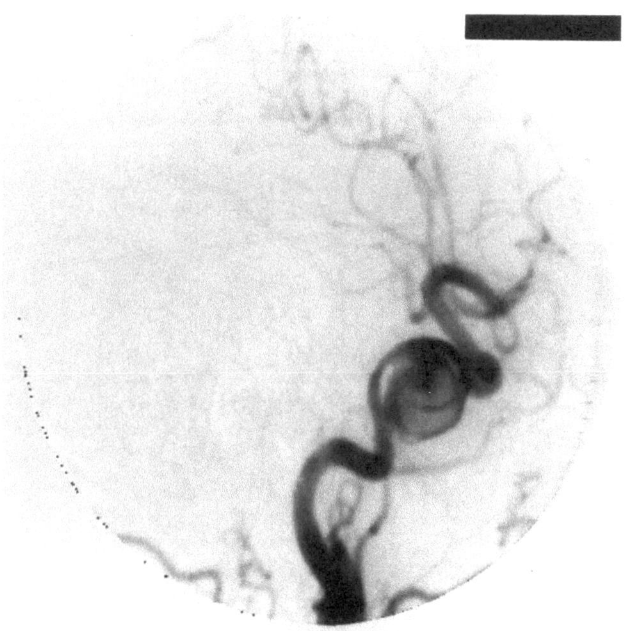

B

FIGURE 8.1. (A) Carotid cavernous fistula with filling of the ophthalmic veins. (B) After balloon occlusion. There is a large aneurysm occupying the cavernous sinus, the source of the spontaneous CC fistula in this case.

from the apex of the petrous bone to the anterior clinoid process.

2. The posterior petroclinoid fold extends from the petrous apex to the posterior clinoid process.
3. The interclinoid fold connects the anterior and posterior clinoid processes.

The anteromedial triangle of Dolenc forms the anterior part of the lateral wall of the cavernous sinus.[4,5] This triangle is defined by three points: the anterolateral part of the pericarotid dural ring, the entry site of the oculomotor nerve in the roof of the cavernous sinus, and the point at which the oculomotor nerve passes over the anterior bend of the intracavernous ICA and enters the superior orbital fissure. Opening this triangle exposes the anterior bend of the intracavernous ICA. The "medial triangle" or Hakuba's triangle, is formed by the anterior rim of the carotid dural ring, the entry site of the oculomotor nerve to the roof of the cavernous sinus, and the anterolateral margin of the posterior clinoid process.[6] This triangle provides more exposure to the horizontal segment of the intracavernous ICA.

Removal of the anterior clinoid process is the first step in approaching structures located in the superior and anterior part of the cavernous sinus.

Lateral Wall of the Cavernous Sinus

The lateral wall of the cavernous sinus consists of two layers of dura mater that separate easily. The inner layer is composed of thin loose connective tissue. The oculomotor and trochlear nerves, and the first and second divisions of the trigeminal nerve course within the two layers of the lateral wall.

In 1965, Parkinson described an area within the lateral wall for approaching the intracavernous ICA.[1] The boundaries of Parkinson's triangle are the lower border of the trochlear nerve superiorly, the upper border of the trigeminal nerve inferiorly, and the dorsum sella and clivus making up the posterior border.

The length of the superior border ranges from 11.0 to 21.0 mm (average 16.4 mm), the inferior margin from 10.0 to 22.0 mm (average 16.5 mm) and the posterior margin from 2.8 to 8.0 mm (average 4.5 mm).[3]

The Medial Wall of the Cavernous Sinus

The superior part of the medial wall of the cavernous sinus participates in the creation of the lateral wall of the sella turcica. The lower or inferior part of the medial wall lies on the lateral surface of the body of the sphenoid bone; thus, the sphenoid sinus lies against the medial wall of the cavernous sinus. Entering the medial wall of the cavernous sinus will usually expose the sphenoid sinus. The carotid sulcus is a bony groove on the lateral surface of the body of sphenoid bone upon which the intracavernous ICA rests. The intracavernous ICA and the second division of the trigeminal nerve may create a bony prominence and bulging into the sphenoid sinus above the lateral wall, especially when the sphenoid sinus is well pneumatized.[7]

The trigeminal ganglion and the first and third divisions of the trigeminal nerve are separated from the

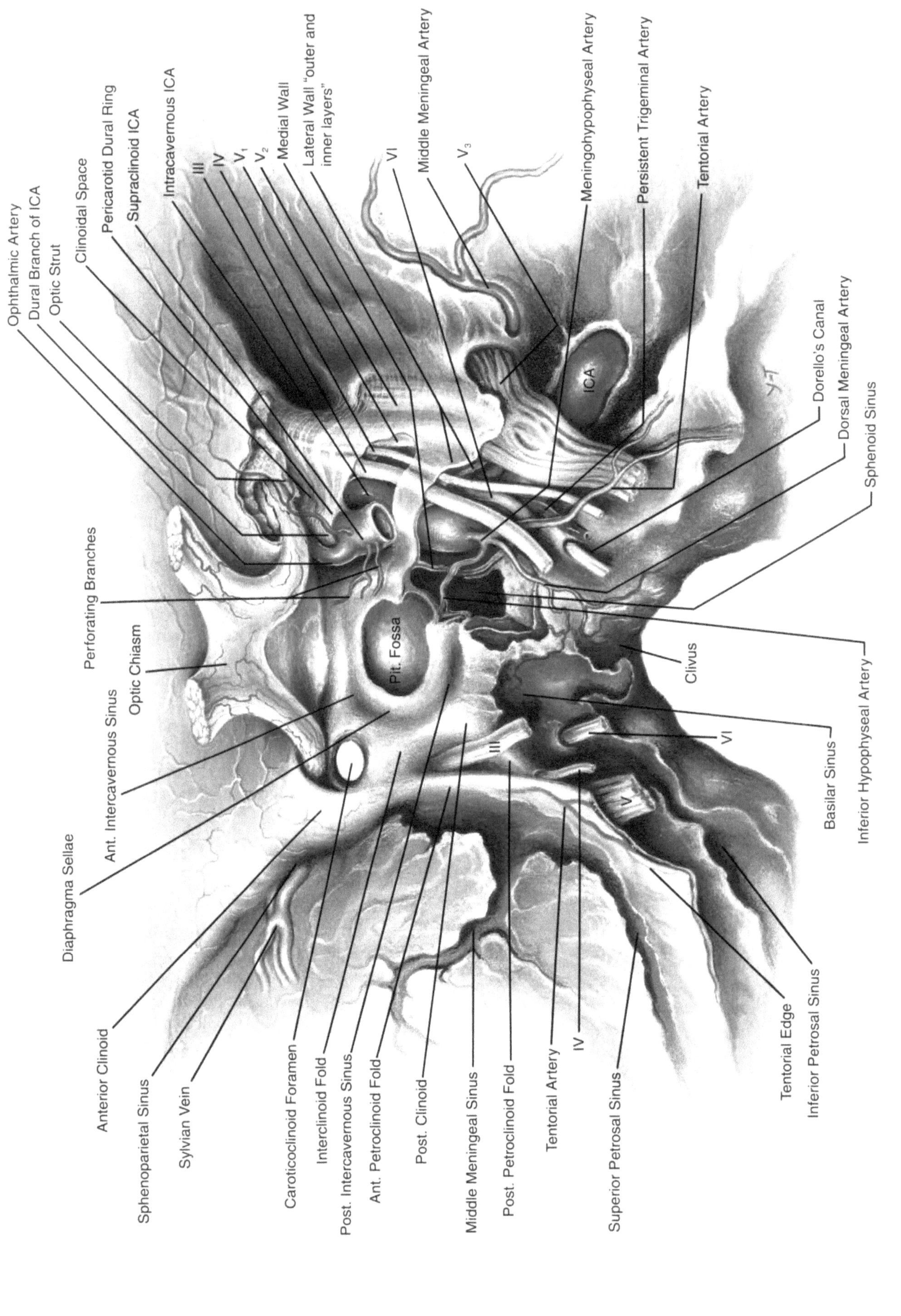
Ophthalmic Artery
Dural Branch of ICA
Optic Strut
Clinoidal Space
Pericarotid Dural Ring
Supraclinoid ICA
Intracavernous ICA
III
IV
V_1
V_2
Medial Wall
Lateral Wall "outer and inner layers"
VI
Middle Meningeal Artery
V_3
Meningohypophyseal Artery
Persistent Trigeminal Artery
Tentorial Artery
ICA
Dorello's Canal
Dorsal Meningeal Artery
Sphenoid Sinus
Perforating Branches
Optic Chiasm
Pit. Fossa
Clivus
Ant. Intercavernous Sinus
Diaphragma Sellae
Basilar Sinus
Inferior Hypophyseal Artery
VI
III
V
Anterior Clinoid
Sphenoparietal Sinus
Sylvian Vein
Caroticoclinoid Foramen
Interclinoid Fold
Post. Intercavernous Sinus
Ant. Petroclinoid Fold
Post. Clinoid
Middle Meningeal Sinus
Post. Petroclinoid Fold
Tentorial Artery
IV
Superior Petrosal Sinus
Tentorial Edge
Inferior Petrosal Sinus

lateral wall of the sphenoid sinus; they do not create bony alterations of the sphenoid sinus.

There may be an inferior extension of the cavernous sinus between the maxillary division fibers and the sphenoid bone. The bone between the sphenoidal sinus mucosa and medial wall of the cavernous sinus is thin or lacking, in rare instances.

Arterial Organization in the Cavernous Sinus

As the ICA leaves the foramen lacerum, it enters the posterior inferior part of the cavernous sinus and then passes upward; after forming the anterior bend, the ICA leaves the cavernous sinus at the medial side of the anterior clinoid process, dorsolateral to the optic canal. The average length of the intracavernous ICA is 18.0 mm.[3]

Rhoton and Inoue[3,8] divided the intracavernous ICA into five segments:

1. The posterior vertical segment is the part of the ICA between its exit site from the foramen lacerum and the beginning of the posterior bend of artery.
2. The posterior bend is distal to the first vertical segment.
3. The horizontal segment of the artery courses forward.
4. The anterior bend turns upward in the anterior part of the cavernous sinus.
5. The anterior vertical segment of the artery, which begins at the end of the anterior bend and passes upward and, after penetrating the roof of the cavernous sinus, passes along the medial side of the anterior clinoid process.

The anterior vertical part of the intracavernous ICA lies close and adjacent to the medial wall of the cavernous sinus. After removal of the anterior clinoid process, the anterior vertical segment of the ICA will be seen through the thin layer of the dura mater, on the medial side of the clinoid space. This part of the artery, which is about 5 mm long, is also called the "clinoidal segment of the ICA."

In some cases the caroticoclinoid ligament extending from the anterior clinoid process to the middle clinoid process may be calcified uniting the anterior and middle clinoid processes by a bony bridge; thus, the distal part of the carotid sulcus will be changed to an ostium called the caroticoclinoid foramen.

The existence of this anomaly, a fibrous, or a bony bridge between the anterior and posterior clinoid process will increase the risk of the ICA injury during removal of the anterior clinoid process in an approach by the cavernous sinus aneurysm. The intracavernous ICA usually causes a prominence into the midportion of the lateral wall of the sphenoid sinus.

On average, the distance between the medial wall of the intracavernous ICA and lateral margin of the pituitary gland is 2.3 mm, but the ICA may protrude medially and lie close to the pituitary gland.[9]

Several small branches arise from the cavernous ICA. The meningohypophyseal artery exists in virtually every case[10] and originates from the dorsal convexity of the posterior bend segment of the ICA. The distance between the origin of this artery from the foramen lacerum ranges from 5.0 to 18.0 mm.[3]

In rare instances, the meningohypophyseal artery and the artery of the inferior cavernous sinus have a common origin. The meningohypophyseal artery divides into three branches. The inferior hypophyseal artery courses medially to supply the posterior pituitary capsule. The tentorial artery passes dorsolaterally to supply the tentorium; this artery is also called the artery of Bernasconi-Cassinari.[11] The dorsal meningeal artery penetrates the dural wall of the posterior part of the cavernous sinus to supply the upper clivus and abducent nerve.[10]

The meningohypophyseal artery gives origin to three branches in 70%, but in 30% one or two of its branches may arise from the ICA directly.

The artery of the inferior cavernous sinus arises from the inferior or lateral surface of the horizontal segment of the intracavernous ICA, 3 to 8 mm distal to the origin of the meningohypophyseal artery. It usually passes above the abducent nerve to supply the inferolateral part of the lateral wall of the cavernous sinus and the region of the foramen ovale and spinosum.

McConnell's[12] capsular artery also originates from the ICA in the cavernous sinus. It arises from the medial surface of the horizontal segment of the ICA approximately 5 mm distal to origin of the artery of the inferior cavernous sinus. This artery is present in 8% to 28% of cases studied. McConnell's capsular artery supplies the anterior and inferior pituitary capsule.

The ophthalmic artery may arise from the intracavernous ICA, passing to the orbital cavity through the superior orbital fissure. When a persistent trigeminal artery exists, it originates from the posterior bend of the

FIGURE 8.2. Superior view of the floor of the anterior, middle, and posterior fossa dissected to demonstrate the branches and supply of the internal carotid artery (ICA) and its relationship to the nerves and osseous anatomy. The optic chiasm has been lifted forward to illustrate the carotid artery as it emerges from the cavernous sinus. Structures in the cavernous sinus and their relation to the carotid artery are shown. The right posterior clinoid process has been drilled away to show the relationship of the inferior hypophyseal artery as it passes superior to the sphenoid sinus. The clinoidal space has also been developed to show the small branches from the ICA as it passes through the dural ring. The two layers of the lateral wall of the cavernous sinus are also shown and in this case, the persistent trigeminal artery is located.

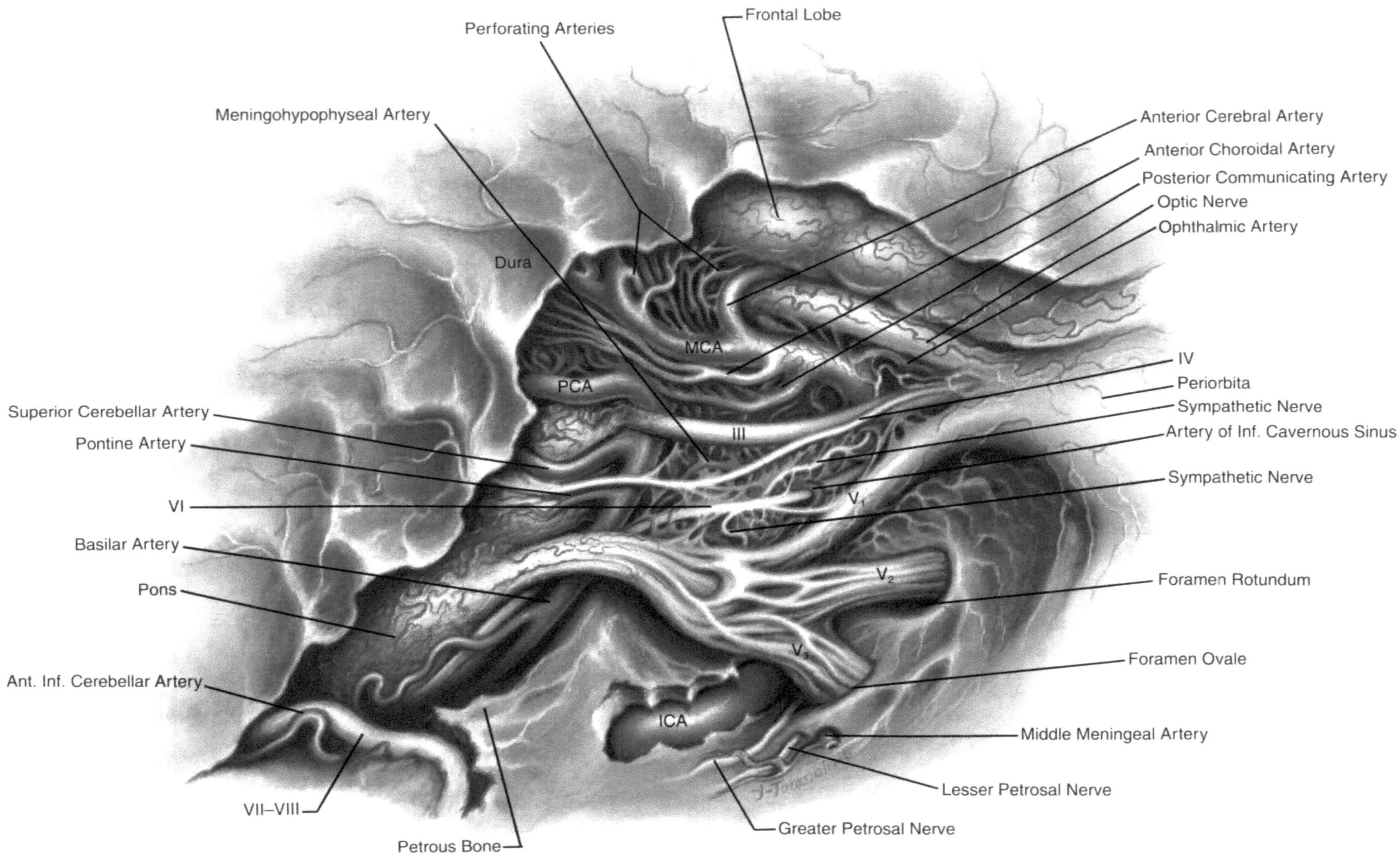

FIGURE 8.3. Right lateral view of the dissected cavernous sinus. The optic nerve and frontal lobe are shown. In the cavernous sinus, the sympathetic plexus surrounding the carotid artery is seen. The small branches that originate from this plexus to pass into the orbit with V_1 and intracranially on the intracranial carotid artery are shown. The meningohypophyseal trunk and its branches and the relationship of the artery of the inferior cavernous sinus to the sixth cranial nerve are illustrated.

intracavernous ICA, usually proximal to the origin of the meningohypophyseal artery. It passes backward, medial to the trigeminal nerve, and penetrates the posterior wall of the cavernous sinus, in the area lateral to the Dorello's canal and medial to the Meckel's cave (Fig. 8.2). It then runs into the interpeduncular cistern, usually inferolateral to the abducent nerve[13] to join with basilar artery between the origin of the superior cerebellar artery and anterior inferior cerebellar artery (AICA).

Neural Structures of the Cavernous Sinus

The oculomotor and trochlear nerves and the first and second divisions of the trigeminal nerve pass through the two layers of the lateral wall of cavernous sinus.

The oculomotor nerve penetrates the roof of the cavernous sinus lateral to the posterior clinoid process; then it courses within the upper part of the lateral wall and passes below the anterior clinoid process to enter the superior orbital fissure.

The trochlear nerve runs forward, below, and medial to the free margin of the tentorium, penetrating the posterior part of the roof of the cavernous sinus, posterolateral to the entrance site of the oculomotor nerve; then it passes through the lateral wall below the oculomotor nerve and enters the superior orbital fissure. The ophthalmic division of the trigeminal nerve passes through the lateral wall of the cavernous sinus, obliquely and upward, to enter the superior orbital fissure. The maxillary branch passes within the two layers of the lateral wall of the cavernous sinus to enter the foramen rotundum. The first and third divisions of the trigeminal nerve are separated from the medial side by the intracavernous ICA; but the second division (maxillary) is adjacent to the medial structures in the anterior and inferior part of the cavernous sinus. Frequently, this division bulges into the lateral wall of the sphenoid sinus.

The abducent nerve enters the posterior part of the cavernous sinus after passing through Dorello's canal, which is formed by the petroclinoid ligament in the upper part and by the superior surface of the petrous apex in its lower part. It passes through the cavernous sinus between the ophthalmic division of the trigeminal nerve and lateral surface of the ICA. It may divide into two or more branches within the cavernous sinus before finally running forward through the superior orbital fissure.

The major part of the fibers of the sympathetic plexus surrounding the intracavernous ICA passes to the abducent nerve and subsequently joins with the first division of the trigeminal nerve to enter the orbit.

Venous Compartments of the Cavernous Sinus

Venous organization in the cavernous sinus is still controversial. There are two opinions: (1) The cavernous sinus is a venous plexus; (2) the cavernous sinus is a trabeculated venous channel.

In relation to the location of the intracavernous ICA, Harris and Rhoton[9] divided the cavernous sinus into four spaces:

1. A medial space between the carotid artery and medial wall of cavernous sinus.
2. A lateral space, which is lateral to the ICA and medial to the lateral wall of the cavernous sinus.
3. An anterior inferior space, which is the space between the anterior bend of the ICA and superior orbital fissure. (This space is narrow posteriorly and has its greatest height anteriorly.)
4. A posterior superior space, which is located behind the posterior bend of ICA. In most cases, this space is smaller than the anterior inferior space.[3]

The cavernous sinus has various venous connections. In the anterior aspect, it communicates with the superior and inferior ophthalmic veins and sphenoparietal sinus. In the lateral aspect, it communicates with the sinus accompanying the middle meningeal artery and with the pterygoid venous plexus via the emissary vein passing through the emissary sphenoidal foramen, which is located medial to the foramen ovale. In the posterior aspect, the cavernous sinus connects to the basilar sinus, which is located in the posterior surface of the dorsum sellae and clivus. The basilar sinus also joins the posterior margins of both cavernous sinuses together. Along the posterior surface, the cavernous sinus communicates with the superior and inferior petrosal sinuses. The superior petrosal sinus runs to the sigmoid sinus and the inferior petrosal sinus terminates in the jugular bulb.

Clinical Features

Jefferson[14] described three classical syndromes that he had observed in patients with aneurysms arising from the cavernous portion of the ICA. In aneurysms arising from the anterior segment of the cavernous sinus, involvement of the first branch of the trigeminal nerve and all of the oculomotor nerves in varying degrees occurred. Aneurysms arising in the middle portions of the cavernous sinus affected the V_1 and V_2, but involvement of the oculomotor nerves was seen less often. In lesions of the posterior cavernous sinus, all branches of the fifth cranial nerve were affected, but oculomotor dysfunction involved muscles supplied by the fourth and sixth cranial nerves (Fig. 8.4). There was relative sparing of the third cranial nerve, due to its anterior entry into the sinus. Because aneurysms most often arise in the anterior portion along the carotid artery, oculomotor disturbances with pupillary abnormalities and diplopia are among the first signs encountered. Aneurysms less than

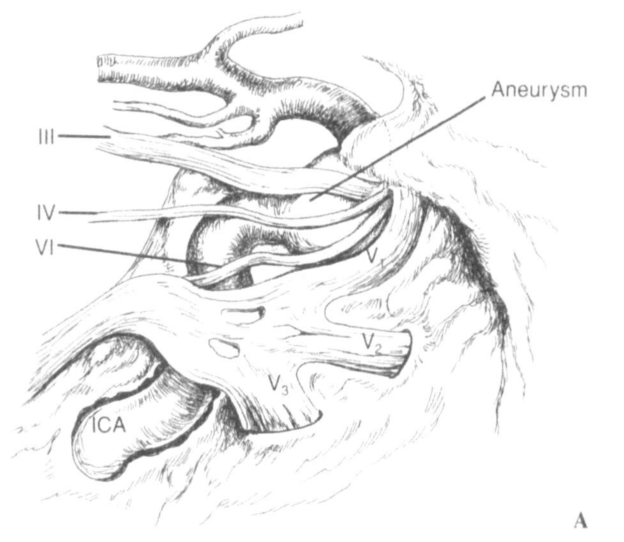

A

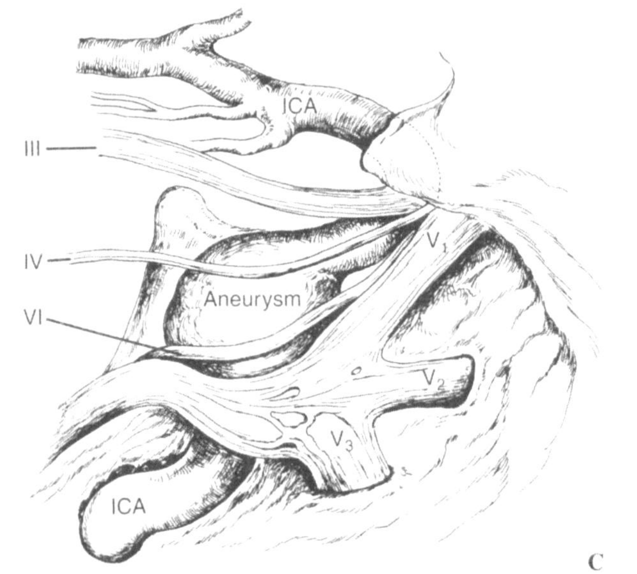

C

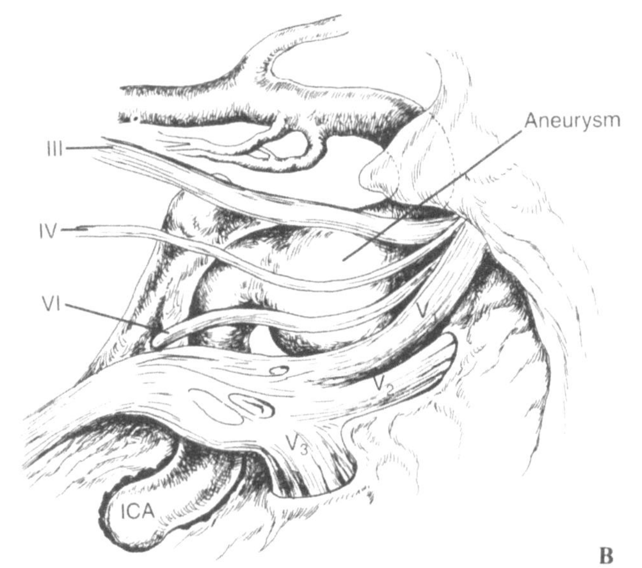

B

FIGURE 8.4. (A) An anterior cavernous sinus syndrome is illustrated. The first division of the trigeminal nerve is compressed out; V_2 and V_3 are spared. The superior division of the oculomotor, trochlear, and abducent nerves are also compressed by this large fusiform aneurysm arising from the internal carotid artery. (B) A middle cavernous sinus syndrome in which both the first and second divisions of the trigeminal nerve are affected is illustrated. In this case, the trochlear and abducent nerves are compressed but the oculomotor nerve is spared. Both first and second divisions of the trigeminal nerves are distorted by the aneurysm. (C) A posterior cavernous sinus syndrome is shown. In this case, all of the trigeminal roots are affected and the abducent nerve is compressed. Any or all ocular motor nerves may be involved by large aneurysms of the cavernous sinus.

1 to 2 cm in diameter rarely produce clinical signs due to their mass effect, but even lesions of this size are known to rupture and produce carotid cavernous sinus fistulae.

SAH from cavernous aneurysms has been noted and reported. The aneurysms usually project into the superior lateral wall and may erode through the dural covering producing SAH upon rupture of the fundus. They may also project into the sphenoid sinus producing massive epistaxis.

Surgical Options

Symptomatic lesions of the cavernous sinus are usually encountered when they attain a size of about 1 cm or more in the greatest dimension. Much depends on the location of the aneurysm within the sinus as to the symptoms produced and the indications for treatment. There are anatomical spaces in the cavernous sinus, especially between the apogee of the first forward curve, that would accommodate an aneurysm of 1 cm or larger without causing any signs of compression.

Based upon the age of onset, clinical signs, and the few anatomical studies from the pathology literature, a degenerative etiology, at least in part, must be considered for this aneurysm. Arteriosclerosis is probably the underlying disorder causing derangement of the arterial wall in most cases. Fusiform dilatations of the cavernous portion of the internal carotid artery occurs commonly in the fifth decade and beyond.

Direct surgical management of fusiform cavernous aneurysms by craniotomy requires special operative skills. Only neurosurgeons thoroughly familiar with the anatomy and surgical approaches to this region should

TABLE 8.1. Surgical alternatives with cavernous sinus aneurysms

Type of aneurysm	Direct operation	Endovascular operation	Test occlusion	Combined operation
Aneurysm < 10 mm with good neck	+	+	+	−
Aneurysm < 10 mm with wide neck	−	±	+	−
Aneurysm > 10 mm	±	+	+	+
Fusiform aneurysm	±	+	+	+

consider direct operation and all the alternatives exercised beforehand.

The configuration of the usual aneurysms that arise from the ICA in the cavernous sinus are, however, appropriate for treatment using endovascular methods. These procedures usually allow preservation of the carotid artery. In those cases in which the carotid artery must be sacrificed, the endovascular approach, with test occlusion, indicates to the surgeon which vessel can be sacrificed safely. Test occlusion is indicated, not only in all endovascular procedures involving the cavernous portion, but also as a preliminary to any direct surgical approach or carotid occlusion procedure and/or trapping. All of these reasons combine to emphasize the need for experience in endovascular therapy and testing by the neurosurgeon. Before the definitive therapy, test occlusion should be carried out for a period of not less than 30 min, evaluating all aspects of carotid artery circulation and neurological function during occlusion. When test occlusion is not tolerated or when blood flow data, measured by either velocity or volume flow determinations, indicate that ischemic problems are likely to arise, modification in therapy is required. The final decision must be predicated on the overall experience of the surgeon or clinic involved. If only an endovascular approach is to be considered, then, this should be attempted without sacrificing the parent artery. Likewise, direct surgical treatment must be structured in order to preserve the artery. Overall, the endovascular approach is preferred because the risk for cranial nerve injury is greatly reduced. Also, the endovascular operation may be abandoned without deficit if the balloon has not been detached in the primary or parent artery. When an occlusion test indicates that the deficits associated with arterial occlusion may be mild or absent and when it is not possible to introduce the balloon into the aneurysm directly, occlusion of the parent artery or a trapping procedure may be acceptable. Conversely, if occlusion testing indicates that the deficit anticipated with a deconstructive operation would be severe and that the balloon cannot be introduced directly into the aneurysm, the endovascular approach should be discontinued. A bypass procedure may be performed before carrying out a subsequent definitive interventional procedure. Further test occlusions are required, however, after maturation of the bypass to confirm its adequacy for protection of the arterial territory in question.

Only cavernous sinus aneurysms that are symptomatic should be considered for either endovascular or direct surgical treatment. Many patients harbor aneurysms in this location for years before they become symptomatic, and many aneurysms reach a stable size and never cause problems. Perhaps some lesions in this location even undergo spontaneous resolution. Because most postmortem examinations do not include this area, the incidence of asymptomatic lesions is not known. Table 8.1 compares the method of treatment for cavernous aneurysms using endovascular procedures, direct operations, test occlusion, and combined approaches.

Technique of Endovascular Surgery for Cavernous Aneurysms

During the past decade, cavernous aneurysms have come more and more frequently to the attention of endovascular therapists.[15,16] Reconstructive operations, in which the ICA is spared, should be pursued in any endovascular procedure involving the cavernous portion of the ICA. However, because of the special configuration of aneurysms in this region, achievement of this goal is not always feasible. Accordingly, the functional significance of the ICA to hemispheric circulation must be known. After test occlusion, the tactics of the endovascular approach may need modification. If the aneurysm is fusiform and the ICA is not essential to neurological function, a deconstructive procedure, may be performed in which the aneurysm and the parent vessel or the parent vessel alone can be occluded with a detachable balloon.

The endovascular approach is best carried out through a common carotid artery puncture. Either of two deconstructive procedures may be employed for fusiform aneurysms. In one of these, the ICA is occluded proximal to the aneurysm. In the other, the aneurysm is occluded along with the ICA. In this procedure, a long balloon is used to occlude the aneurysm at its origin and along all or a greater part of the fusiform segment. This lessens the risk of bleeding or growth of the lesion due to back pressure.

Acute occlusion may be carried out. In this case, the balloon is immediately detached after inflation and left in place. The effect of blood flow and pressure tends to force the balloon upstream distally. This may lead to subtotal occlusion with distal embolization into the middle cerebral artery (MCA) and its terminal branches, either by the balloon or by clot in the aneurysm.

Delayed occlusion may be preferred, in which case the balloon and catheter are left in place in the carotid artery. The balloon is later deflated sequentially over a 7- to 10-day interval as thrombus replaces the balloon and catheter. The delayed occlusion procedure, with the proximal end of the catheter fixed in the neck by a suture, prevents proximal migration of the balloon until after the thrombus has become well fixed (Fig. 8.5). With delayed occlusion, a few drops of contrast material are allowed to leak from the balloon each day for several days until the balloon is completely deflated. Then angiography is carried out to ensure that occlusion is complete. At this point, the catheter and balloon may be safely withdrawn.

In deconstructive procedures, the balloon extends along the longest axis of the aneurysm, beyond the orifice, and back into the main channel of the ICA, blocking it permanently. In this way, the balloon cannot become displaced by pressure or flow. If more than one balloon is required to completely block an aneurysm from the circulation, these balloons must be impacted tightly so that no movement is possible. Blood volume and pressure must be maintained and clinical parameters assessed at frequent intervals after deconstructive procedures to recognize ischemia early. Even when the balloon test occlusion indicates low risk for the development of these complications, postoperative monitoring may be used to indicate embolic complications. The two major hemodynamic problems relate to reduction in flow in the distal branches of the ICA and thromboembolic complications related to distal embolization. The blood pressure must be maintained in a normal to slightly hypertensive state, and coagulation must be controlled by the administration of aspirin or heparin.

Reconstructive operations are done in patients harboring aneurysms that have a good neck that can be entered easily and safely from the ICA. The goal for reconstructive operations, in which the carotid artery is spared, is to place the balloon along the longest axis of the aneurysm permitting simultaneous occlusion of the orifice and fundus (Fig. 8.6). Otherwise, the balloon may be displaced and become free in the aneurysm cavity. Technically, occlusion with balloons or coils is not usually difficult for aneurysms in this location. Absence of tortuosity of the ICA facilitates the maneuver, especially when the aneurysm occurs proximal to the siphon. Manipulations and test occlusions may be carried out relatively safely proximal to the major communicating arteries. If the diameter of the aneurysm orifice is half

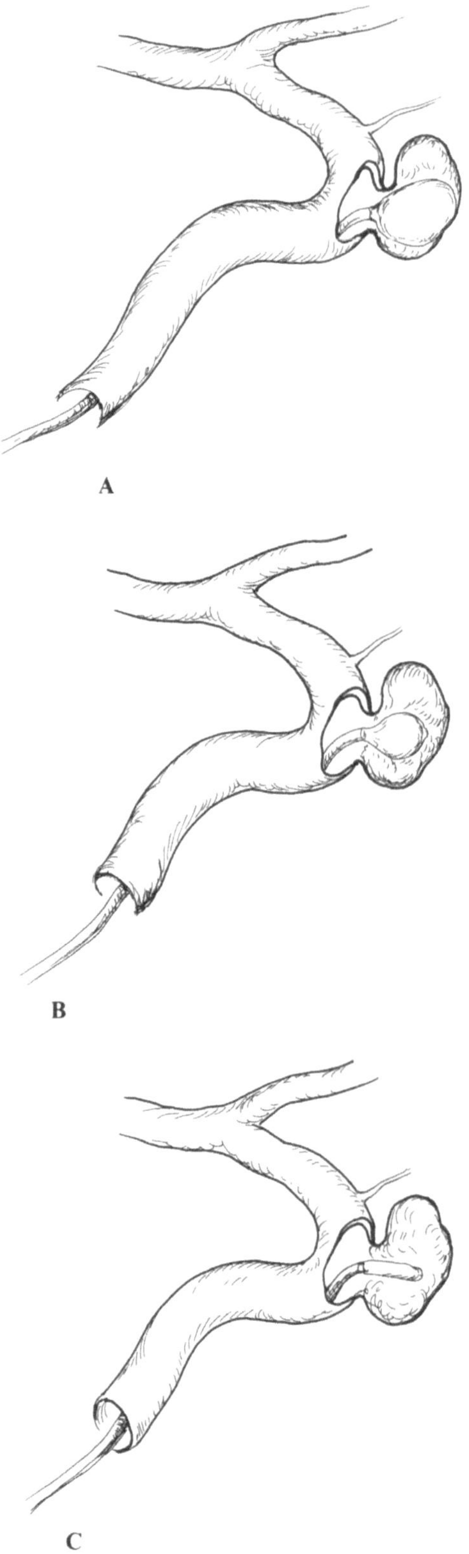

FIGURE 8.5. (A) A balloon has been introduced into the aneurysm through the orifice. As thrombus forms, the balloon is intervally deflated. (B) Thrombus continues to develop as the balloon is deflated. Finally, the balloon is deflated and withdrawn leaving the thrombus to fill the aneurysm. (C) The balloon and catheter are then withdrawn.

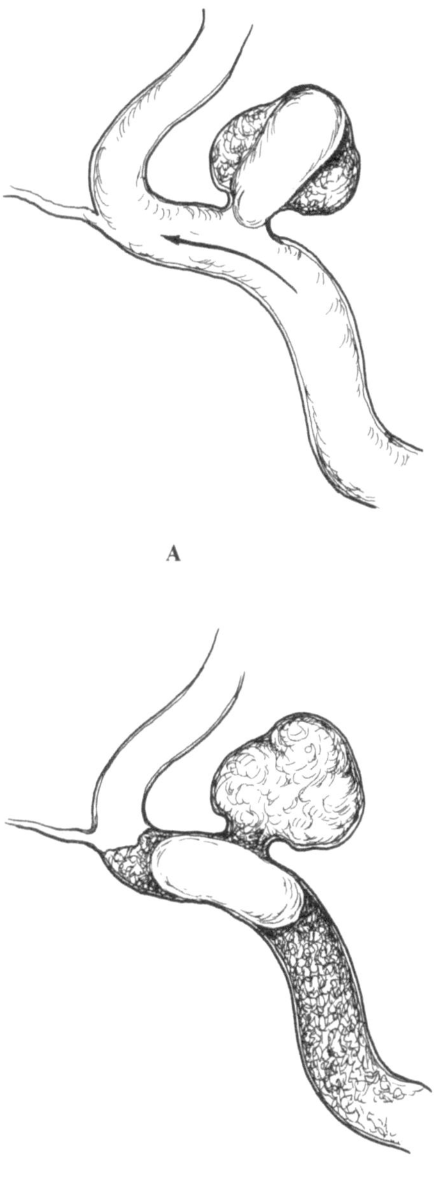

A

B

FIGURE 8.6. Reconstructive (A) and deconstructive (B) occlusion of cerebral aneurysms involving the cavernous sinus. The balloon has been placed opposite the aneurysm orifice and the carotid artery occluded. This is prolonged occlusion of a cavernous sinus aneurysm.

that of the ICA or more, there is usually no difficulty in introducing the balloon into this orifice. If the orifice is smaller than half the diameter of the parent artery, a helper balloon may be placed above the aneurysm to direct the primary balloon into the smaller orifice. In the case of large or giant aneurysms, one balloon may not be sufficient to produce satisfactory occlusion. Liquid contrast material is preferred for inflating the balloons, allowing some leakage through the latex and later shrinkage of the aneurysm, after thrombosis has occurred. It is rarely impossible to produce occlusion of a giant aneurysm with balloons placed sequentially into the fundus. Preferably, three or more balloons of varying sizes should be introduced into the cavity without inflation. All balloons are then inflated to slowly obliterate the cavity from the most distal site proximally. The last balloon to be totally inflated projects into the orifice and occludes it, hopefully without compromise of the parent artery. Then all balloons are detached sequentially (Fig. 8.7). Total occlusion of some aneurysms may not be required or possible. Even partial occlusion may result in shrinkage, freeing cranial nerves from compression (Fig. 8.8).

Direct Surgical Approaches

Surgical approaches to the cavernous sinus focused originally not at the aneurysm, but toward the ICA from which the aneurysm arose. These procedures were first applied to the common and internal carotid arteries in the neck, generally to treat cranial nerve dysfunction associated with a mass lesion in the cavernous sinus, namely the ICA aneurysm. Carotid artery ligation became a standard among neurosurgeons for management of cavernous aneurysms. The operation was usually applied to symptomatic patients who complained of facial pain, ptosis, or ophthalmoplegia. The operation produced the desired effect of thrombosis and exclusion of the aneurysm from the arterial circulation, but, in some cases, subsequent growth of the lesion and even rupture occurred after indirect surgical approaches. The most serious complication of the procedure was ischemic lesion in the territory of the occluded internal carotid artery.

In 1939, Dandy[17] introduced the trapping procedure in which the ICA in the neck and the intracranial ICA were both ligated, thus trapping the aneurysm in the intervening segment. This procedure effectively excluded the aneurysm from the circulation, but did not address the issue of ischemic changes in the hemisphere in the territory of the affected ICA. The incidence of ischemic complications after carotid artery ligation depends on many factors, including the collateral circulation. In the Cooperative Aneurysm Study, there was a 59% incidence of ischemic complication for abrupt ligation of the ICA and a 32% incidence of ischemic complication with acute ligation of the common carotid artery.[18] Ischemic complications occurred in 41% of those undergoing gradual occlusion of the ICA and in 24% undergoing gradual occlusion of the common carotid artery. Virtually, all of the ischemic complications occurred during the first 7 days after progressive closure of the artery. This figure may have included those patients who deteriorated from vasospasm or other ischemic disorders. Even so, in

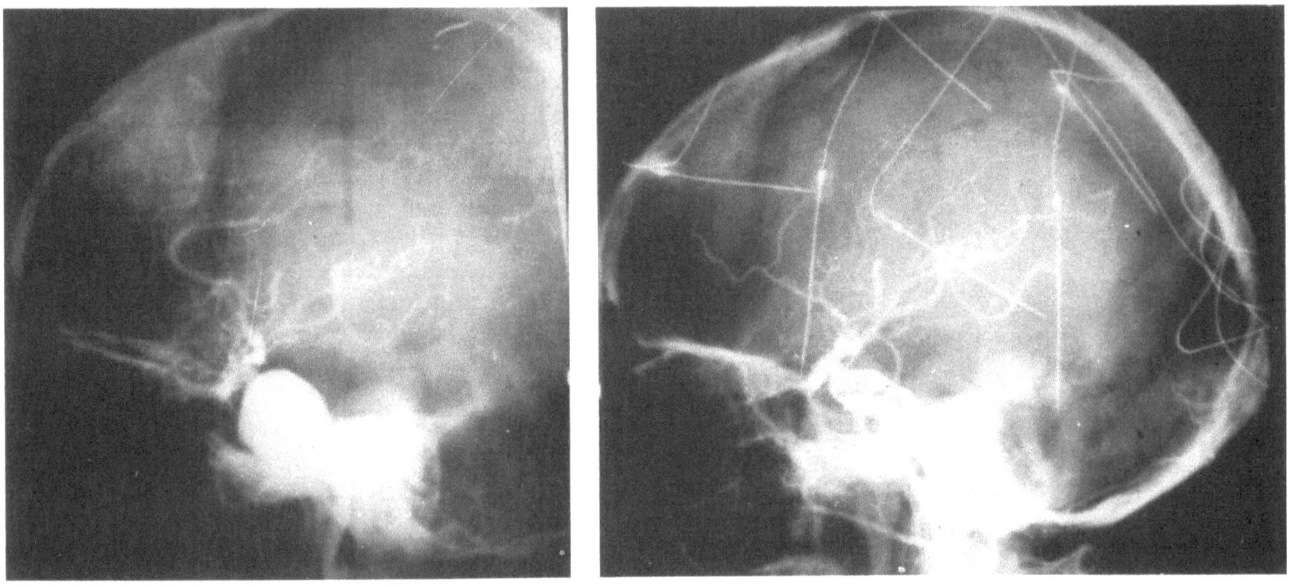

A B

FIGURE 8.7. A large aneurysm of the cavernous sinus (A) has been treated by the introduction of three balloons into the cavity (B). An initial balloon was placed in the aneurysm followed by two additional balloons. These were subsequently manipulated until they were in proper position, inflated, and detached simultaneously.

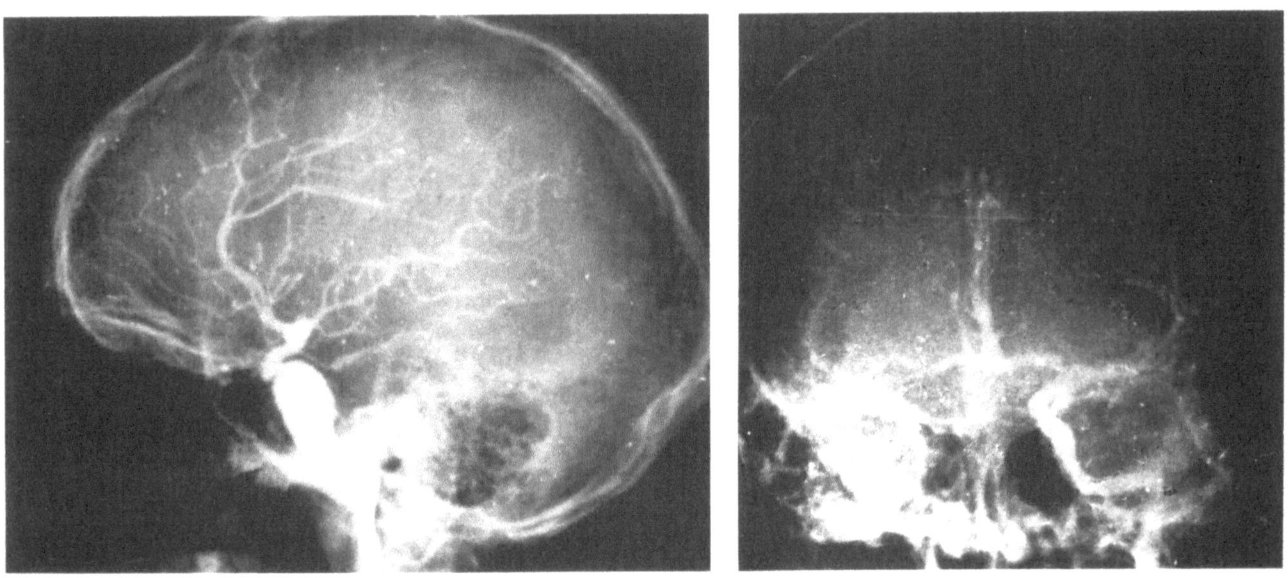

A B

FIGURE 8.8. (A) Deconstructive endovascular procedure in which a fusiform aneurysm of the cavernous sinus has been occluded. (B) Good collateral blood flow in the hemisphere after the deconstructive procedure.

patients judged suitable for carotid occlusion, a 21% incidence of temporary and a 5% incidence of permanent ischemic deficits occurred. Thus, Spetzler and Carter[19] suggested that extracranial–intracranial (EC-IC) bypass graft be used to improve the safety of parent vessel ligation. This procedure carried low risk and seemed to be effective in preventing ischemic complications. These authors reported only one case of ischemic deficit among 23 patients treated with combined bypass and gradual occlusion. However, the EC-IC bypass carries only 20 to 60 ml of blood per minute, leading Al-Mefty and co-workers[20] to suggest the use of a bypass graft and shunt method. An external intrapetrous supraclinoid carotid shunt of Dacron or a saphenous vein graft may be used.

Parkinson[1] and Taptas[21,22] described eloquently the anatomy of the cavernous sinus, indicating a possible surgical approach for lesions arising in this location. Hypothermia and cardiac arrest were further advised for lesions in this area. Johnston[23] described a case in which bilateral aneurysms of the cavernous sinus were treated using Parkinson's descriptive approaches. Dolenc[24] employed similar approaches in three cases. In two of these cases, the aneurysm was successfully clipped and, in another case, the artery was repaired primarily with suture. Dolenc suggested exposure of the intradural portion of the ICA and proximal control at this level. The optic canal was opened and the anterior clinoid process drilled away in order to provide anterior exposure. Before reflection of the dural margins, the cranial nerves contained in the lateral superior wall must be dissected free. Bleeding may be controlled along the lateral border of the cavernous sinus by packing. Ohmoto and co-workers[5] exposed the intracavernous carotid artery for treatment of five large and giant aneurysms and for two cases of an intracavernous aneurysm arising from the anterior knee. They also exposed the ICA in the neck and performed a pterional craniotomy. The dura overlying the roof of the optic canal and the anterior clinoid process were excised together with the falciform fold. The optic canal was unroofed, and a total anterior clinoidectomy was performed. This exposed the superior margin of the superior orbital fissure. The optic strut was then removed along with the ring of dura covering the carotid artery. The edges of the cavernous sinus were advanced using blunt dissection and oxidized cellulose employed to control bleeding. They then opened the lateral wall of the cavernous sinus along the anterior margin of the third cranial nerve. This exposed the cavernous portion of the ICA and aneurysms that arise along its anterior knee.

In 1990, Dolenc[25] reviewed his further experience with direct cavernous sinus surgery. At that time, he recognized the good results that had been obtained in endovascular management of aneurysms arising in the cavernous sinus and that this treatment carried fewer complications than the direct surgical approach.

Direct surgical treatment should be applied only to cavernous sinus aneurysms that have produced SAH, which cannot be treated effectively with endovascular methods. Direct surgery may also be justified in patients whose collateral circulation is so poor that an endovascular occlusion of the parent artery would not be accepted without intolerable deficits.

In the superior intradural approach, the superior wall of the sinus is exposed through a frontoparietal or pterional craniotomy. The dura is opened along the anterior margin of the exposure. The sylvian fissure must be opened and the frontal and temporal lobes separated to expose the roof of the sinus. The roof is bounded laterally by the dural fold along the medial edge of the tentorium and oculomotor nerve, anteriorly by the anterior clinoid process and the falciform dural fold, medially by the pituitary gland and stalk, and posteriorly by the posterior clinoid process and dorsum sellae. The ICA emerges from the anterior part of the roof of the cavernous sinus medial to the anterior clinoid process and posterolateral to the optic canal. To enter the cavernous sinus, the posterior edge of the planum sphenoidale and the base of the anterior clinoid process are drilled away. The dural flap overlying the optic nerve and clinoid process are incised in a curve and reflected over the ICA posteriorly. The optic canal forward to the roof of the orbit is unroofed. The oculomotor nerve passes below the anterior clinoid process and must be protected during the drilling process. The carotid artery and aneurysms that arise from it must also be protected. Exposure of the roof of the ethmoidal and sphenoid sinuses during the drilling process may be unavoidable. Removal of the anterior clinoid process opens a small triangular space called the clinoid space lined by dura surrounding the anterior clinoid process. The ring of dura that surrounds the carotid artery and separates it from the cavernous sinus must be excised. Usually, cranial nerves are found at the lateral surface of the aneurysm covered by a thin reflection of dura making up the lateral wall. The oculomotor nerve may cross the anterior knee of the ICA and aneurysm. The second division of the fifth cranial nerve may also be found medially. Sympathetic fibers are also present. The ICA must be exposed proximally for control.

Cavernous aneurysms may be approached laterally and superiorly. The superior approach involves removing the anterior clinoid process, with medial displacement of the optic nerve after the canal has been drilled. This is suitable for small aneurysms projecting medially. However, a large intracavernous aneurysm may require a lateral approach combined with the superior approach (Fig. 8.9).

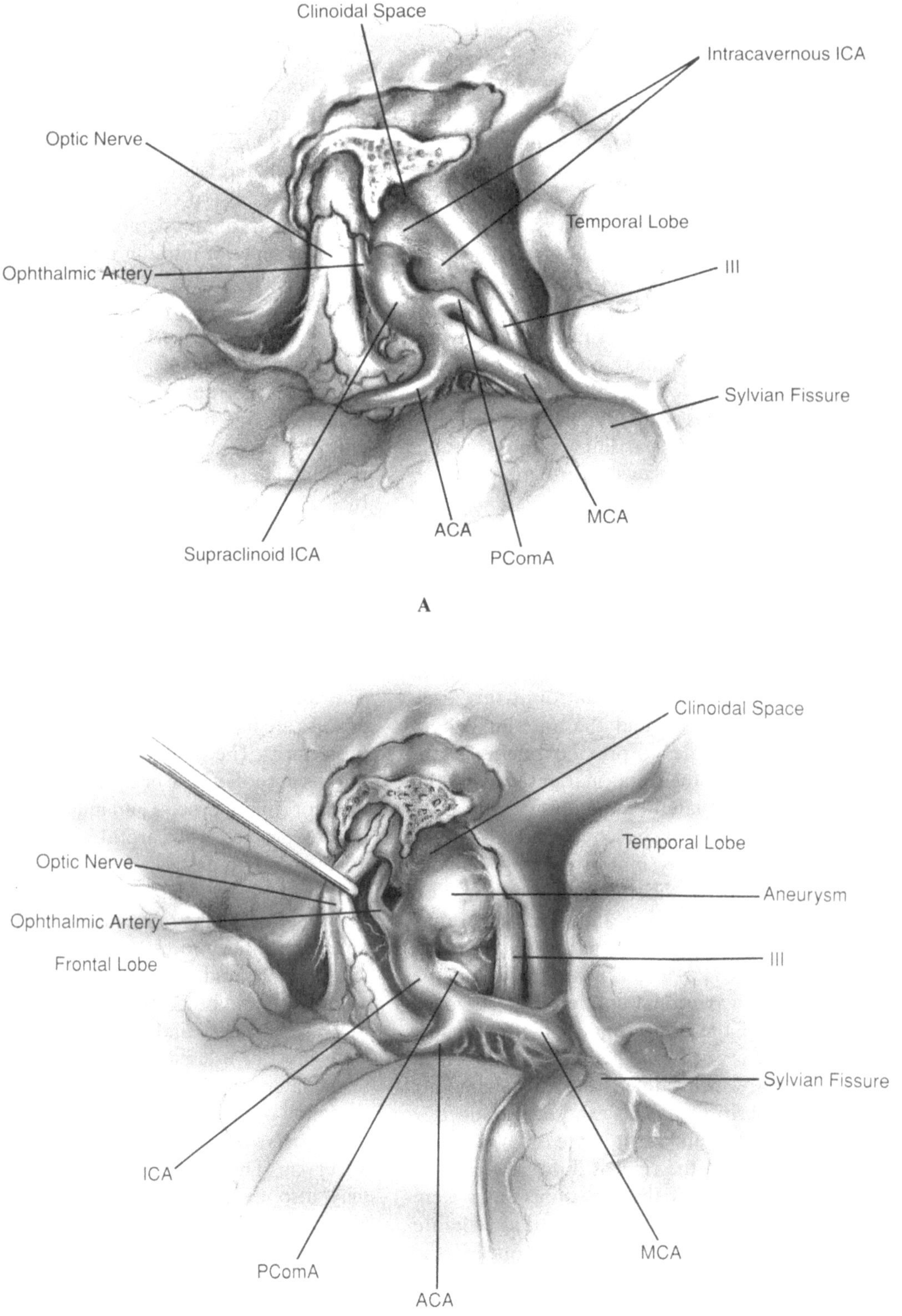

FIGURE 8.9. (A) A right pterional craniotomy with superior and lateral entry into the cavernous sinus is illustrated. The anterior clinoid process has been drilled away to open the clinoidal space inferiorly. (B) The anteromedial triangle of the lateral wall is shown. This triangle provides entry to the intracavernous internal carotid artery (ICA) in its most anterior knee. (C) Aneurysms usually arise from the posterior aspect of the carotid artery in this loop. ACA, anterior cerebral artery; MCA, middle cerebral artery; PComA, posterior communicating artery.

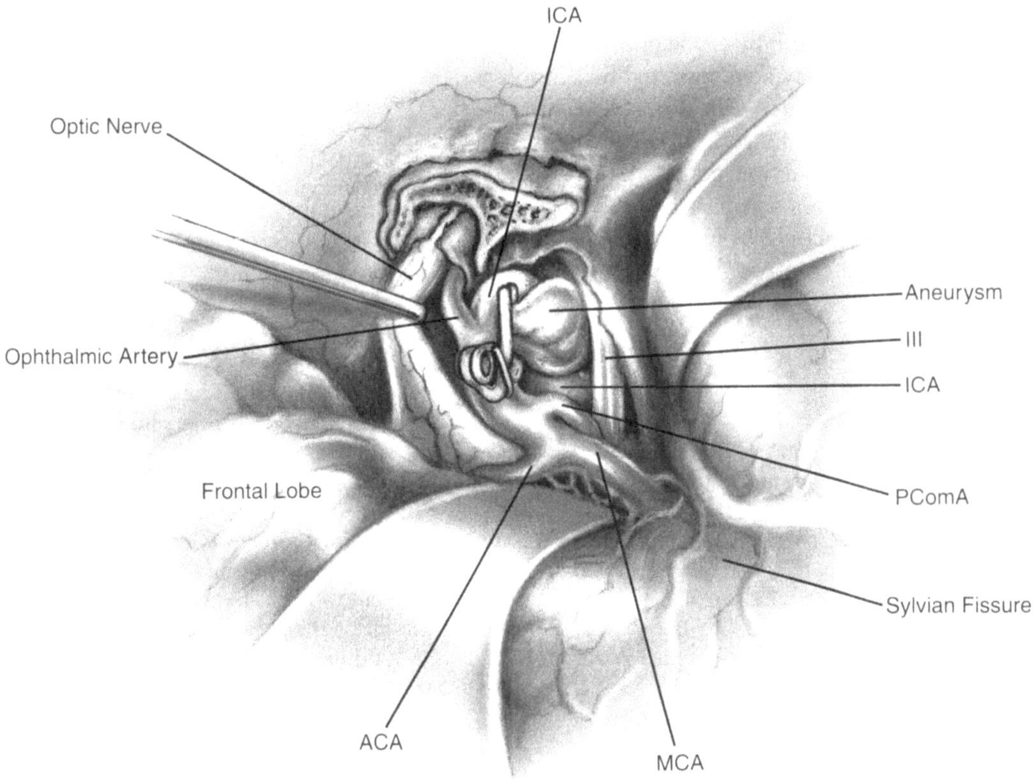

C

FIGURE 8.9 (*continued*)

The dura is reflected posteriorly, and the anterior clinoid process and the frontal bone overlying the optic nerve are drilled away until the optic nerve can be freely mobilized. The anterior clinoid process must be drilled medially until the optic strut has been removed. This exposes the ophthalmic artery and the ring of dura or dura propria, which surrounds the entrance of the ICA into the subarachnoid space. After excision of the dural ring, the ICA can be followed into the cavernous sinus and the anterior knee can be visualized through the medial wall of the cavernous sinus. The wall can be excised along the third cranial nerve and the cavernous sinus entered at this level. Surgical sponge or collagen sponge may be used to control bleeding. The knee of the ICA must be visualized because the aneurysm usually arises in the internal surface of this knee. If the aneurysm is large, it may partly obscure the knee, and it may be covered with cranial nerves III, V, and VI. These must be separated from the dome of the aneurysm in order to expose the neck. Proximal control is essential with this lesion. The ICA in the neck may be isolated and an umbilical tape and a Rumel tourniquet placed around it. This obviates the need for drilling the petrous portion of the ICA, and proximal control is achieved much more easily and quickly than by drilling the petrous portion of the temporal bone intracranially, as has been advocated. A balloon catheter may be introduced percutaneously into the ICA to also provide proximal control should this be needed.

The clips should be applied along and parallel to the long axis of the carotid artery when possible. This usually means that an acutely angled clip must be used. A fenestration permits preservation of flow in the ICA while successfully occluding the neck of the aneurysm in some cases.

Conclusion

Direct approaches to cavernous sinus aneurysms are rarely called for. The unruptured lesion is fairly benign. Only when progressive mass threatens to destroy vision or ocular motility or when pain is the indication, should surgery be considered. Even then, endovascular methods are usually safer and more successful. Deconstructive procedures are usually accepted, but preocclusion testing with clinical transcranial doppler (TCD) or cerebral blood flow (CBF) monitoring assures tolerance for the procedure.

When a cavernous sinus aneurysm has bled into the

subarachnoid space or when an aneurysm is unsuitable for an endovascular operation by virtue of intolerance of the arterial sacrifice that may be required, direct clipping is possible and feasible under very controlled circumstances. The cavernous sinus is a small structure. It tolerates dissection or retraction poorly. Cranial nerve injury is not a complication but part and parcel of this approach. The decision should be made to enter directly only after all other alternatives have been given due consideration.

References

1. Parkinson D. A surgical approach to the cavernous portion of the carotid artery. Anatomical studies and case report. *J Neurosurg*. 1965;23:474–483.
2. Knosp E, Muller G, Pernsezky A. The paraclinoid carotid artery: anatomical aspects of a microneurosurgical approach. *Neurosurgery*. 1988;22:896–901.
3. Inoue T, Rhoton AL, Theele D, Barry ME. Surgical approaches to the cavernous sinus: a microsurgical study. *Neurosurgery*. 1990;26:903–932.
4. Dolenc VV. *Anatomy and Surgery of the Cavernous Sinus*. Vienna and New York: Springer-Verlag; 1989.
5. Ohmoto T, Nago S, Mino S, Ito T, Honma Y, Fujiwara T. Exposure of the intracavernous carotid artery in aneurysm surgery. *Neurosurgery*. 1991;28:317–324.
6. Hakuba A, Matsuoka V, Suzuki T, Komiyama M, Jin TB, Inoue V. Direct approaches to vascular lesions in the cavernous sinus via the medial triangle. In: Dolenc VV, ed. *The Cavernous Sinus, A Multidisciplinary Approach to Vascular and Tumorous Lesions*. Vienna and New York: Springer-Verlag; 1987:272–284.
7. Fujii K, Chambers SM, Rhoton AL. Neurovascular relationships of the sphenoid sinus. A microsurgical study. *J Neurosurg*. 1979;50:31–39.
8. Rhoton AL, Inoue T. Microsurgical approaches to the cavernous sinus. *Clin Neurosurg*. 1991;37:391–439.
9. Harris FS, Rhoton AL. Anatomy of the cavernous sinus. A microsurgical study. *J Neurosurg*. 1976;45:169–180.
10. Weir B. *Anatomy of the Internal Carotid Artery, Aneurysm Affecting the Nervous System*. Baltimore: Williams and Wilkins; 1987:308–311.
11. Day AL, Rhoton AL Jr. Aneurysms and arteriovenous fistulae of the intracavernous carotid artery and its branches. In: Youmans JR, ed. *Neurological Surgery*. Philadelphia: WB Saunders; 1982:1764–1785.
12. McConnell EM. The arterial blood supply of the human hypophysis cerebri. *Anat Rec*. 1953;115:175–203.
13. Merry GS, Jamieson KG. Operative approach to persistent trigeminal artery producing facial pain and diplopia. Case report. *J Neurosurg*. 1977;47:613–618.
14. Jefferson G. On the saccular aneurysms of the internal carotid artery in the cavernous sinus. *Br J Surg*. 1938;26: 267–302.
15. Alexander LF, Benashvili GM, Zubkov YN. Endovascular treatment of giant internal carotid artery aneurysms (abstract). Proceedings of the 17th International Joint Conference on Stroke and Cerebral Circulation; Phoenix, Arizona, USA; 1992:2.
16. Fox AJ, Vinuela F, Pelz DM, Peerless SJ, Ferguson GG, Drake CG, Debrun G. Use of detachable balloons for proximal artery occlusion in the treatment of unclippable cerebral aneurysms. *J Neurosurg*. 1987;66:40–46.
17. Dandy WE. The treatment of internal carotid aneurysms within the cavernous sinus and the cranial chamber. Report of three cases. *Ann Surg*. 1939;109:689–711.
18. Locksley HB. Report on the Cooperative Study of Intracranial Aneurysms and Subarachnoid Hemorrhage. Section V, Part I and Part II. Natural history of subarachnoid hemorrhage, intracranial aneurysms and arteriovenous malformations. Based on 6368 cases in the Cooperative Study. *J Neurosurg*. 1966;25:219–239, 321–368.
19. Spetzler RF, Carter LP. Revascularization and aneurysm surgery: current status. *Neurosurgery*. 1985;16:111–116.
20. Al-Mefty O, Khalil N, Elwany MN, Smith RR. Shunt for bypass graft of the cavernous carotid artery: an anatomical and technical study. *Neurosurgery*. 1990;27:721–728.
21. Taptas JN. Intradural and extradural ICA (letter-to-editor). *J Neurosurg*. 1979;51:877–878.
22. Taptas, JN. The so-called cavernous sinus: a review of the controversy and its implications for neurosurgeons. *Neurosurgery*. 1982;11:712–717.
23. Johnston I. Direct surgical treatment of bilateral intracavernous internal carotid artery aneurysms. Case report. *J Neurosurg*. 1979;51:98–102.
24. Dolenc V. Direct microsurgical repair of intracavernous vascular lesions. *J Neurosurg*. 1983;58:824–831.
25. Dolenc VV. Surgery of vascular lesion of the cavernous sinus. *Clin Neurosurg*. 1990;36:240–255.

9
Supraclinoid Aneurysms

Aneurysms in this location make up 40% of all aneurysms reported in major clinical series and 24% in anatomical studies. The supraclinoid carotid artery has a complex relationship with the structures that surround it, including the optic nerve, the third cranial nerve, the base of the temporal and frontal lobes, and the cavernous sinus from which it arises.

These aneurysms may be classified in a number of ways, but, traditionally, they are grouped according to their origin from the internal carotid artery (ICA) and the branch near to where they originate. Also, they are classified according to the wall of the ICA from which they originate and the nearest branch junction. Yasargil[1] further subdivided the carotid ophthalmic artery aneurysms into distal medial wall aneurysms, superior wall aneurysms, and inferior wall aneurysms.

Sengupta et al.[2] classified ophthalmic aneurysms based on their relationship to the anterior clinoid process. Eighty-five percent arose medial to the anterior clinoid process and the remainder from the lateral wall. The dome of the aneurysm projected superiorly in 38%, anteriorly in 8%, and posteriorly in 54%. In a study of 2699 aneurysms, Sahs[3] found that 5% of the aneurysms arose from the ophthalmic segment. Apparently, ophthalmic aneurysms have less tendency to bleed, and a substantial portion become giant-sized. In Sahs' series, 75% were over 10 mm in diameter, and over 50% were giant aneurysms.

Yasargil[1] has classified aneurysms of the posterior communicating artery (PComA) as anterolateral, superolateral, posterolateral, posterior (supratentorial), posterolateral infratentorial (infratentorial), and posteromedial inferior in location.

Of all unruptured aneurysms that arise from the supraclinoid portion of the ICA, cranial nerve dysfunction is perhaps the most common focal neurological deficit. When the aneurysm is located near the ophthalmic artery, the second cranial nerve is most often involved. Those located near the PComA most often involve the third cranial nerve, especially if they arise from the posterior or posterolateral wall. Involvement of these cranial nerves is dependent on two major factors: compression and circulatory disorders in the nerve proper.

Anterior choroidal and bifurcation aneurysms project superoposteriorly and inferolaterally in relation to the carotid artery. These aneurysms project near the uncus, and, since they are above the tentorium, they do not contact the third cranial nerve. The aneurysm arises near many short branches of the ICA, and these branches may be found in the fundus or dome of the aneurysm. Carotid bifurcation aneurysms are located superiorly, posteriorly, and inferiorly, and they rarely affect cranial nerves.

Microanatomy of the Supraclinoid Internal Carotid Artery

In 1664, Thomas Willis[4] described the anatomy of the cerebral vasculature. The intradural or supraclinoid portion of the ICA originates as the artery penetrates the anterior portion of the roof of the cavernous sinus and emerges inferomedial to the anterior clinoid process. As the artery enters the supraclinoid space, it courses within the carotid cistern until it bifurcates. The cistern is surrounded by the anterior clinoid process and orbitofrontal lobule superiorly, the roof of the cavernous sinus inferiorly, the wall of the chiasmatic cistern medially, and the free margin of the tentorium and temporal lobe laterally.

The anterior inferior wall of the carotid cistern commonly has a loose attachment to the roof of the cavernous sinus, and approximately 1 or 2 mm of the ICA between the carotid cistern and cavernous sinus may be naked.[1]

Liliequist's membrane usually consists of two layers between the inferior wall of the carotid cistern and superior portion of the interpeduncular cistern. The carotid cistern contains the supraclinoid ICA, the origin

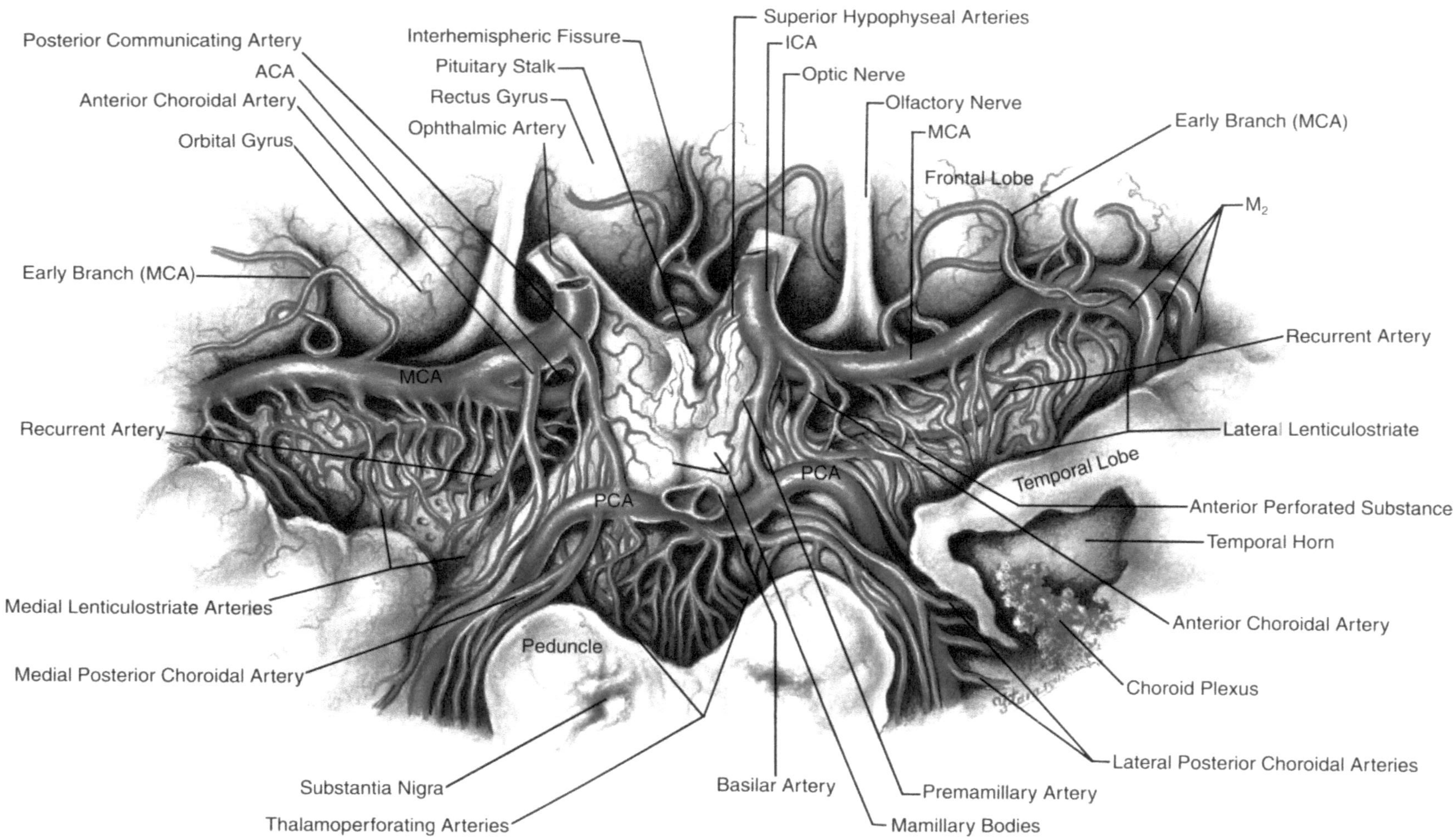

FIGURE 9.1. Basal view of the circle of Willis demonstrating the important small branches affecting the supraclinoid portion of the internal carotid artery (ICA) and the posterior circulation. The superior hypophyseal branches are shown leaving the posterior surface of the internal carotid artery to supply the infundibulum and hypothalamic area. The premamillary arteries are shown originating from the posterior communicating artery. These vessels are also known as anterior thalamoperforating arteries and supply the area between the mamillary body and optic tract. In addition, they supply the anterior thalamus. MCA, middle cerebral artery.

of the PComA, the anterior choroid artery (AChA), and the superior hypophyseal artery and the small branches to the dural covering of the anterior clinoid process (Fig. 9.1).

The supraclinoid ICA emerges below the optic nerve, and then passes posterosuperior to lie lateral to the optic nerve. The artery passes beneath the anterior perforated substance and medial to the sylvian fissure, at which point it divides into the anterior and middle cerebral arteries.

The length of the supraclinoid ICA varies from 14.0 to 25.0 mm, and the average diameter of the artery is 5.0 mm at the proximal part and 4.1 mm in its distal prebifurcation segment. Anomalies of the supraclinoid ICA, including hypoplasia and aplasia of one or both arteries, and abnormal anastomosis via the base of the skull and transsellar area have been reported.[1,5] The autonomic plexus covers the artery. Vasa vasora are present only in the portion proximal to the origin of the ophthalmic artery,[1] but in atherosclerotic cases may extend to the bifurcation of the ICA.

Based on its relationship to the origin of the ophthalmic artery, the supraclinoid ICA may be divided into three segments[6]:

1. The ophthalmic segment lies between the origin of the ophthalmic artery adjacent to the roof of the cavernous sinus and the origin of the PComA. The length of this segment varies from 6.0 to 15.0 mm and is the longest segment of the supraclinoid ICA.
2. The communicating segment lies between the origin of the PComA and the origin of the AChA and is the shortest segment. Rhoton et al.[7] report its length as 1.5 to 9.0 mm.
3. The length of the choroidal segment (between the origin of the AChA and the ICA bifurcation) measures 2.5 to 10.0 mm.

Major Branches of the Supraclinoid ICA

The ophthalmic artery is the first major branch of the supraclinoid ICA. The artery commonly arises at a right angle to the most proximal portion of the supraclinoid ICA, and immediately turns forward and parallel to the ICA (Fig. 9.2).

The artery arises from the ICA below the optic nerve and 2.0 to 10.0 mm medial to the anterior clinoid process[6]. The site of its origin varies from as far as 5.0 mm anterior to 7.0 mm posterior to the tip of the anterior clinoid process. Ordinarily, the artery originates from the ICA anterior to the tip of the anterior clinoid process.

The ophthalmic artery originates from the intradural ICA at a point where the artery leaves the roof of the cavernous sinus in 83%, it originates within 1 mm of this site in 7%, it is partly intradural and partly extradural in 2%, and from the intracavernous portion of the ICA in 8% of the cases.[8]

The artery arises from the superomedial surface of the ICA in 78% and from the middle third of the superior surface in 22%. The ophthalmic artery enters the optic canal immediately after it originates from the ICA in 14%, but in 86% of cases there is a segment of the ophthalmic artery approximately 3.0 mm long exposed proximally to the optic foramen.[9]

The caliber of the ophthalmic artery at its origin is 0.4 to 2.0 mm and it lies inferior to the optic nerve in 60%, medial in 27%, and lateral in 13%; as it passes forward through the optic canal to enter the orbit, it commonly courses anterolaterally.[6] Gibo et al.[6] reported small perforating arteries arising from the ophthalmic artery in two of the 50 ophthalmic arteries examined. These fine branches passed posteriorly to the optic nerve, optic chiasm, and pituitary stalk.

Posterior Communicating Artery

The PComA originates commonly from the midportion of the supraclinoid ICA. The average length of the ICA between the origin of the ophthalmic artery and the origin of the PComA is 9.6 mm, and the distance between the origin of the PComA and the carotid bifurcation is about 9.7 mm. The artery originates from the posteromedial surface of the supraclinoid ICA in 44%, the posterior surface in 30%, the posterolateral surface in 22%, and the medial surface in 4%.[6]

The PComA passes posteromedially below the tubercinerum above the sella turcica, close to the dural covering of the posterior clinoid process; it then joins the posterior cerebral artery (PCA) at the point above and medial to the oculomotor nerve. In the fetal type of PComA, it may course posterolaterally to the oculomotor nerve. In some cases, the artery may attach to the dura of the posterior clinoid process, making its release difficult in some aneurysm operations.

The PComA is suspended from the walls of the cisterns by arachnoid bands, and a sleeve of the arachnoid encases the artery which is continuous with the arachnoid sleeve of the oculomotor nerve.[8] The visualization of the arachnoid compartment of the PComA is feasible after opening Liliequist's membrane. This membrane encloses the superior border of the interpeduncular cistern.

In some cases, the PComA may be seen easily through the opticocarotid triangle. This triangle is formed by the optic nerve medially, the supraclinoid ICA laterally, and the ACA posteriorly.

The average diameter of the PComA varies from 0.4 to 4.0 mm, and the average length from 5.0 to 18 mm. The PComA is a common site of anomalies in the circle of

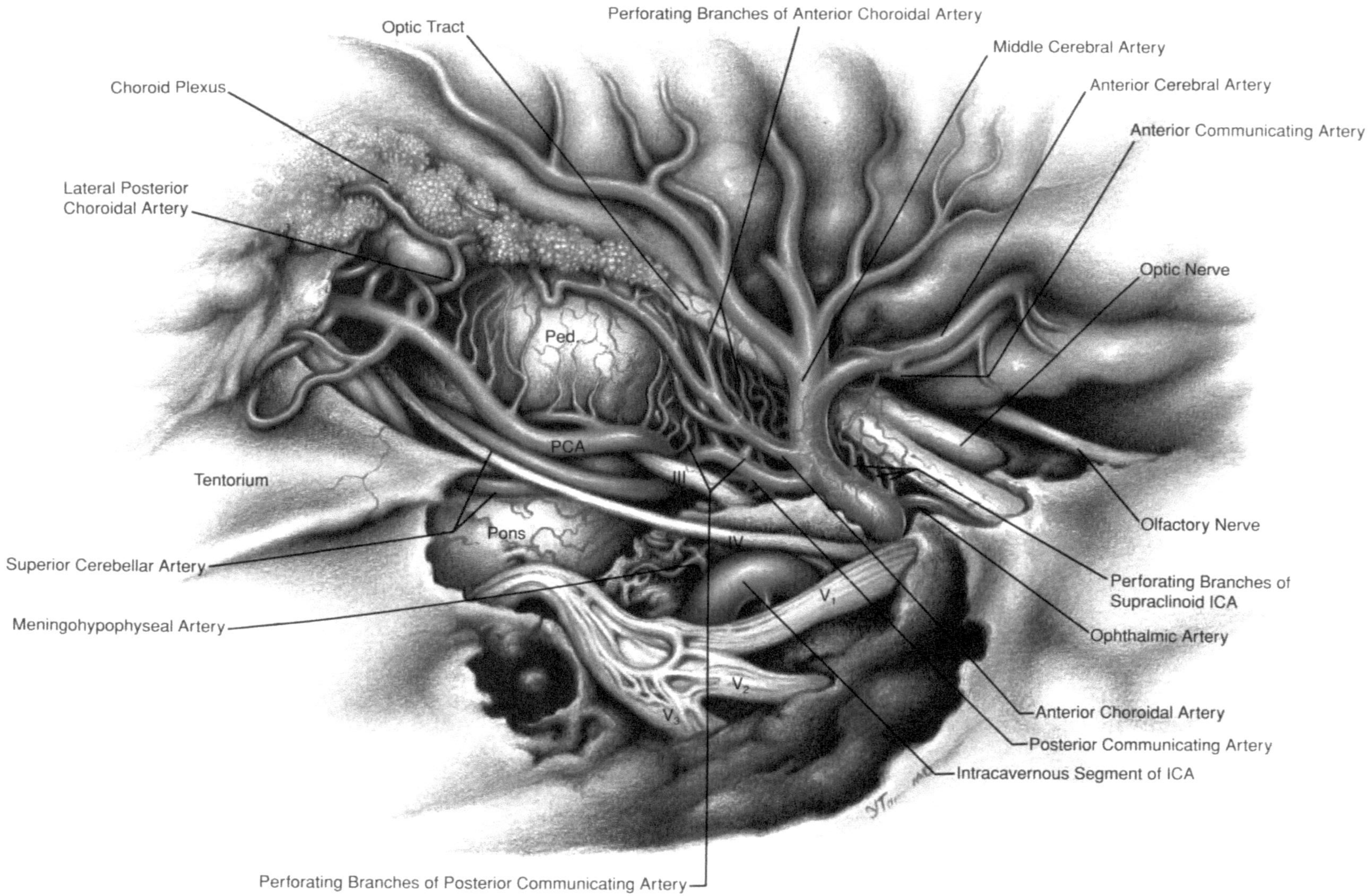

FIGURE 9.2. Lateral view of the supraclinoid portion of the internal carotid artery is shown. The cavernous sinus has been opened to show the course of the ICA beneath the dural folds. This figure demonstrates the perforating arteries and small branches that originate from the ophthalmic artery and the ICA just as it enters the intracranial cavity. Penetrating arteries that originate on the anterior choroidal and posterior communicating arteries are shown. The meningohypophyseal trunk in the cavernous sinus is illustrated.

Willis. During the third stage of Padget's[10] classification (7–12 mm, 31- to 33-day-old embryo) the internal carotid arteries supply the posterior circulation through the PComA. At stage 4 (12–14 mm or 34–36 days old) vertebral arteries have formed and the PComA begins to regress in the posteroanterior direction.[10–12]

The direction of regression of the PComA may explain the presence of the infundibular widening "junctional dilation" at the origin of the artery. Hassler and Saltzman,[13] reported the presence of infundibular dilation in 6.5% of normal angiograms.

There are three types of embryologic patterns in the PComA: (1) a fetal type, in which the caliber of the artery is more than the ipsilateral PCA; (2) an intermediate type, in which both arteries have the same caliber; and (3) an adult type, in which the caliber of the PComA is less than that of the PCA.

In the fetal type, the proximal PCA (P_1) is usually hypoplastic. The incidence of the fetal-type PComA is 15% to 40%. A large PComA is more frequently seen in children than adults.[1]

In Yasargil's[1] report, the PComA was one-third to one-half the size of the ipsilateral PCA in 67.5%, it was equal in caliber to the PCA in 8%, and it was larger than the PCA in 24.5% of the cases. Unilateral and bilateral hypoplasia of the PComA is a common variation in the circle of Willis.[14–16]

Two to 14 perforating arteries originate from the PComA.[1,7,8] They usually arise 2.0 to 3.0 mm from the origin of the PComA. Their diameter varies from 0.1 to 0.6 mm. These small arteries mostly arise from the anterior half of the PComA.[1] Usually, the perforating branches arise from the superior surface of the PComA and pass superomedially to terminate in the tubercinerum, pituitary stalk, mamillary bodies, optic chiasm, optic tract, posterior perforating substance, and interpeduncular fossa.

These branches provide blood supply to the posterior hypothalamus, anterior thalamus, posterior limb of the internal capsule, and subthalamus.

The largest branch of these perforating arteries commonly arises from the middle portion of the PComA to enter the floor of the third ventricle between the mamillary body and optic tract; it is called the anterior thalamoperforating or premamillary artery.

In some cases one or more perforating branches may lie parallel to the PComA. This configuration may be confused with duplication of the PComA, and care must be taken to preserve these perforating arteries during aneurysm surgery.

Anterior Choroidal Artery

The AChA originates from the posterior surface of the supraclinoid ICA, 1.0 to 5.0 mm distal to the origin of the PComA, and 2.0 to 8.0 mm proximal to the ICA bifurcation. In one study, the origin of the AChA in comparison to the origin of the PComA was located laterally in 94%.[7] The AChA is the first branch next to the origin of the PComA in 60% to 68%, but in the remaining cases there are one to three perforating arteries arising from the ICA between the origin of the PComA and origin of the AChA, usually coursing to the anterior perforated substance.[6,7,17]

The initial course of the AChA is behind the ICA and lateral to the optic tract, but it immediately passes posteromedially, below or along the medial side of the optic tract to reach the lateral margin of the cerebral peduncle. The average length of this arterial segment is 12.0 mm. At the point of the anterior margin of the lateral geniculate body, the artery passes posterolaterally, crossing the optic tract. This part of the artery lies within the crural cistern and then passes to a location posteromedial to the uncus. The AChA then courses laterally across the wing of the ambient cistern and finally enters the choroidal fissure and joins the choroid plexus within the supracorneal cleft of the temporal horn immediately posterior to the knee of the temporal horn. The artery continues from this point as a single artery in the medial border of the choroid plexus close to the branches of the lateral posterior choroidal artery, which originates from the posterior cerebral artery; then it courses within the choroid plexus along the floor of the lateral ventricle. It may also extend to the foramen of Monro. The AChA is divided to the cisternal and plexal segment. The cisternal segment is located between the origin of the artery and the choroidal fissure. The average length of this portion of artery is 15 to 35 mm. The diameter of the AChA is 0.7 to 2 mm. Rhoton and associates[7] reviewed the 1421 AChAs that were reported in several articles between 1907 and 1979. The artery originated from the supraclinoid ICA in 97%, from the middle cerebral artery (MCA) in 1%, from the PComA in 1%, and from the ICA bifurcation in 1% of cases. The AChA was duplicated in 4% of cases studied by Saeki and Rhoton.[17] Aplasia of the AChA is extremely rare. Four to 18 perforating arteries originate from the AChA. The caliber of these arteries is from 0.1 to 0.8 mm. The AChA sends branches to the optic tract in 100%, cerebral peduncles in 98%, the uncus in 88%, lateral geniculate body in 74%, anterior perforated substance in 48%, the tip of the temporal lobe in 38%, the hippocampus-dentate gyrus and fornix in 22%, and to the pulvinar in 10%.[7] The perforating arteries arising from the cisternal segment of the AChA, pass laterally in 49%, medially in 30%, superiorly in 16%, and inferiorly in 5%.

The superior branches mostly pass to the anterior and posterior perforated substances, and the proximal group of these branches supplies the medial two-thirds of the globus pallidus and the genu of the internal capsule. The distal group, which originates from the AChA beside the lateral geniculate body, supplies the inferior half of the posterior limb of the internal capsule, the retrolenticular fibers of the internal capsule, and the origin of the optic radiation.

The medial perforating arteries, originating from the cisternal segment of the AChA, supply the substantia nigra, part of the ventroanterior and ventrolateral nuclei of the thalamus, and the anterolateral part of the lateral geniculate body. The lateral and inferior perforating arteries, enter the uncus and temporal lobe to supply the anterior part of the hippocampus, fascia dentata, and amygdaloid nucleus.

The plexal branches of the AChA usually divide and enter the medial border of the choroid plexus of the temporal horn. Sometimes the branches to the choroid plexus originate from the AChA before entering the choroid fissure. There is a well known anastomosis between the branches of the AChA and branches of the PComA, PCA, MCA, and the supraclinoid ICA. The branches of the AChA anastomose with the branches of the lateral posterior choroidal artery on the surface of the choroid plexus; they also anastomose with the branches of the PCA on the lateral surface of the lateral geniculate body and on the temporal lobe near the uncus.

Occlusion of the AChA during vascular surgical procedures has been associated with varying degrees of contralateral hemiplegia, hemianesthesia, and hemianopsia, but in some patients occlusion of the AChA may be tolerated without major complication.

Perforating Branches of the Supraclinoid ICA

About 3 to 16 (average 8.2) small perforating arteries originate directly from the supraclinoid ICA in addition to those arising from the ophthalmic, PComA, and anterior choroidal branches.

The superior hypophyseal arteries are a group of perforating branches that most commonly originate from the posteromedial aspect of the ophthalmic segment of the ICA. They course below the optic nerve, within the carotid and chiasmatic cistern,[8] and terminate on the pituitary stalk and gland, the optic nerve, the optic chiasm, and the floor of the third ventricle. They number one to five. The superior hypophyseal arteries anastomose with similar arteries from the opposite side and with the inferior hypophyseal arteries.

The infundibular arteries are a group of perforating branches that originate from the PComA to terminate on the infundibulum.

The superior hypophyseal and infundibular arteries pass medially to the ventral surface of the optic chiasm and anastomoses around and along the pituitary stalk to form the circuminfundibular anastomosis.[6]

The ascending branches of this arterial plexus supply the inferior surface of the optic chiasm, the median eminence, and the tubercinerum. Some of the descending branches of this plexus are short and penetrate the infundibulum to form capillaries that end at the sinusoids extending down the stalk. Other descending branches are larger and pass down the surface of the pituitary stalk to end on the anterior lobe of the pituitary gland. The superior hypophyseal and the infundibular arteries supply the stalk and the anterior lobe of the pituitary gland, the inferior hypophyseal artery provides blood supply to the posterior lobe, and the capsular artery supplies the capsule of the pituitary gland.

Perforating arteries originating from the communicating segment of the supraclinoid ICA were seen in 40% of the cadaver specimens examined by Gibo and associates.[6] They found one to three of these branches arising from the posterior wall of the ICA. These branches terminate on the optic tract, the premamillary part of the floor of the third ventricle, the optic chiasm, the infundibulum, and the anterior perforated substance.

The choroidal segment of the supraclinoid ICA is the most frequent site of origin of perforating arteries. They originate most commonly from the posterior surface of the ICA between the origin of the AChA and ICA bifurcation. Their number varies from one to nine, and they enter the anterior perforated substance, the optic tract, and the uncus.

Clinical Signs

Headache, described in the retroorbital area, is a common presentation. Others present with visual loss, either in one eye or both. Ferguson and Drake[18], found visual disorders in 32% of their cases. In some patients, the visual loss occurred in both eyes.

Day[19] defined two types of aneurysms that may arise near the ophthalmic segment. The ophthalmic artery aneurysm arises superiorly and projects superomedially toward the lateral half of the optic nerve, just distal to the ophthalmic artery origin. The lateral aspect of the nerve is usually uplifted and displaced medially. The superior hypophyseal artery aneurysm arises from the ventromedial surface of the ICA near the posterior aspect of the carotid ring in close association with the perforating arteries entering the sella. These lesions may appear purely ventral on lateral angiography. The aneurysm may extend and erode the wall, creating a deformity in the lateral sella wall. This is the paraclinoid variant. This variant is not usually associated with visual symptoms since expansion occurs lateral to the chiasm. Ophthalmic aneurysms cause medial displacement of the nerve against the sharp falciform ligament, located laterally. Thus, the early visual field loss is in the inferior nasal quadrant. A superior temporal quadrant defect in the opposite eye may occur if the knee of Wildbrand is compressed. Large aneurysms arising from the superior hypophyseal segment may project medially where they impact upon the chiasm, causing bitemporal field defects. Day has succinctly described the visual defects associated with aneurysms arising in this segment. Unilateral field loss is almost always attributable to an aneurysm.

Unruptured aneurysms of the AChA usually produce no clinical signs. Aneurysms of the AChA may attain large size before they produce symptoms, which may consist of convulsive seizures, often involving the temporal lobe. The clinical signs caused by aneurysms occupying this arterial segment depend upon many variables, including whether they have ruptured, the rate of bleeding, the size of the hematoma produced, and its location. In 80% of patients, subarachnoid hemorrhage (SAH) is the only variant. Others have cerebro-SAH with hematoma formation.

In Yasargil's[1] series, subdural hematomas were encountered in 17 of 23 patients with hemorrhage. In eight of these, the hematoma was located exclusively in the subarachnoid space, while in nine it also involved cerebral substance.

Subarachnoid Hemorrhage

When hemorrhage is massive, clots may form in the basal cisterns. Usually, clots involve the interpeduncular system and ambient cisterns, but they may involve their counterpart on the contralateral side. Clinical signs depend greatly on the massiveness of the clot in the basal cistern, which may be responsible for both vasospasm and hydrocephalus. The clot usually projects more toward one side, which may explain the unilateral vasospasm that is occasionally seen. In high-grade patients, the hematoma usually dissects into the basal cisterns, producing vasospasm in the vertebrobasilar system. In 60% of the patients, the clinical course is stable, and patients remain compensated in low clinical grade throughout their acute interval. In 20%, however, complications such as hydrocephalus and vasospasm intervene. Clinical condition deteriorates into stupor, and, in approximately 20%, coma is present, the patient deteriorates due to intracranial hypertension, and herniation may occur. Patients arriving severely ill and moribund may further deteriorate during the next few days as complications manifest. To manage these complications effectively, prompt and accurate diagnosis is essential.

Cerebro-SAH Hemorrhage

Cerebro-SAH with hematoma formation creates a distinctive computed tomography (CT) pattern in patients with supraclinoid aneurysms. The hematoma develops in the frontal lobe and is directed toward the frontal horn of the lateral ventricle into which it may rupture, especially with aneurysms that arise from the anterior surface of the ICA and the carotid artery bifurcation. Aneurysms that project posteriorly produce hematomas that dissect into the temporal horn, sylvian fissure, and temporal lobe proper. Cerebro-SAH characteristically produces higher-grade patients in poorer neurological condition than do aneurysms that are associated with SAH only. Those associated with small cerebro-SAH hematomas, less than 50 ml, may be less severely affected, however. Patients with larger hematomas, measuring greater than 100 ml, are always in higher grades with stupor or coma. Both generalized and focal neurological signs appear. Of those producing focal cortical or subcortical pressure, speech disorders, hemiparesis, and hemianopsia may appear. Mild hemorrhages into the subarachnoid space may produce only headaches and third cranial nerve deficits.[20] Yasargil[1] found 43% to also involve the third cranial nerve when the aneurysm had ruptured.

Surgical Options

Because of difficulties that have been occasioned by location and size, a large number of surgical approaches and techniques have been devised for management of aneurysms arising from the supraclinoid segment. Since this is the most common aneurysm considered for direct surgical clipping, many variations are seen. In the best configuration of anatomy and good clinical grade, the results of clipping of aneurysms of the supraclinoid segment are excellent. The choice of any particular operation depends on many factors, including the size of the aneurysm, its projection from the parent artery, the condition of the parent vessel, and the aneurysm neck.

The results of surgery in this region are not always as successful as suggested by first impression, particularly when the lesion to be obliterated is large or giant, or if it occurs in older individuals. Aneurysms in this location, especially when associated with stiffness or friability of the parent artery, comma may result in tearing of the aneurysm from its origin or tearing into the trunk of the parent artery. Aneurysms arising from the PComA junction may actually arise in a location that makes clipping difficult because of their proximal takeoff in relation to the anterior clinoid process or the cranial base. Aneurysms arising medially along the carotid surface and projecting beneath the optic nerve or chiasm may present an especially difficult challenge for aneurysm neck exposure. All these difficulties combined make occlusion of the ICA, after preocclusion testing, more appropriate and safer for some aneurysms in this segment.

Evaluation of the collateral circulation is an important

adjunct in planning surgery for aneurysms in this location. Test occlusion is safe and reliable for assessing adequacy of the collateral circulation of the supraclinoid segment. For this, a number of procedures have proved successful. Balloon occlusion with clinical testing, balloon occlusion with single photon emission computed tomography (SPECT) and/or clinical testing and blood flow measurements, and both balloon occlusion with transcranial Doppler (TCD) sonography and Matas/TCD have been used effectively to lower the risk of ischemic deficits after permanent occlusion. Occlusion of aneurysms in this location using coils and/or balloons may be preferred when direct surgical access is limited by the cranial base or contiguous eloquent structures. Both balloon catheters and tracker catheters may be employed with relative ease along the supraclinoid segment. Using these methods, the functional significance of the parent vessel may be estimated, the relationship of the parent vessel to the orifice evaluated, and the size of the aneurysm neck measured in relation to the balloon or other device that will be introduced into it. However, the choice of the operative procedure, either direct or indirect, and the many variants of each depend mainly on the patient's condition, the stage in the disease, the patient's age, and the experience of the surgeon. During the acute hemorrhagic period, endovascular or direct operations may be employed with consistently good results in compensated patients. Only in patients with significant intracranial hematomas is emergency operation warranted with evacuation of the clot, decompression of the brain, and clipping of the aneurysm. During the so-called cold phase, all methods, including endovascular and direct, may be employed with much better success rates. Table 9.1 compares the methods of treatment for supraclinoid aneurysms using endovascular procedures, direct operations, test occlusion, and combined approaches.

TABLE 9.1. Surgical alternatives with supraclinoid aneurysms

Location of aneurysm	Direct operation	Endovascular operation	Test occlusion	Combined operation
Ophthalmic				
Small	+	+	−	±
Large	±	+	+	±
Giant	±	+	+	±
Posterior communication, anterior choroidal				
Small	+	−	±	−
Large	±	+	+	+
Giant	±	+	+	+
Bifurcation				
Small	+	+	+	−
Large	+	+	+	+
Giant	+	+	+	+

Multiple Aneurysms

The surgical tactics for managing intracranial aneurysms in various locations are described in their respective chapters. Aneurysms occurring on multiple vessels of the arterial tree, however, also require unique management skills and philosophy. The following tactics are listed here although, admittedly, multiple aneurysms may be found proportionately in much greater frequency on other vascular segments.

1. The aneurysm responsible for the SAH must be excluded from the arterial circulation.
2. The largest aneurysm visible is commonly the aneurysm responsible for SAH.
3. A surgical approach should be developed to permit the exclusion of the most dangerous aneurysms from the arterial circulation, provided that the operative exposure entails reasonable risks.
4. Following recent SAH, dissection along the arterial tree may precipitate cerebral vasospasm and other complications.
5. Secondary operations on nonbleeding aneurysms may be carried out later, when the patient's condition is stable.
6. Multilobular aneurysms rupture and bleed more frequently than smooth, round-walled aneurysms. These should be treated after the aneurysm responsible for SAH. The risk of rebleeding and death from this cause must be weighed in each case against the risk associated with the operative clipping. Small aneurysms, less than 5 mm in diameter, especially if found in older individuals, may not need operative clipping.

Direct Approaches

Frontal, frontotemporal, and frontolateral approaches have been employed for aneurysms arising from the supraclinoid portion of the ICA. In 1930, Dott[21] described a frontal approach to a giant aneurysm, first diagnosed angiographically. In 1932, Trevani[22] described a wide temporal approach to what he thought was tumor, which later was found to be a giant supraclinoid aneurysm. In 1938, Dandy,[23] perhaps the first to use a metallic clip for neck occlusion of an aneurysm, described a frontolateral approach. More recently, pterional approaches have been favored with some variation in technique offered by individual surgeons. This approach has been described in Chapter 6.

Orbitocranial approaches have also been used for exposing aneurysms of the ophthalmic segment. Since the ophthalmic aneurysm is partly covered by the clinoid process, high-speed air drills are required for better viewing of the neck in relationship to its parent vessel. In patients with supraclinoid aneurysms that project superiorly, controlling the proximal circulation in the ICA is also a necessity to prevent massive bleeding, should premature rupture occur. The proximal ICA may be managed in a number of ways also. If the aneurysm arises distally on the supraclinoid segment, temporary clipping of the intracranial ICA may be achieved. Distal clipping, beyond the aneurysm, of the A_1 and M_1 may also be required. Proximal control for aneurysms that arise beneath the clinoid process and are obscured by this structure must be managed using other methods. Transcutaneous pressure applied to the ICA in the neck or surgical exposure of the ICA in the neck with temporary placement of umbilical tapes is preferred but, the ICA may be occluded in the neck by percutaneous placement of a balloon catheter. Tamaki and co-workers[24] describe an interesting method in which a "trapping" evacuation technique was employed. In this method, the catheter also contains a lumen to which suction may be applied, evacuating the parent artery and aneurysm. To provide decompression for a giant aneurysm, Scott[25] employed a double-lumen occlusion balloon catheter. The distal carotid artery is temporarily clipped proximal to the PComA. The trapped vessel segment, including the aneurysm, is decompressed by aspiration through the catheter. This maneuver collapses the aneurysm, allowing easier dissection and clipping. Among 12 patients, there was one complication consisting of monocular blindness.

Percutaneous techniques, although less invasive, carry an inherent risk for thromboembolic and hemorrhagic complications and for complications related to dissections.

Ophthalmic Aneurysms

The ophthalmic segment aneurysm may occupy the anteromedial triangle of the cavernous sinus. Exposure of these aneurysms requires extensive bony openings, preferably from an intradural approach. To unroof and completely free the optic nerve from its canal and displace it medially, the approach must begin in the floor of the frontal fossa along the medial surface of the nerve. The nerve should be moved for the exposure of aneurysms whose origin is the medial surface of the carotid artery, especially if they arise in the cavernous sinus.

Good relaxation is essential and a spatula should be placed between the frontal lobe and the high-speed drill. In some cases, the spatula must be used to isolate and cover the medial surface of the aneurysm and drilling of the optic canal; all loose material, such as strings and cotton pledgets, must be removed before the drill is used. We use a Midas Rex drill with a diamond point. In order to insulate the shaft, a red rubber catheter of appropriate size is passed over the shaft of the drill, cutting the catheter on a slant so that only the drill point will be exposed. The shaft is covered by the red rubber catheter and is therefore less apt to enwrap loose tissue or suture.

The initial incision into the frontal fossa dura is

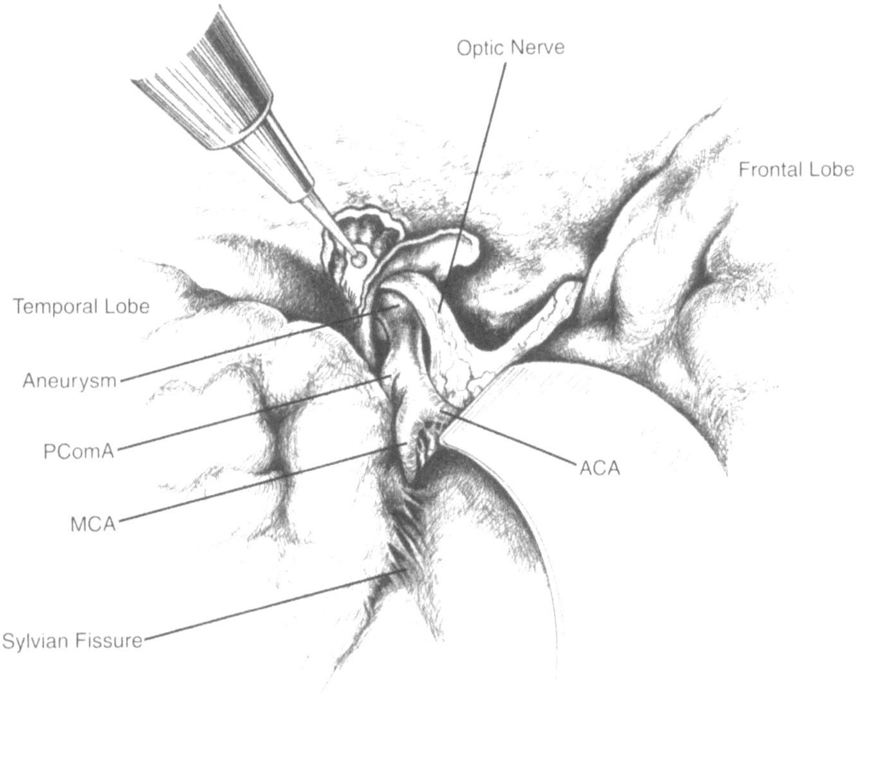

FIGURE 9.3. Pterional view of a left internal carotid artery aneurysm arising from the ophthalmic segment. The dura overlying the optic canal has been incised to create a semicircular flap that covers the aneurysm and optic nerve while the anterior clinoid process and optic canal are drilled. The optic canal is opened superiorly, laterally, and medially so that the nerve can be displaced medially to expose the aneurysm. The dural flap covers and protects these structures during the drilling. ACA, anterior cerebral artery; PComA, posterior communicating artery.

lunar shaped, beginning laterally over the lateral portion of the carotid artery, swinging anteriorly for about 1.5 cm, and then posteriorly again over the medial border of the optic nerve. This half-moon–shaped piece of dura is then reflected posteriorly, covering the aneurysm and carotid artery. The optic canal should be drilled first, extending as far as possible into the frontal floor. Medially, the optic strut separating the nerve from the carotid artery should be removed in its superior one-third. Drilling the anterior clinoid process invariably causes bleeding from major venous channels that drain into the cavernous sinus. Small pieces of collagen sponge may be placed into these vessels using up pointing forceps, effectively controlling bleeding. Any remaining fragments of bone representing the anterior clinoid process or optic canal can be removed with a small punch and microcurettes.

The proximal part of the optic nerve is covered by a dural fold, the falciform ligament; this serves to protect the nerve from the drill. The diamond burr generates heat, however, and it is necessary to keep it well irrigated during the drilling process. The drilling exposes the proximal 5 to 6 mm of the optic nerve in the canal. Afterward, the drilling is extended laterally, toward the lateral border of the clinoid process (Fig. 9.3). The superior border of the cavernous sinus may extend to this region. After severing the anterior attachment of the clinoid to the frontal floor, the remaining loose pieces can be dissected free with curettes and sharp microdissectors. The carotid ring comes into view after the last portions of the canal and clinoid are removed. This ring makes up the superior boundary of the cavernous sinus. It surrounds the artery obliquely. A ring of bone, representing a connection between the anterior and middle clinoid process may surround the carotid as it becomes intradural, but the posterior wall is ordinarily made up by the cavernous sinus. The artery may also be covered by periosteum as it emerges. The third cranial nerve abuts and may groove the carotid as it enters the cavernous sinus anteriorly. If the cavernous sinus is entered during drilling or dissection, bleeding may be controlled easily with Gelfoam and by elevating the head. Occasionally, the bleeding can be so brisk as to suggest aneurysm rupture.

Clips should ultimately be placed parallel to the parent artery with the blades directed posteriorly toward the branches. Clip blades that are forced forward and anteriorly are more apt to cause carotid artery compromise (Fig. 9.4). Wide opening of the optic canal allows medial displacement of the optic nerve but without undue traction, thus exposing those medial aneurysms that arise from the superior hypophyseal artery junction. Still, some of these aneurysms must be clipped from a more superior approach, using a fenestrated clip passed over the carotid artery.

Occasionally, the cavernous sinus must be opened to clip an aneurysm that partly arises in this structure. The ophthalmic artery and the superior hypophyseal artery both emerge in close association with the ring of folded dura, usually slightly above it. The dura may be extremely thin at the base of this ring and the anterior loop of the ICA may be visualized in the anteromedial triangle. Aneurysms that arise from the ophthalmic artery junction almost invariably project superiorly while elevating the anterior lateral aspects of the optic nerve (Fig. 9.5).

For aneurysms that arise deep in the cavernous sinus, the superior wall may be advanced slightly over the cavernous sinus with cautery and coagulation. Avateen (collagen) sponge and Surgicel effectively stop bleeding if the head is elevated slightly, allowing the cavernous sinus adjacent to the artery to be opened and compressed downward. Minor venous bleeding can thus be controlled simultaneously as the neck of the aneurysm is further developed for clipping.

Posterior Communicating Artery Aneurysms

The typical aneurysm in this location arises with a small neck that projects laterally or posterolaterally, leaving the carotid artery slightly distal to the takeoff of the posterior communicating branch. Atypically, the neck may arise from the circumference of the ICA or, alternatively, the aneurysm may be fusiform. The dome ordinarily extends laterally or posterolaterally toward the free margin of the tentorium. The dome may come to rest either below (usual) or above this free margin, but, alternatively, the free margin may divide the aneurysm into lobes. Usually, the third cranial nerve plays some role in the anatomical relationships of the PComA aneurysm. It may rest on the dome, splayed and flattened, or above or below the main mass. The dome may extend and be covered by the cortex of the medial temporal lobe.

The surgical approach must be tailored to accommodate any peculiar anatomical relationships of the aneurysm to the brain and to the status of the anticipated operative field. In the acute case, within a few days of SAH onset, tightness, edema, and fresh hematoma in the subarachnoid pathways should be expected. Spinal drainage with the option of direct ventricular drainage should be considered and opening of the sylvian fissure in its anterior extent may be required to visualize the aneurysm. The surgeon should be prepared to extend the patient's head in order to better visualize the contents of the basal cisterns. Retractors should first be placed along the base of the frontal lobes, and the frontal lobe should

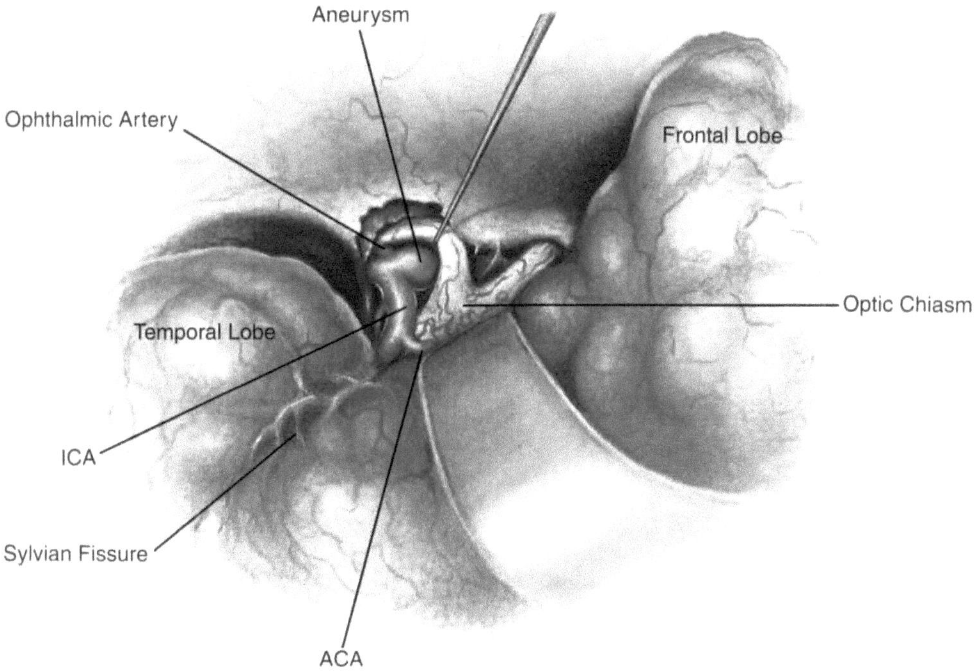

A

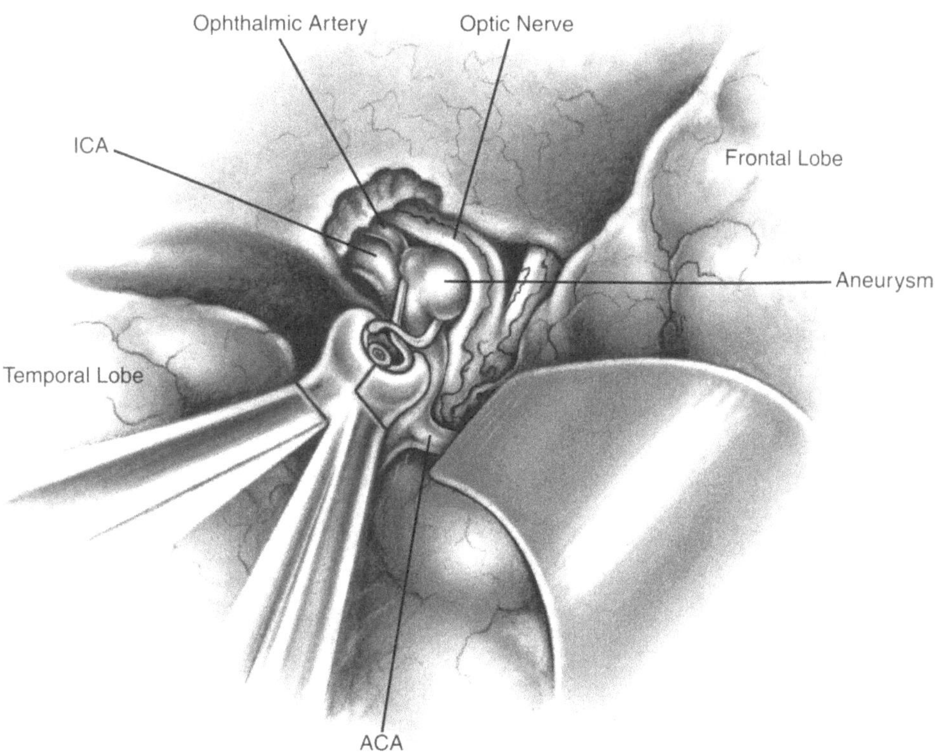

B

FIGURE 9.4. (A) Aneurysm of the ophthalmic segments projecting medially and inferior to the left optic nerve, the most common position for aneurysm in this location. The ophthalmic artery is visualized after the anterior clinoid process and optic nerve have been exposed. The dural ring surrounding the carotid artery must be removed to demonstrate this anatomy. (B) Further isolation of the aneurysm results in application of a clip, which should be placed parallel to the internal carotid artery. Preferably, the clip blades project posteriorly to permit adequate viewing.

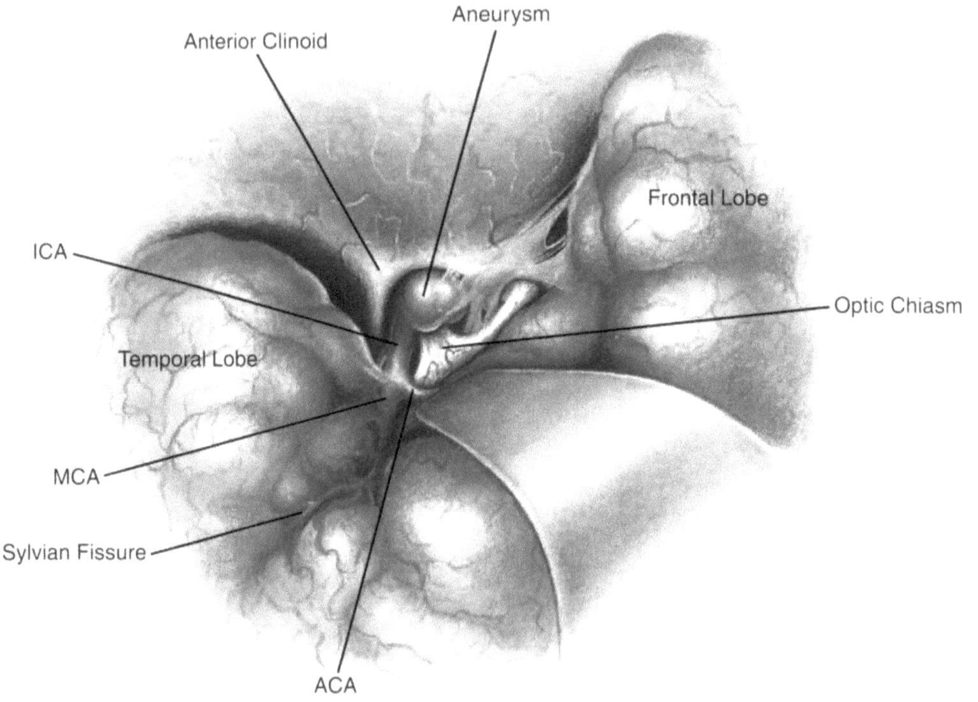

A

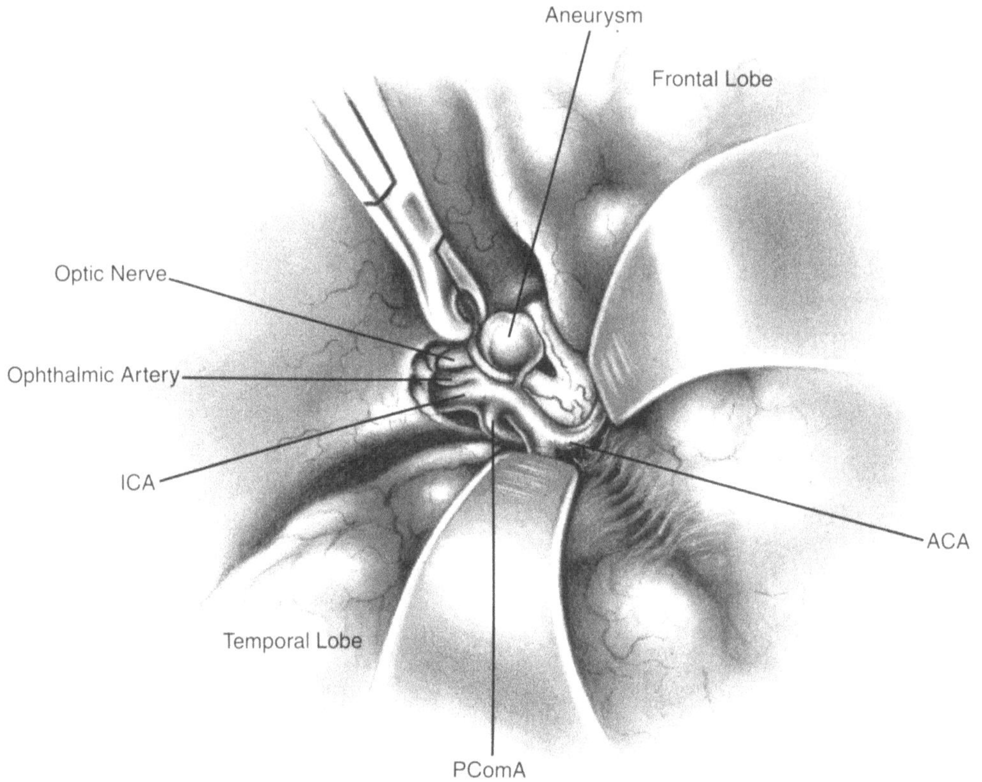

B

FIGURE 9.5. (A) An aneurysm arising from the superior ophthalmic segment and extending superior to the left optic nerve is shown. The anterior clinoid partly covers the dome of the aneurysm and must be removed to adequately expose the neck. (B) Superior ophthalmic segment aneurysm after removal of the anterior clinoid process. The clip blades do not approximate after release.

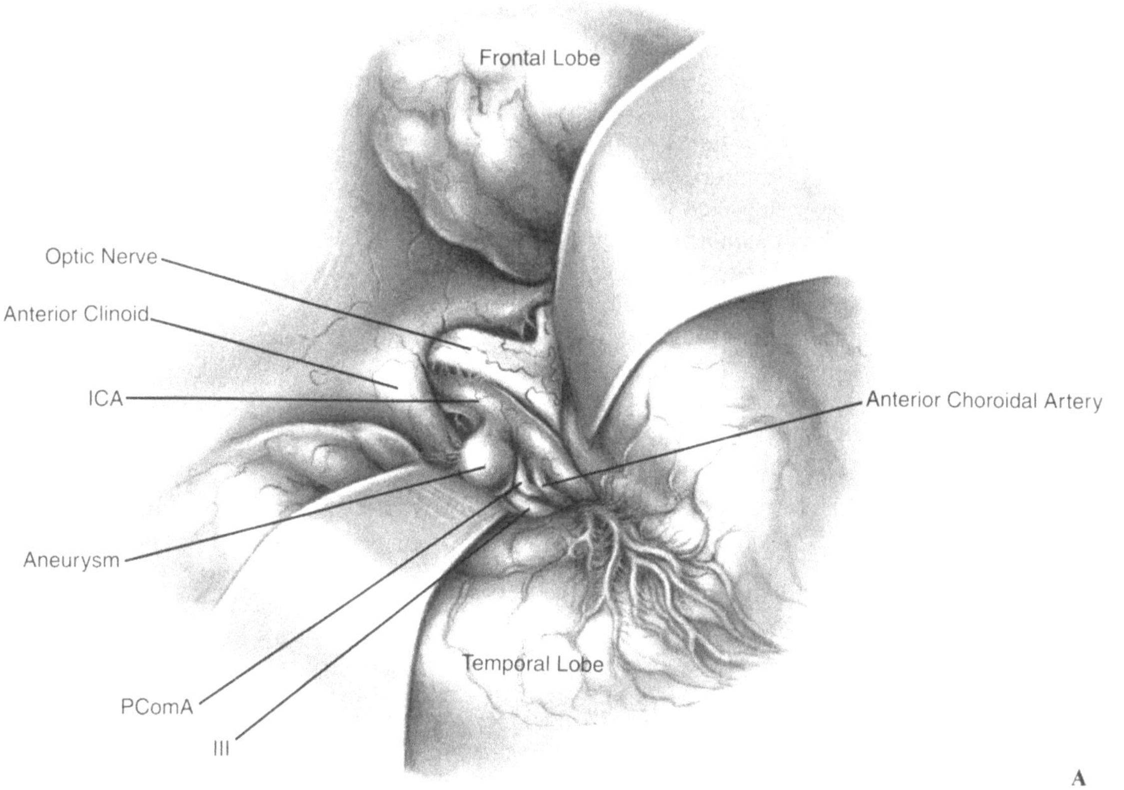

A

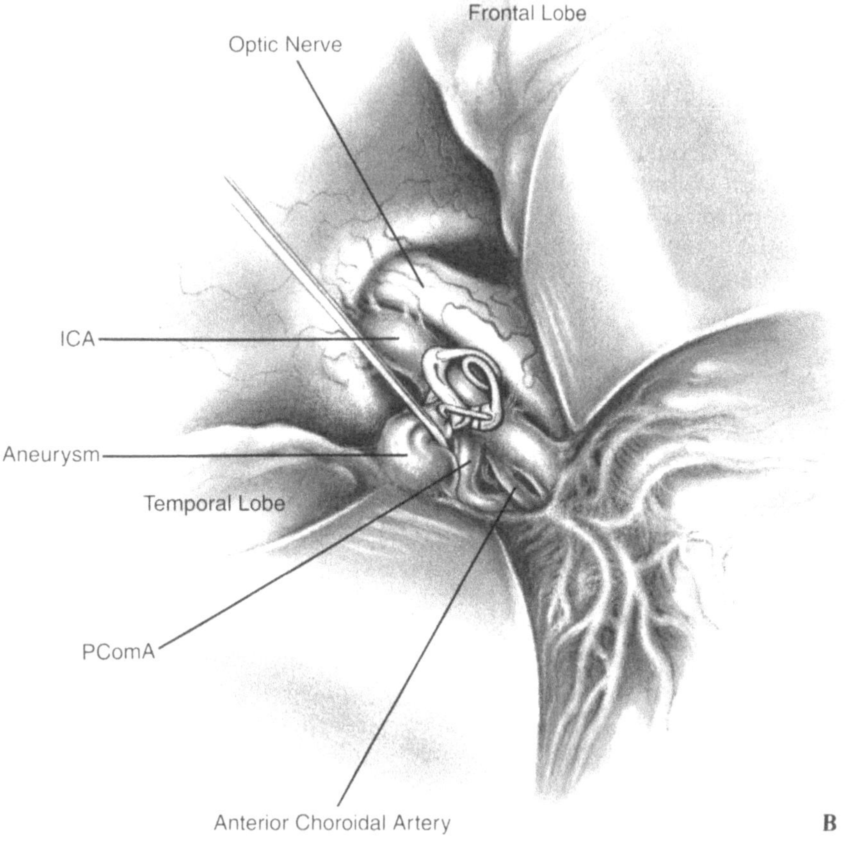

B

FIGURE 9.6. (A) Pterional craniotomy and exposure of an aneurysm arising from the posterior communicating segment of the ICA. The anterior choroidal artery arises a few millimeters distally. The third cranial nerve is usually in contact with the dome of the posterolateral projecting aneurysm. (B) The aneurysm has been dissected free of the posterior communicating branch and the clip applied along the neck.

be elevated until the olfactory nerve can be identified. Moving posteriorly along the olfactory nerve, the entry of the optic nerve into the optic canal can be seen with only a few millimeters of dissection. Using fine bipolar coagulation forceps, the arachnoid covering the optic nerve is opened and cerebrospinal fluid (CSF) allowed to escape. The optic nerve can be distinguished from the ICA by its more yellow color and the presence of vessels along its surface. The arachnoidal opening is extended with microscissors into the prechiasmatic cistern, achieving further decompression. Brain retractors can now be placed in the sylvian crease, which may require opening in the patient with brain tightness. Self-retaining retractors free a hand so that both traction and dissection can be carried out simultaneously, while the assistant only applies the suction, which has been adjusted to the lowest setting. This retractor should be placed more laterally to expose the dorsal surface of the ICA. The optic nerve, anterior clinoid process, and carotid artery form a W at the cranial base. Using the microbipolar cautery, the arachnoid is opened along the dorsal surface and retracted laterally to visualize the lateral and posterior surface of the carotid artery.

Temporary clipping of the proximal carotid artery may be used to avert premature rupture of the aneurysm. However, since an unknown quantity of dissection is still a major probability at this point, mild reduction in mean arterial blood pressure to 60 to 70 mm Hg usually provides a more pliant artery and aneurysm, thus avoiding the risk of ischemic complications associated with prolonged clipping. The aneurysm should not be touched until both sides of the neck have been adequately exposed. Using microdissectors and suction, gentle retraction is placed on the neck to discover the position of the PComA branch and the third cranial nerve. The fundus is spared any dissection until all of the proximal neck and parent artery have been isolated. Temporary clips may be applied to the proximal ICA if needed or if further dissection will be required.

A straight or angled clip is usually needed to isolate the aneurysm neck and spare the PComA branch. In applying the clip, the blade may butt against the cranial base beneath the aneurysm, preventing full enclosure of the neck (Fig. 9.6). In such cases, an angled clip with a "knee" may pass around it and extend along the floor parallel to the artery. The clip blade should be just long enough to encompass the neck without extending far into the interpeduncular fossa. The aneurysm should be soft enough to allow manipulation of the neck and proximal fundus to visualize the PComA and the third cranial nerve. If either is involved in the clip, it should be gently opened until the vessel/nerve can be extracted. Occasionally, the nerve will be found to be flattened along the surface of the fundus. Its recovery does not seem to be contingent upon removal from this compromising attachment.

After the clip has been applied, the fundus should be inspected for pulsations. Opening the fundus is not necessary to demonstrate complete separation from the arterial circulation.

Anterior Choroidal Artery Aneurysms

Aneurysms of the AChA are located posteriorly, inferiorly, and laterally to the origin of this vessel. Commonly, the aneurysm in this location involves the artery itself, and this becomes much more complex when there are multiple origins of the AChA. Also, the approach to this aneurysm may lead to damage of the sixth cranial nerve because the dome of this aneurysm may project toward the entry of the sixth cranial nerve into the cavernous sinus. The AChA may also be damaged or injured by aneurysms and by surgical treatment of aneurysms that involve the PComAs since the AChA may project along its course quite near to the PComA. A pterional approach may be used for this aneurysm. A wide opening of the sylvian fissure is to be recommended because often this aneurysm will attach itself to the lateral surface of the temporal lobe. Retraction of the temporal lobe therefore may precipitate premature bleeding from the vessel or aneurysm. The ICA and its branches must be well visualized and dissected free prior to the application of a clip. Also, because of the juxtaposition of this aneurysm to the sixth cranial nerve, this structure should be visualized before clipping (Fig. 9.7).

Aneurysms of the Carotid Artery Bifurcation

Aneurysms in this location make up less than 10% of all those that occur on the anterior circulation. Although this aneurysm occasionally projects slightly toward the anterior cerebral artery, virtually all these aneurysms project superiorly or slightly posterior from the bifurcation point. These aneurysms are located at the point where the carotid artery and the cisterns of the lamina terminalis and sylvian fissure meet. The perforating vessels usually lie on the deep aspect of the aneurysm. In approaching aneurysms at this location, opening the sylvian fissure is usually required. The fissure is covered, in part, by the superficial sylvian vein. The orbital basal part of the frontal lobe may partly encase the aneurysm (Fig. 9.8).

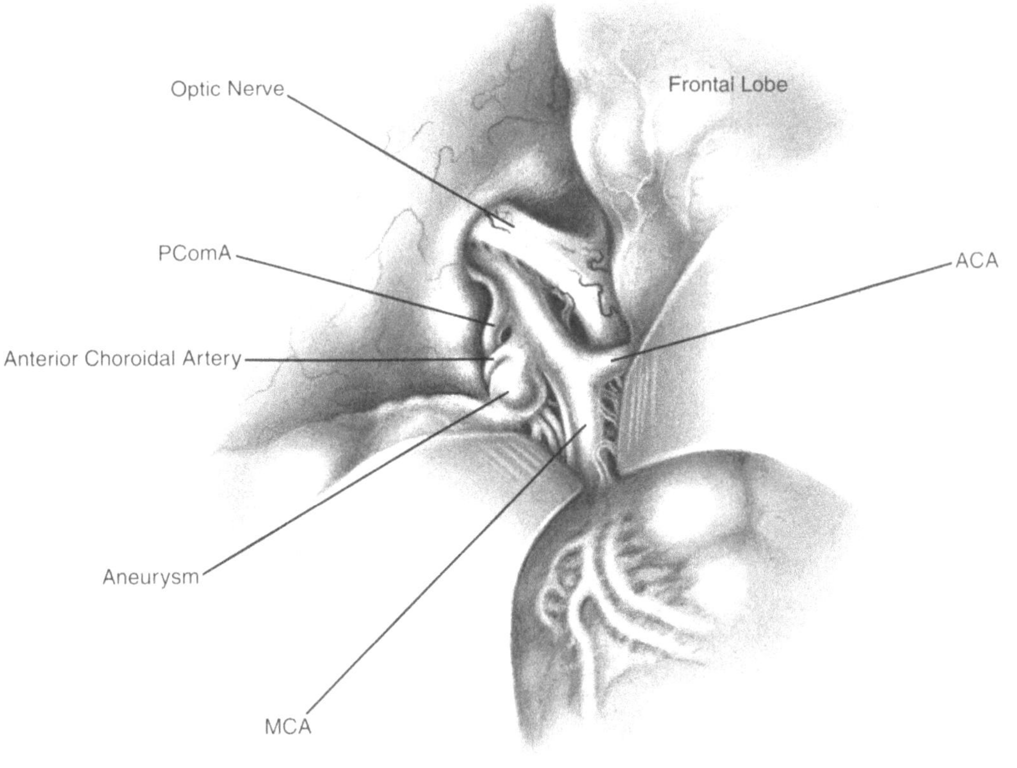

A

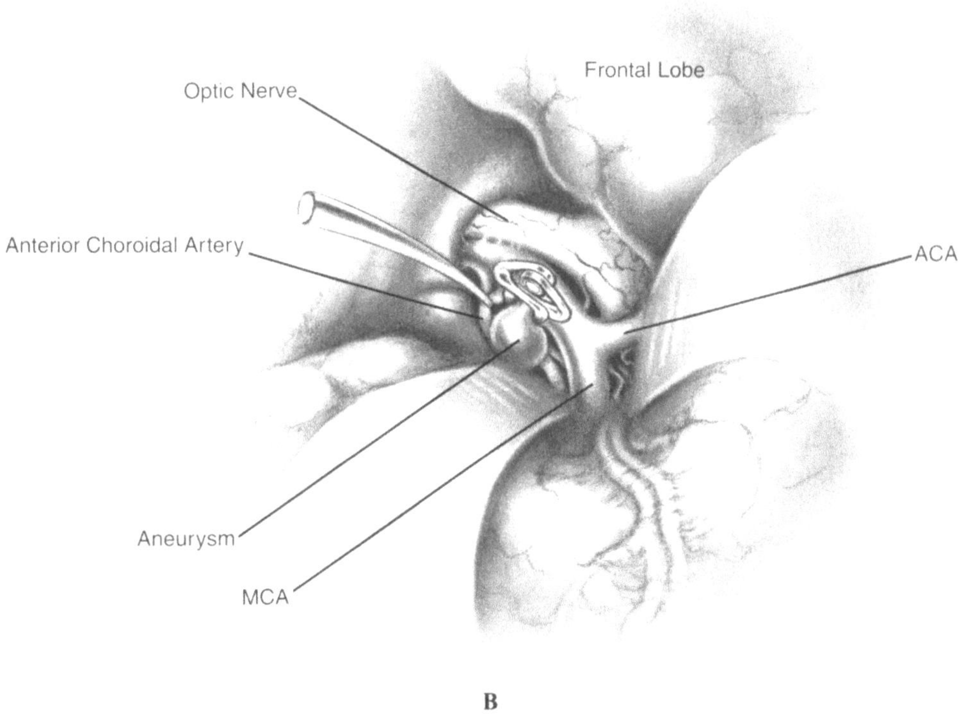

B

FIGURE 9.7. (A) Anterior choroidal artery aneurysm arising from the junction with the ICA. Distal anterior choroidal branches pass posterior to the dome of the aneurysm. (B) After retracting the anterior choroidal artery to identify the artery and its distal branches, a clip is applied.

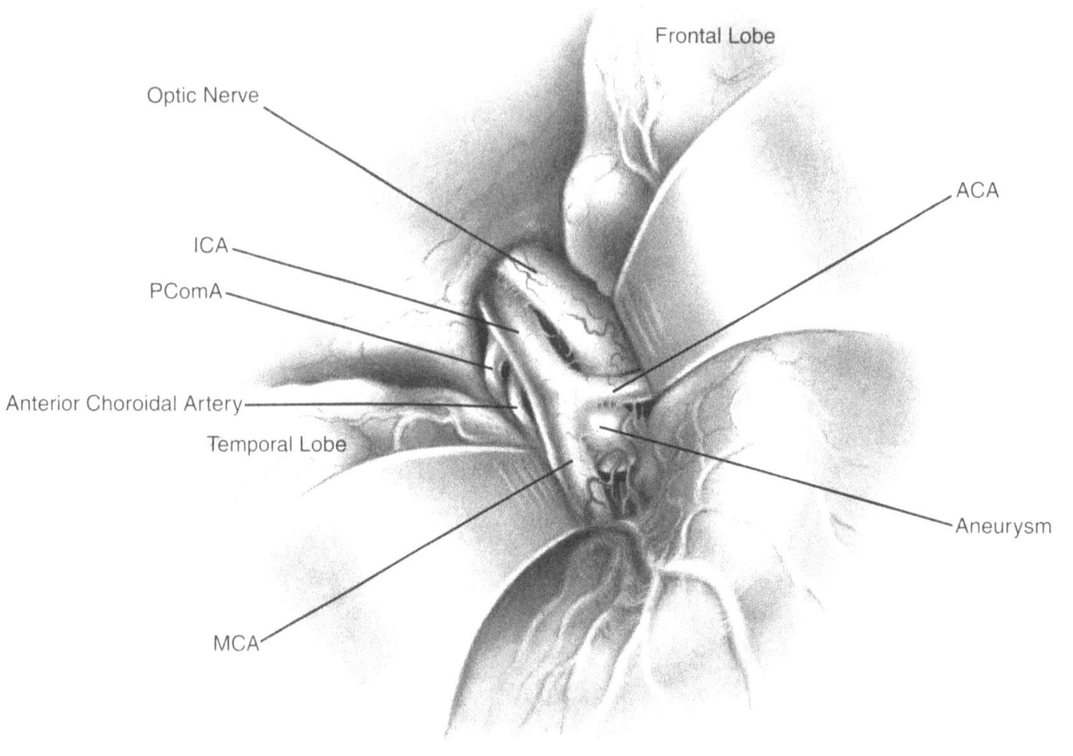

A

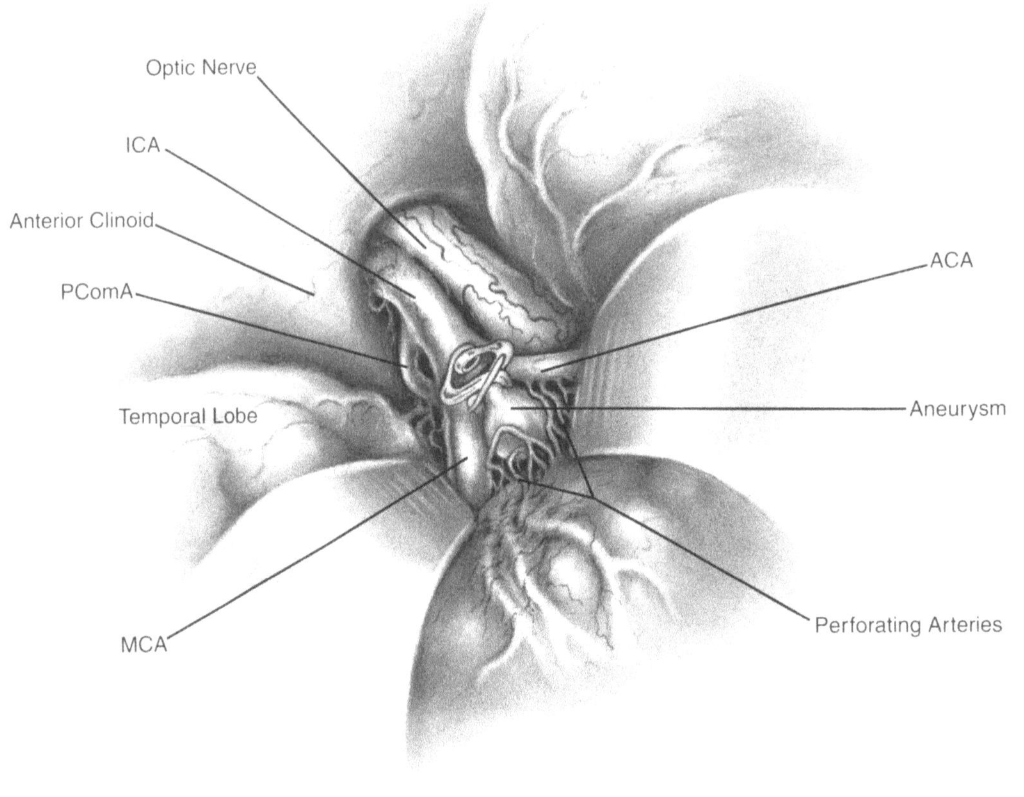

B

FIGURE 9.8. (A) Pterional approach to a left bifurcation aneurysm is shown. The aneurysm arises from the junction of the A_1 and M_1 branches. (B) The important perforating vessels that originate along the posterior surface of the internal carotid artery at the bifurcation are shown after application of a clip.

Endovascular Operations for Supraclinoid Aneurysms

The supraclinoid aneurysm is perhaps the best suited of all aneurysms for management using the innovative techniques recently developed. Aneurysms of the supraclinoid portion of the ICA arise preferentially at certain sites (i.e., at the takeoff of the ophthalmic, posterior communicating, or anterior choroidal artery branches or at the bifurcation). Aneurysms at each site must be evaluated individually, however, for endovascular therapy. Before the surgeon elects an endovascular procedure over a direct approach or decides on a specific endovascular operation, the functional significance of the parent artery from which the aneurysm arises must be estimated. The terminal distribution of the artery and any neurological deficit that would result from its closure must be anticipated. All possible complications must be kept in clear focus. Of importance to the outcome are the results of occlusion of an ophthalmic artery or the short branches of any major artery that may supply the internal capsule, midbrain, or thalamus. During the endovascular procedure, termination of the operation may be necessary in order to avert complications, and test occlusions are therefore an important part of the endovascular procedure.

Prior to any operation being contemplated, the endovascular surgeon, like the direct surgeon, must have a clear understanding of the hemodynamics of the arterial tree. He must know if vasospasm is present, if good collateral circulation is present, and if there are distal infarcts or abnormalities in cerebral blood flow. Prior to definitive occlusion of the aneurysm, all complications of the acute period must be dealt with individually. Hydrocephalus, syndrome of inappropriate antidiuretic

A

B

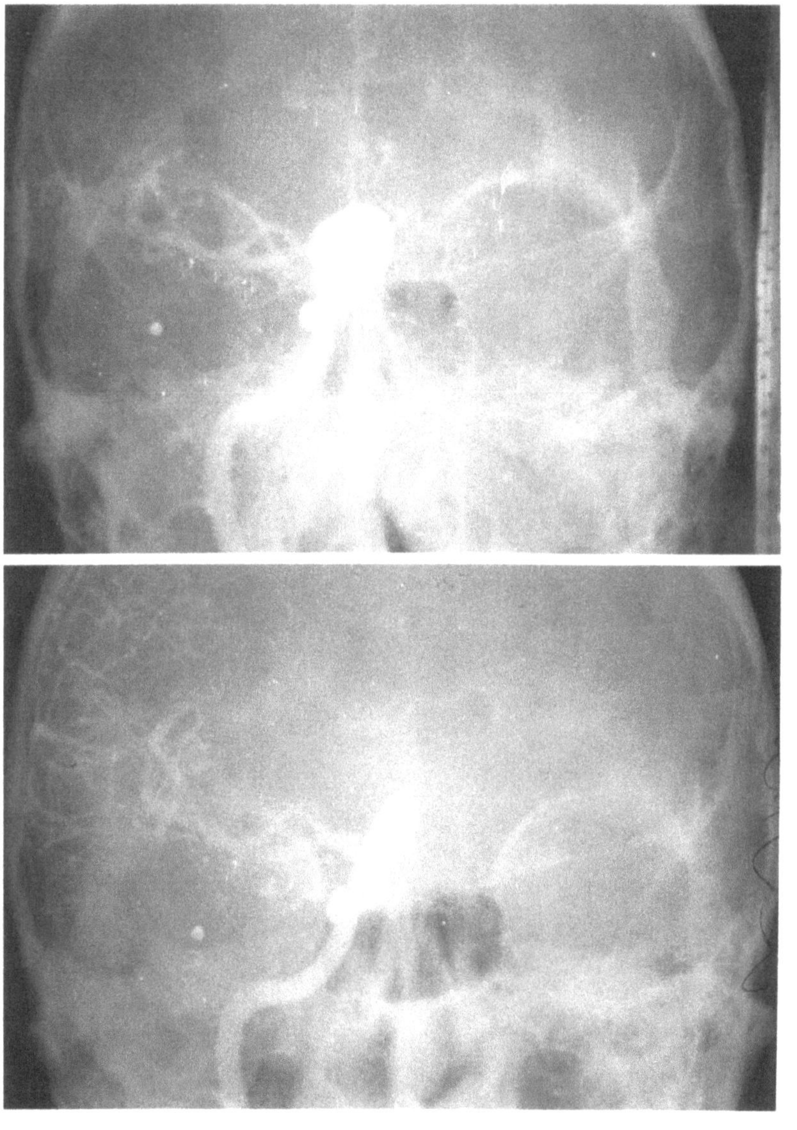

FIGURE 9.9. (A) Ophthalmic artery aneurysm projecting superiorly. (B) The aneurysm has been filled with a balloon.

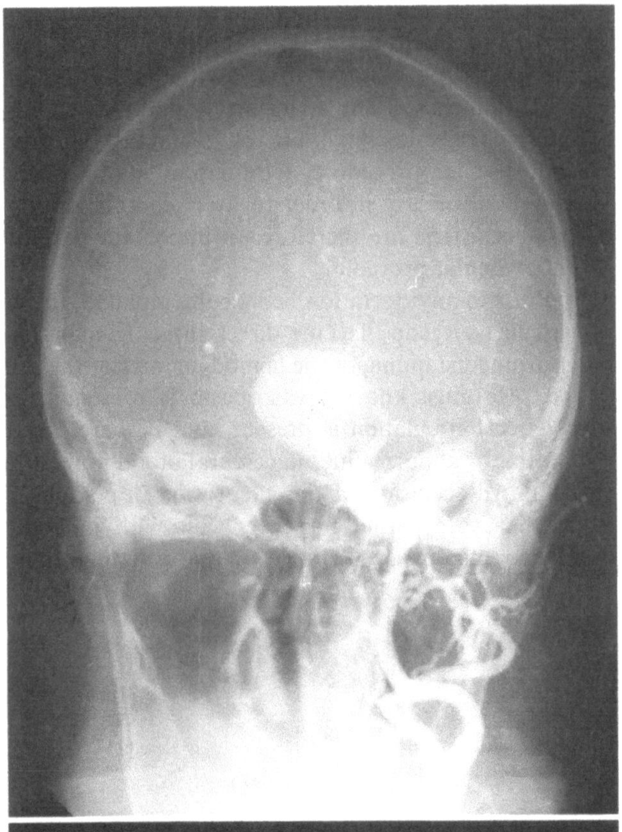

A

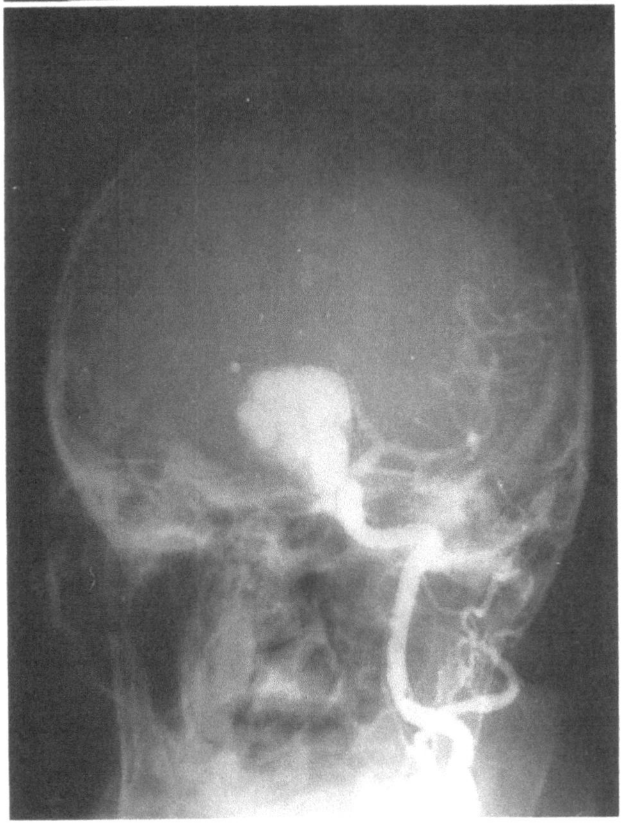

B

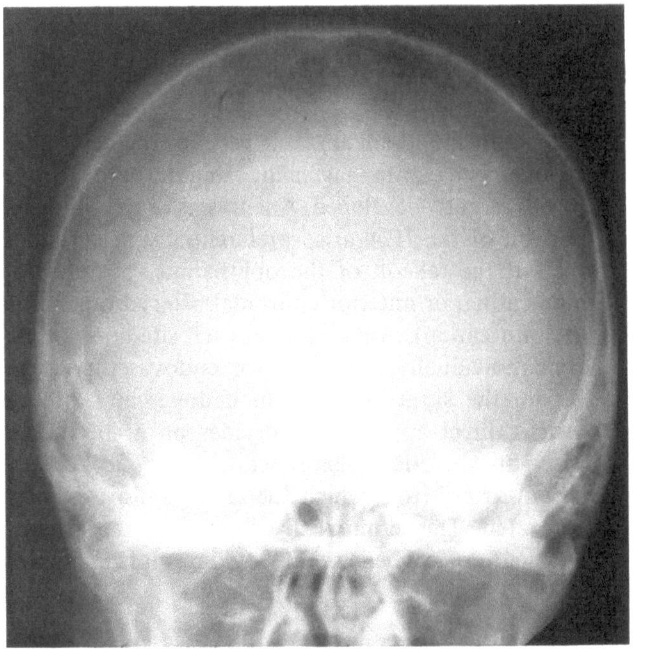

FIGURE 9.10. (A) Giant aneurysm of the ophthalmic segment. (B) Seven balloons have been introduced into the aneurysm cavity. (C) The balloons are shown, excluding the aneurysm from the circulation.

hormone (SIADH), brain edema, intracerebral hemorrhage, and all the other complications of SAH must be managed in order to prepare the patient for the endovascular procedure. Otherwise, when treating a patient in poor neurological grade, as in the direct surgery, worsening of complications may be expected. Before deciding on a procedure for definitive occlusion, the structure of the aneurysm, its size, its relationship to the parent vessel, its relationship to other brain structures nearby, and the size of its neck are all important parameters to be considered.

Techniques

For approaches to the supraclinoid aneurysm, a cervical carotid artery puncture is the preferred route. The introduction of a catheter (onto which is fixed a detachable balloon) into the supraclinoid portion of the carotid artery is usually not difficult. However, catheters may be directed more easily into aneurysms that project medially from the ICA than those projecting laterally or inferiorly. In this location, the use of helper balloons or methods whereby the direction of blood flow is altered are not usually necessary. Those aneurysms arising from the ICA bifurcation are in a direct line of flow, and balloon catheters naturally progress along the arterial wall toward this lesion.

If the orifice of the aneurysm projects toward the

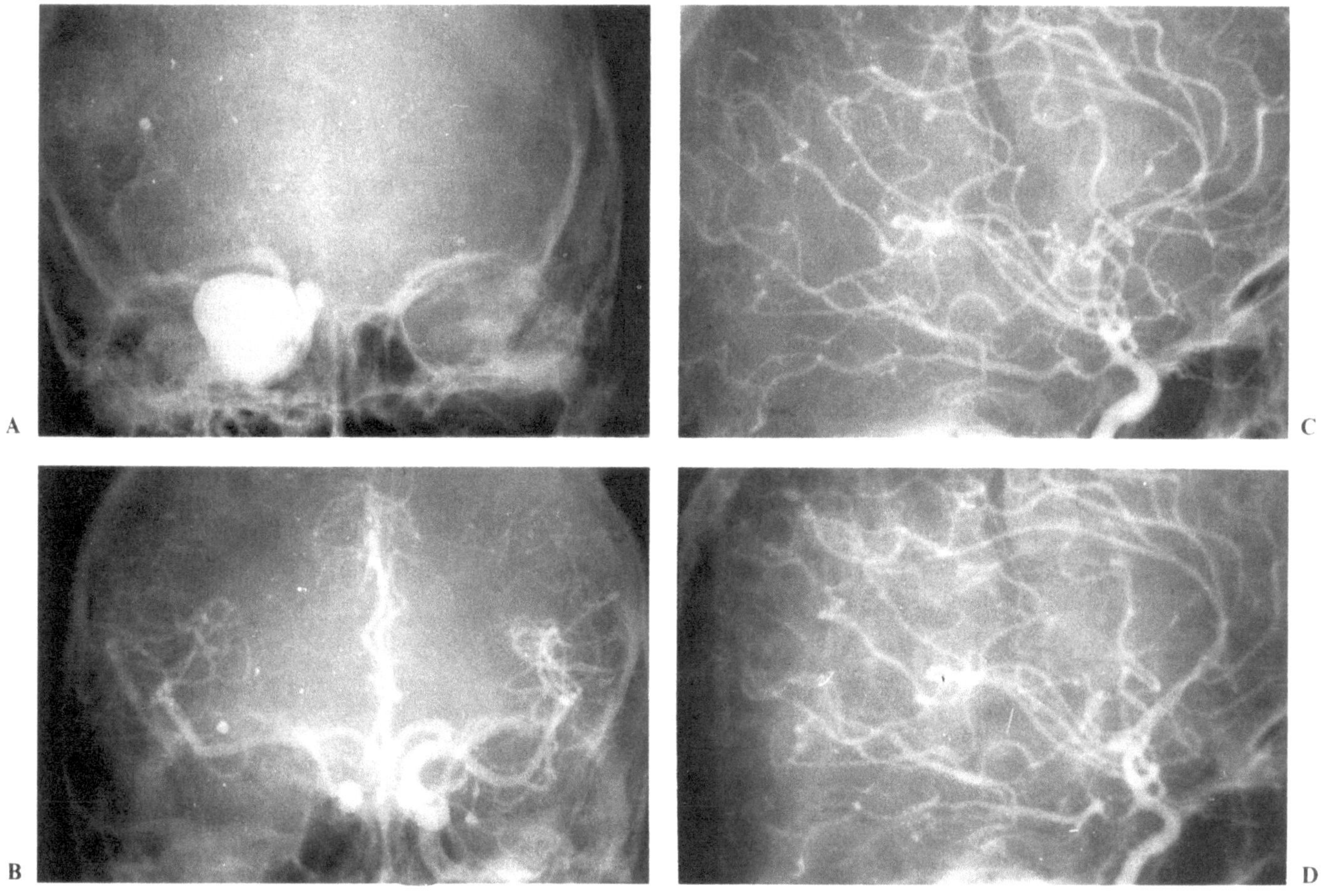

FIGURE 9.11. (A) Giant aneurysm of the ophthalmic segment of the internal carotid artery. (B) A balloon has been placed in the internal carotid artery blocking the orifice of the aneurysm. (C) Contralateral cerebral circulation showing displacement of the anterior cerebral circulation by the giant aneurysm before endovascular occlusion. (D) The contralateral circulation has been restored to a normal pattern 3 months following endovascular occlusion of the aneurysm.

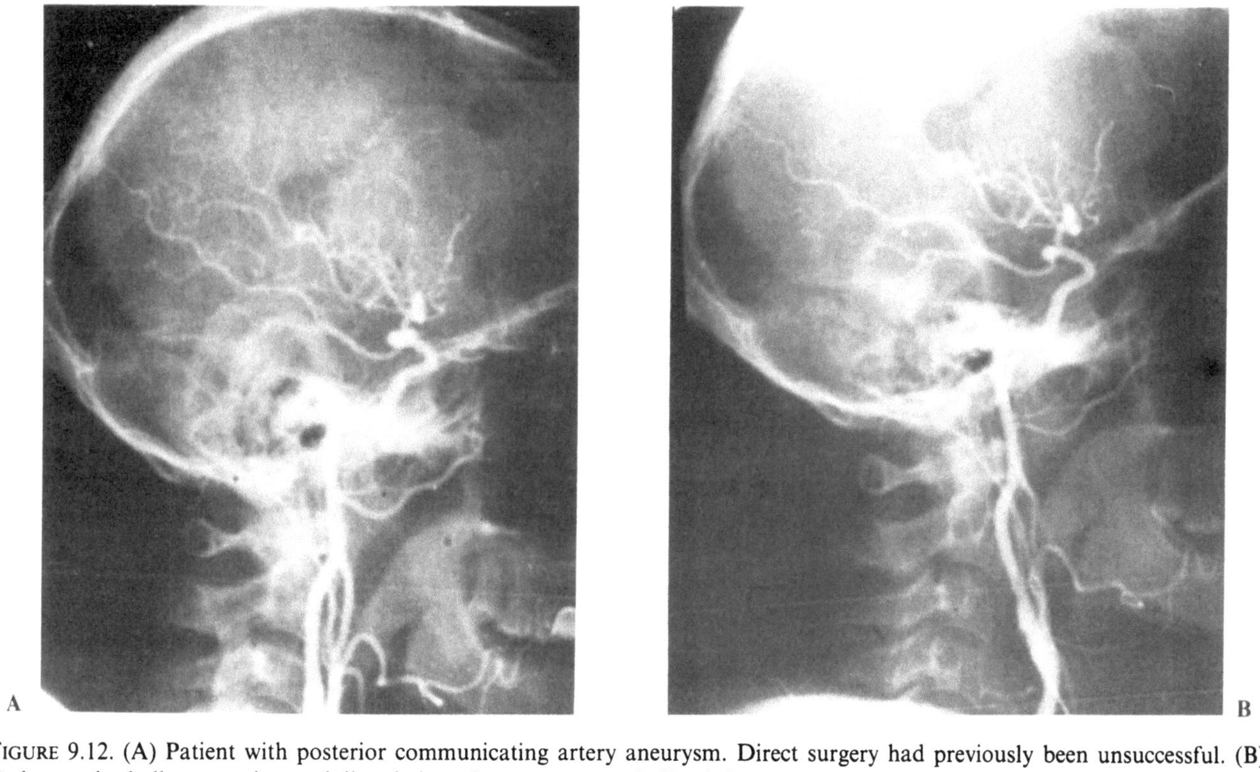

FIGURE 9.12. (A) Patient with posterior communicating artery aneurysm. Direct surgery had previously been unsuccessful. (B) Endovascular balloon was inserted directly into the aneurysm excluding it from the circulation.

origin of the A_1 or M_1, the position and direction of travel of the balloon catheter must be altered. More difficult still, are arterial aneurysms that arise along the posterior surface of the ICA, such as those that arise near the ostium of the PComA. The balloon tends to migrate anteriorly and medially along the surface of the carotid artery because it is filled with contrast material that is lighter than blood. To introduce the balloon into an aneurysm with a posterior location, adjunctive measures, such as occlusion of the contralateral ICA with the finger, turning of the head to either side, and a helper balloon, are needed.

ICA aneurysms often consist of two or more lobules. They may also be elongated, or otherwise irregular. When dealing with aneurysms that are multilobulated, it is imperative that the balloon be interposed along the longest trajectory to the distal fundus, simultaneously blocking the orifice. Aneurysms originating with long thin necks must be handled in a different manner. In this case, a balloon may be introduced and partially inflated, leaving the uninflated portion remaining in the neck. The balloon must be specially trained to inflate distally and retain some uninflated portion proximally. The distal portion of the balloon must be inflated first and the proximal portion left uninflated in the neck, causing thrombosis within the aneurysm later. Giant aneurysms that produce their symptoms by virtue of their mass, should preferably be filled with a soft material so as not

A

B

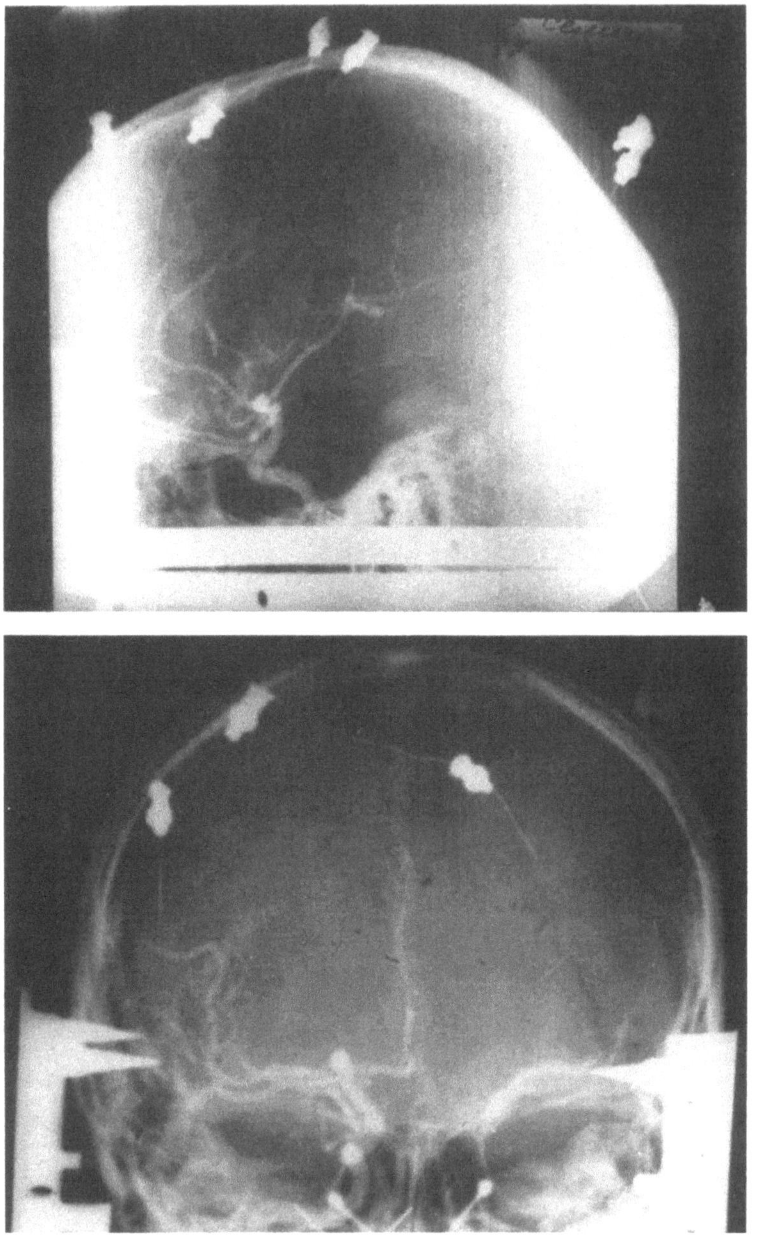

FIGURE 9.13. (A) Bifurcation aneurysm before and (B) after occlusion with endovascular balloon.

to increase the mass effect. Contrast material is effective in this regard because it leaks from the balloon gradually over time as the aneurysm shrinks in volume. On the other hand, small aneurysms may also be filled with a hardening material such as silicone or hema.

In dealing with aneurysms with a wide neck or orifice, the use of helper balloons makes detachment safer. Otherwise, as the catheter is extracted, the balloon may be pulled into the orifice of the parent artery, obstructing it. The helper balloon holds gently against the primary balloon, keeping it well placed within the orifice during attachment.[26] Some examples of endovascular occlusion of supraclinoid aneurysms using endovascular methods are shown in Figs. 9.9–9.13.

Conclusions

There are many options for managing aneurysms of the supraclinoid segment. The choice depends on the size and configuration of the lesion, its location, its relationship to the hemorrhage, and most importantly, the expertise and experience of the aneurysm team. Quality preoperative studies with test occlusion render decision-making easier and more accurate. Both endovascular and direct clipping can be difficult, and complications occur far too often in most accessible anatomical location. Unfortunately, the supraclinoid arteries are most susceptible to plaque formation, making vessel rupture a major complicating feature of either approach.

References

1. Yasargil MG. *Microneurosurgery.* New York: George Thieme, Verlag; 1984;1:56–71.
2. Sengupta RP, Gryspeerdt GL, Hankinson J. Carotid–ophthalmic aneurysms. *J Neurol Neurosurg Psychiatry.* 1976;39:837–853.
3. Sahs AL. Observations on the pathology of saccular aneurysms. In: Sahs AL, Perret GE, Lockley HB, Nishioka H, eds. *Intracranial Aneurysms and Subarachnoid Hemorrhage—A Cooperative Study.* Philadelphia, PA: JB Lippincott, 1969:22–36.
4. Willis T. Cerebri anatome nervorum que description, et usus. *Amestelodami.* 1664.
5. Smith RR, Kees CJ, Hogg AJ. Agenesis of the internal carotid artery with an unusual primitive collateral. *J Neurosurg.* 1972;37:460–461.
6. Gibo H, Lenkey C, Rhoton Al Microsurgical anatomy of the supraclinoid portion of the internal carotid artery. *J Neurosurgery.* 1981;55:560–574.
7. Rhoton AL, Fuji K, Faadd B. Microsurgical anatomy of the anterior choroidal artery. *Surg Neurol.* 1979;12:171–187.
8. Weir B. *Aneurysm Affecting the Nervous System.* Baltimore, MD: Williams & Wilkins; 1987;317–320.
9. Harris FA, Rhoton AL Jr. Microsurgical anatomy of the cavernous sinus. A microsurgical study. *J Neurosurg.* 1976; 45:169–180.
10. Padget DH. The development of the cranial arteries in the human embryo. *Contr Embryol Carnet Inst.* 1948;32:205–261.
11. Truemper EJ, Fisher QA. Cerebrovascular embryology and anatomic variation. In: Newell D, Ward R, eds. *Transcranial Doppler.* New York: Raven Press; 1992:231–282.
12. Vincetelli F, Caruso G, Grisoli F, Rabehanta P, Adriamamonjy C, Gouaze A. Microsurgical anatomy of the cisternal course of the perforating branches of the posterior communicating artery. *Neurosurgery.* 1990;26: 824–831.
13. Hassler OG, Saltzman G-F. Angiographic and histologic changes in infundibular widening of the PComA. *Acta Radiol Diagn.* 1963;1:321–327.
14. Alpers BJ, Berry RG, Paddison RM. Anatomical studies of the circle of Willis in normal brain. *Arch Neurol Psychiat.* 1959;81:409–418.
15. Riggs HE, Rupp C. Variations in form of circle of Willis. *Arch Neurol.* 1963;8:8–14.
16. Stopford JSB. The arteries of the pons and medulla oblongata. Part I. *J Anat Physiol.* 1916;50:131–163.
17. Saeki N, Rhoton AL Jr. Microsurgical anatomy of the upper basilar artery and the posterior circle of Willis. *J Neurosurg.* 1977;46:563–577.
18. Ferguson GC, Drake CG. Carotid–ophthalmic aneurysms: visual abnormalities in 32 patients and the results of treatment. *Surg Neurol.* 1981;16:1–8.
19. Day AL. Clinicoanatomic features of supraclinoid aneurysms. *Clin Neurosurg.* 1990;36:256–74.
20. Suzuki J, Kodama N, Fujiwara S. Surgical treatment of internal carotid–posterior communicating aneurysms: From experience of 213 cases. In: Suzuki J, ed. *Cerebral Aneurysms.* Tokyo, Japan: Neuron; 1979:256–262.
21. Dott NM. Intracranial aneurysms: cerebral arterioradiography: surgical treatment. *Edinburgh Med J.* 1933;40:219–234.
22. Trevani E. Ein als parasellarer Tumor operiertes aneurysma der Arteria carotis interna. *Dtsch Z Chir.* 1932;237: 534–535.
23. Dandy WE. Intracranial aneurysm of internal carotid artery cured by operation. *Ann Surg.* 1938;207:654–659.
24. Tamaki N, Kim S, Ehara K, Asada M, Fujita K, Taomoto K, Matsumoto S. Giant carotid–ophthalmic artery aneurysms: direct clipping utilizing the "trapping evacuation" technique. *J Neurosurg.* 1991;74:567–572.
25. Scott JA. Occlusion balloon suction decompression of supraclinoid carotid aneurysms: work in progress. *Neuroradiology.* 1991;33(suppl):152.
26. Pasqualin A, Battaglia R, Scienza R, De Pian R. Italian cooperative study of giant intracranial aneurysms: 4. Results of treatment. *Acta Neurochir Suppl (Wien).* 1988;42: 65–70.

10
Anterior Cerebral and Anterior Communicating Artery Aneurysms

Patients with anterior cerebral artery (ACA) and anterior communicating artery (AComA) aneurysms make up one third of all those presenting with subarachnoid hemorrhage (SAH). In autopsy material, the incidence is lower, perhaps because the small lesion is not recognized as easily on gross dissections as it is on good quality angiograms. Aneurysms in this location may be subclassified according to their projection in relationship to the A_1, A_2, and AComA. Yasargil[1] described six subsets: an anterior projection, a superior projection, a posterior projection, a posterior inferior projection, an inferior projection, and a complex aneurysm in which the AComA becomes part of the aneurysmal mass. Nathal et al.[2] classified aneurysms into three types, based on their projection. Roughly one-third project directly posteriorly from the anterior communicating (type 1), 58.4% project anteriorly and superior to the A_2 vessels (type 2), and, in type 3, the aneurysm projects inferiorly and anterior to the A_2 branches.

Microvascular Anatomy

Because of the high incidence of ACA aneurysms and the component vascular channels supplying the deep nuclei of the forebrain, a thorough knowledge of this system is essential to the operating surgeon. The anterior cerebral arterial complex is first seen in the 12- to 14-mm embryo, 34 to 36 days old (Padget's fourth stage).[3] The two anterior cerebral arteries originate from the primitive olfactory artery, and, in the fifth stage (16–18 mm, 39–41 days old) both ACAs are small and well defined.

The ACA arises from the medial surface of the internal carotid artery (ICA) bifurcation and lies medial to the sylvian fissure, lateral to the optic chiasm, and immediately inferior to the anterior perforated substance. It usually courses with a posterior superior convex curve above the optic chiasm and under the thick arachnoid membrane covering the olfactory trigone to enter the lateral part of the lamina terminalis cistern, joining the ACA from the opposite side to create the AComA. This occurs just anterior to the lamina terminalis.

After connecting, the ACA passes in the interhemispheric fissure ascending in front of the lamina terminalis making another curve between the rostrum and genu of the corpus callosum and then passes along the corpus callosum. It lies in the pericallosal cistern and passes around the splenium to become fine and tortuous terminal branches ending in the choroid plexus of the third ventricle (Fig. 10.1).

Classification of the ACA Segments

The ACA has been segmented by a number of anatomists. Fischer[4] divided the ACA finally into five segments, A_1 through A_5. The A_1 segment lies proximal to the AComA and the A_2 through A_5 segments lie distal to the AComA.

Proximal A_1 Segment

This part of the artery is a segment between its origin at the ICA proximal to the AComA. The A_1 is smaller in comparison to the middle cerebral artery (MCA) in 71% of the cases studied, but the two arteries are about equal size in 24%. In 5%, it may actually be somewhat larger than the MCA.[1] This occurs especially when some anomaly is present. The average length of this segment is 12.7 mm and it courses above the optic chiasm in 70%. In 30%, it courses over the ipsilateral optic nerve. The normal diameter of the A_1 varies between 1 and 4 mm. In about 80% of the cases, there is asymmetry between the two A_1 segments.[5] Hypoplasia or aplasia may also be present. Riggs and Rupp[6] noted hypoplasia of the A_1 segment on one side in 7% of the cases studied. The A_1 segment hypoplasia has been also associated with AComA aneurysms. This incidence has been reported at 85% by Wilson et al.[7] True aplasia is rare. Severe hypoplasia may appear as aplasia on an angiogram subject to dispute at the time of surgical procedures.

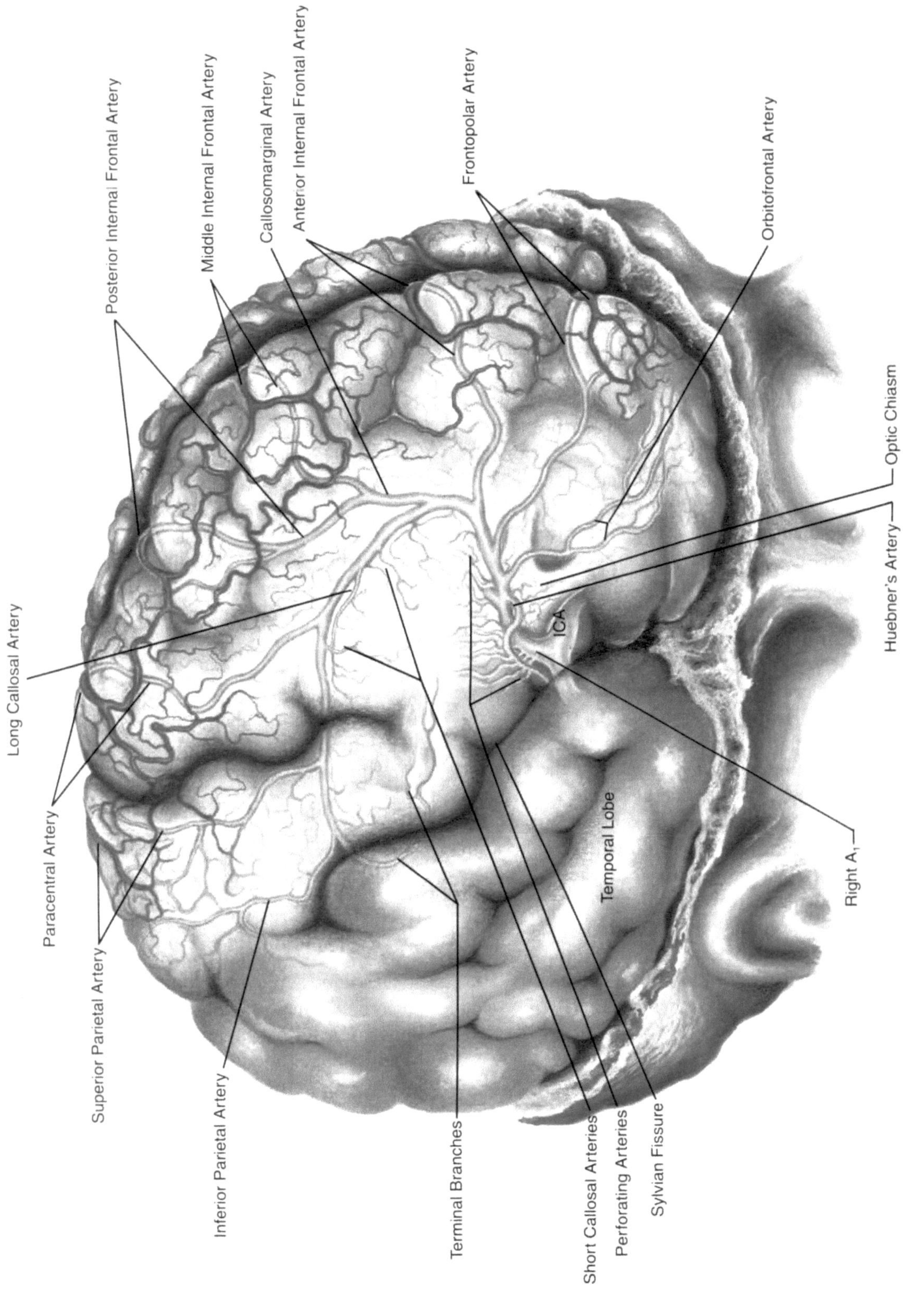

FIGURE 10.1. **Right anterolateral view of the superficial branches of the anterior cerebral circulation along the cortical surface. The deep branches of the anterior cerebral artery are depicted transparently through the cortex.**

Von Mitterwallner[8] reported an incidence of 0.3% and Yasargil[1] reported the A_1 aplasia in 0.5% of 200 cadaver brains. The ACA may deviate from its normal course. An abnormal course in which the ACA passes beneath the optic nerve has been reported in nine cases.[5] Maurer et al.[5] reported a case of perforation of the optic tract by the A_1 segment. The duplication in a portion of the A_1 was found in 4% of hemispheres studied by Perlmutter and Rhoton.[9]

The Perforating Branches of the A_1 Segment

Several small branches arise from the A_1, mostly laterally and from the proximal portion. The average number varies from five to eight. They arise from the superior surface in 54%, from the posterior surface in 32%, from the inferior surface in 9%, and from the anterior surface in 5%.[9] Yasargil[1] reported the posterior inferior surface as the most common site for origination of these branches. Perforating arteries from the A_1 segment supply the septum pellucidum, the medial portion of the anterior commissure, the pillar of the fornix, the optic chiasm, the paraolfactory area, the anterior limb of the internal capsule, the anterior inferior part of the striatum and the anterior hypothalamus.

The diameter of the perforating arteries varies from 0.1 to 1 mm. Commonly (46%), one of these arteries may arise as a stem originating from the A_1 segment and take a course similar to that of the recurrent artery of Heubner, terminating in the medial part of the anterior perforated substance.[1] If the lateral striate arteries are small, this artery will become thicker and supply the lateral portion of the anterior perforated substances. In 41% of the cases, the perforating branches of the A_1 terminate in this region; the dorsal surface of the optic chiasm or suprachiasmatic portion of the hypothalamus may be the terminating site in 29%, the optic tract in 11%, the inferior surface of the frontal lobe in 10%, the sylvian fissure in 5%, the optic nerve in 2%, and between the cerebral hemispheres in 2%.[9]

The Anterior Communicating Artery

The AComA is formed as an arterial plexus in the 16- to 18-mm embryo (stage V).[3] The artery joins and connects the two ACAs. In the 24-mm embryo (stage VI), the median callosal artery arises from this plexiform network. By the time of birth, the plexus has regressed to be replaced by a single channel, the AComA. The length of the AComA varies between 0.1 and 3.0 mm and forms a single channel in about 75% of cases studied.[1,8] Anomalies of the artery, including a reticular pattern, duplication, triplication, fenestration, loop formation, and a bridge, may be seen. Perlmutter and Rhoton[9] reported a duplicated AComA in 30% and triplication in 10% of the cases studied. Yasargil[1] found duplication in 20.5% and triplication in 18.5% of 200 cadaver dissections. The AComA may be hypoplastic in 3% to 16%.[10] Gomes and co-workers[10] reviewed 12 reports and found the accessory AComA in 7% to 42% of cases.

Perforating Branches of the Anterior Communicating Artery

The AComA gives rise to several important perforating channels. The number varies between 1 and 11; most arise superiorly (54%) and on the posterior surface 36% of the AComA.[9] The caliber varies from 250 to 500 μm. In some cases, a main trunk that divides into several small branches as well as other small branches may be present. The medial callosal artery is a rare anomaly in this area and may be mistaken at the time of surgery for a main trunk of A_2. The average angle between the AComA perforating branches and the A_2 segment in the sagittal plane is 30° to 180°, but in 70% of the cases studied by Vincentelli and Lehman[11] it was 90° to 120°. This angle is important in planning surgical approaches to AComA aneurysms. Most of the perforating branches terminate in the suprachiasmatic area and the remainder pass dorsally along the surface of the optic chiasm anterior perforating substances, and frontal lobes (Fig. 10.2). Four anatomical groups are supplied by these important perforating branches:

1. The lamina terminalis and hypothalamus.
2. The anterior commissure, trigone, septum pellucidum, and paraolfactory gyrus.
3. The subcallosal region, and the anterior part of the cingulate gyrus.
4. The area beyond the genu of the corpus callosum.

The blood supplying group II has the richest collateral pattern. Damage to the AComA perforating branches may cause severe impairment in septocommissural and hypothalamic function, including endocrine dysfunction and memory impairment.

The Distal Anterior Cerebral Artery

This portion of the ACA may be referred to as the postcommunicating or A_2 segment. The term *pericallosal artery* has been applied to that portion of the ACA distal to the origin of the callosomarginal branch, but Perlmutter and Rhoton[12] reported that the callosomarginal branch may be absent in up to 18% of cases. Thus, it is preferable to apply the term *pericallosal artery* to all of the distal ACA, beginning at the AComA level.

The distal ACA is situated in the interhemispheric

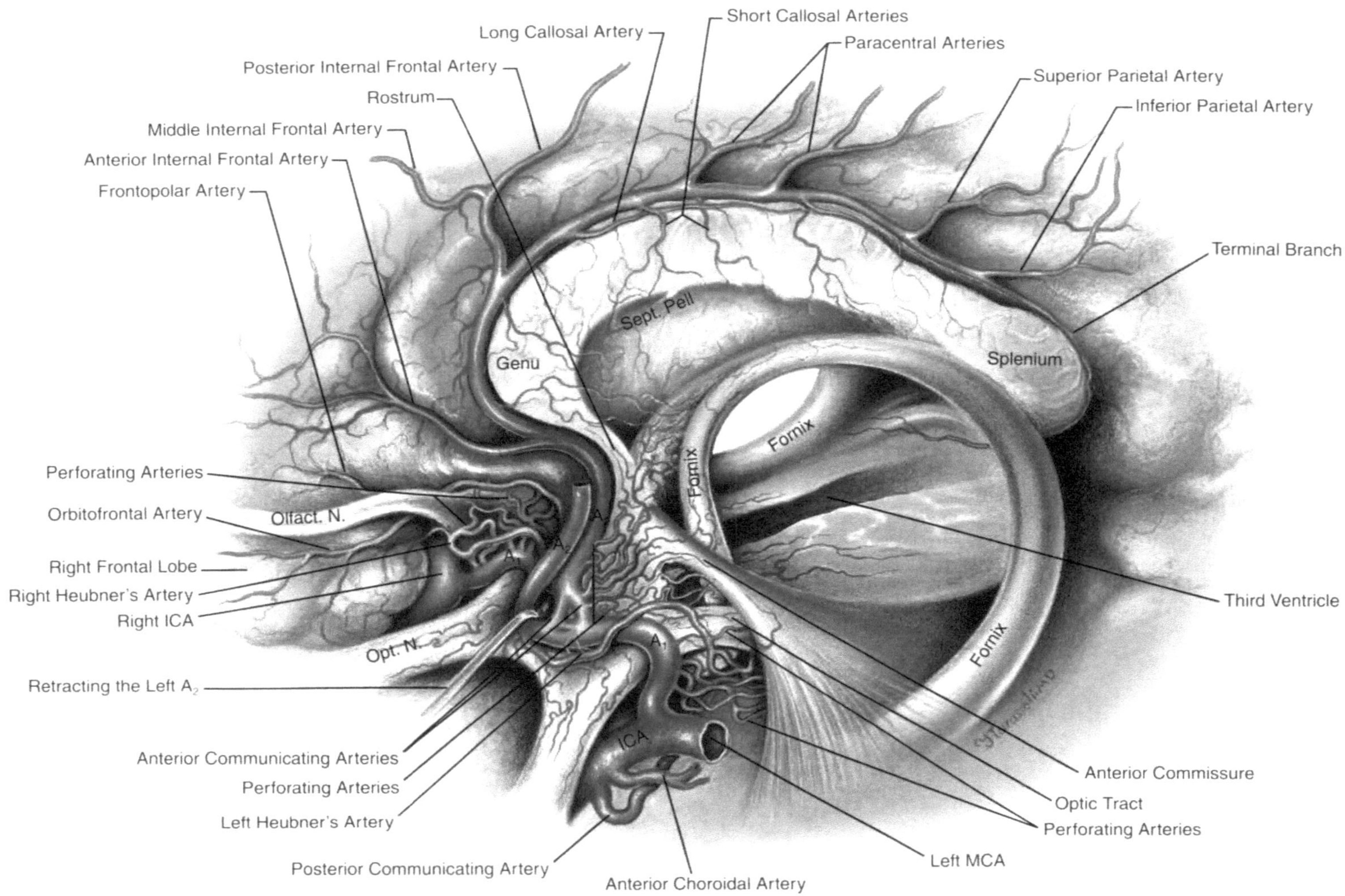

FIGURE 10.2. Left anterolateral view of the deep and penetrating branches of the A_1 and A_2 segments. The superficial cortex has been removed to illustrate the supply of the deep structures. The left A_2 branch has been retracted forward to demonstrate the posterior hypothalamic perforators and in this case, the fenestrated AcomA. There are many variations in the origin of these penetrating branches. ICA, internal carotid artery; MCA, middle cerebral artery.

fissure ascending in the lamina terminalis cistern, and it passes over the genu, above the body of the corpus callosum in the pericallosal cistern. Its terminal branches pass below the splenium and terminate in the choroid plexus of the third ventricle. In 90% of the cases, the ACAs have an equal caliber. Because the width of the anterior portion of the falx cerebri (in the sagittal plane) is narrower than its posterior portion, the entire course of the pericallosal artery (except its posterior part) and the proximal part of the callosomarginal artery are situated below the free edge of the falx cerebri. The anterior segment of the artery can be displaced from the midline by a unilateral mass, serving as a useful angiographic sign. The distal ACA may be further classified into four segments, A_2 through A_5.[4] The A_2 segment begins at the origin of the AComA and passes anteriorly and superiorly, terminating at the junction of the rostrum and genu of the corpus callosum. The A_3 segment passes around the genu of the corpus callosum and ends where the artery turns posteriorly above the genu. The A_4 and A_5 segments may be separated just behind the coronal suture in the lateral view.

Several abnormalities involving the distal ACA segments have been described. The median callosal artery, also called the third A_2 or the triplication of the ACA, usually arises from the posterior inferior surface of the AComA and passes around the genu of the corpus callosum. Its length varies, occurring in 2% to 20%.[1,9,10] A single azygous ACA supplying both hemispheres has also been found. The azygous artery has been demonstrated angiographically in 0.2% and in up to 5% in cadaver specimens.[1] The distal ACA may send branches to the contralateral hemisphere; this happened in 64% of cases studied by Perlmutter and Rhoton.[12]

The Branches of the Distal Anterior Cerebral Artery

The Recurrent Artery of Heubner

This artery was first described by Heubner in 1872. It originates from the ACA and makes a backward course on the ipsilateral ACA, terminating in the anterior perforated substance. The artery originates along the proximal A_2 in 78%, from the A_1 in 14%, and at the level of the AComA in 8%.[9] However, others found the artery of Heubner in a more proximal position. The caliber varies from 0.2 to 2.9 mm and the length varies from 12 to 38 mm.[9,13] This artery usually passes anterior and superior to the A_1 segment extending past the proximal portion of the MCA, terminating in the lateral aspects of the anterior perforated substances, medial to the sylvian fissure. Most commonly, it has a main trunk but before penetration divides into terminal branches. Heubner's artery has several important perforating branches, the average number being four to six. In addition to penetrating the anterior perforated substances, 20% of these branches pass to the inferior surface of the frontal lobe, including the area lateral to the olfactory sulcus and gyrus rectus. These branches supply the anterior part of the caudate nucleus, the anterior third of the putamen, the tip of the outer segment of the globus pallidus, and the anterior limb of the internal capsule, along with the hypothalamus. Occlusion of the recurrent artery of Heubner may lead to hemiparesis with brachial dominance due to impairment of blood supply to the anterior limb of the internal capsule and aphasia in the dominant hemisphere. It may also cause paralysis of the face and tongue because of the location of all of these fibers in the anterior limb of the internal capsule.

Perforating Branches of the Distal Anterior Cerebral Artery

Four to eight small branches may originate along the proximal part of the A_2 segment, close to the AComA. These branches usually terminate in the lamina terminalis, the anterior forebrain below the corpus callosum, and in the optic chiasm. They provide blood supply to the anterior hypothalamus, the medial portion of the anterior commissure, the pillar of the fornix, and the septum pellucidum.

Cortical Branches of the Distal ACA

The medial surface of the cerebral hemispheres, especially the anterior portion, are supplied by the cortical branches of the ACA. The medial surface of the frontal lobes, the cingulate gyrus, the paracentral lobule, the precuneus, and a portion adjacent to the parietooccipital fissure are supplied by these branches. On the basal surface, the olfactory tract and bulb, the gyrus rectus, and the medial part of the orbital gyrus are supplied by the cortical branches. On the lateral surface, they supply the superior frontal gyrus and beyond the superior frontal sulcus, the precentral gyrus, and the postcentral gyrus.

The callosomarginal artery is a primary division of the distal ACA, although it may be absent. When it is present, it usually originates from the A_3 segment and courses superior to the cingulate gyrus. It gives rise to several small cortical branches supplying the medial frontal lobes, premotor, motor, and sensory areas. The paracentral and internal frontal arteries are most frequently cortical branches arising from the callosomarginal artery.

The Orbitofrontal Artery

Perlmutter and Rhoton[12] found that the orbitofrontal artery is the smallest of the cortical branches of the distal ACA originating from the A_2 segment and passes forward on the basal surface of the frontal lobe toward the anterior fossa floor. It is usually the first cortical branch of the distal ACA and it often supplies small branches to the olfactory tract and bulb, gyrus rectus, and the medial parts of the orbital gyrus along with the small part of the frontal pole.

The frontopolar artery normally originates from the A_2 segment passing forward and inferior along the medial surface of the frontal lobe supplying the medial and lateral surfaces of the frontal pole.

The anterior internal frontal artery originates from the A_2–A_3 segment of the distal ACA ascending on the medial surface of the frontal lobe. It supplies the anterior portion of the superior frontal gyrus. This artery may also arise from the callosomarginal artery.

The middle internal frontal artery frequently arises from the A_3 segment as a branch of the callosomarginal artery and, after ascending in the medial surface of the frontal lobe, supplies the medial and lateral surface of the middle part of the superior frontal gyrus. This is the most frequent cortical branch arising from the callosomarginal artery.

The posterior internal frontal artery takes off from the A_3 or A_4 segment and usually passes beyond the cingulate gyrus. It enters the precentral sulcus to partly supply the posterior third of the superior frontal gyrus, a portion of the cingulate gyrus, and the anterior portion of the paracentral lobule.

The paracentral artery arises from the A_4 segment or the callosomarginal artery and arises anterior to the marginal limb of the cingulate sulcus. It then passes to a superior position to supply the premotor, motor, and somatic sensory area around the paracentral lobule.

The superior parietal artery usually arises from the A_5 segment passing beyond the marginal limb of the cingulate sulcus, sending a branch to this area. It also supplies portions of the cuneus.

The inferior parietal artery is the last cortical branch of the distal ACA and usually arises from the A_5 segment or the callosomarginal artery. Sometimes it is absent. When present, it supplies the anterior portion of the precuneus and parts of the cuneus. The terminal branches of the distal ACA usually anastomose with the splenial branches of the posterior cerebral artery (PCA).

The callosal branches of the distal ACA provide a primary blood supply for the corpus callosum. There are two types of callosal branches: long and short penetrating branches.[12] The short callosal arteries are small perforating branches that arise directly from the pericallosal artery and penetrate the corpus callosum to supply the rostrum, genu, body, and splenium. These small branches also pass through the corpus callosum and supply the septum pellucidum, anterior commissure, and anterior pillar of the fornix. They average about seven in number.

The long callosal arteries originate from the pericallosal artery and pass parallel to the parent artery lying between it and the corpus callosum. After a short course, they give several penetrating branches to the corpus callosum.

Clinical Features

Unruptured aneurysms in the A_1, AComA, and A_2 region rarely produce symptoms unless they are large. Giant aneurysms produce symptoms by cortical irritation (seizures), by involvement of the visual pathways and optic nerves, and by involvement of the hypothalamus. Nearly 10% of patients with aneurysms of the AComA that rupture also develop the syndrome of inappropriate secretion of the antidiuretic hormone (SIADH) due to direct injury of the hypothalamus.

Large ACA and AComA aneurysms may be associated with visual field loss. AComA aneurysms usually cause symmetric compression of one or both optic nerves, with the eye contralateral to the parent artery being most often affected. Classical bitemporal hemianopsia also occurs.[14]

Patients with AComA aneurysms also develop disconnection syndromes characteristic of anterior corpus callosal lesions. Memory loss, disorientation, perceptual problems, decreased initiative, and inconsistent muscle control are associated. There is usually a left–right conflict and asymmetric left–right performance consistent with the disconnection pattern.

Ruptured Aneurysms

Hemorrhagic presentation is the most common manifestation of aneurysms in this region. Symptoms may be attributable to hemorrhage into the ventricular system and intracerebral substance as well as to classical subarachnoid hemorrhage.

Subarachnoid Hemorrhage

In the milder forms of hemorrhage, there may be only an admixture of blood with cerebrospinal fluid (CSF). With more extensive hemorrhage, however, clots are found in the basal cisterns, and these may dissect around the cerebral cortex, filling the cisterns and the ventricular system.

Among patients who present with acute SAH, approximately 60% are stable in grade 1 (Hunt and Hess grades

I and II) (compensated). The remaining 40% respond poorly due to their hemorrhage.[15] The initial onset in patients who are awake and alert and can relate a good history indicates that headache, of short duration and sudden in onset, is the predominant symptom. The headache is usually poorly localized, but eventually the patient describes some radiation toward the occipital region. It is associated with vomiting, and occasionally there are brief periods of loss of consciousness in alert patients. Some patients experience transient episodes of paraparesis or monoparesis involving one of the lower extremities.

During the first week, headache is persistent and associated with meningeal signs. These symptoms diminish toward the end of the first week. In approximately 20% of these grades 1 and 2 patients, symptoms reappear toward the end of the first week, usually manifested by lethargy, low-grade fever, disorientation, and increased nuchal rigidity. In some, focal neurological deficits of a mild nature may be detected.

Some patients with these complications of the hemorrhagic period progress into a subcompensated state (grade III Hunt and Hess). From day 7 until the end of the first month, a period of high risk for patients with recent SAH occurs. Those who have no symptoms during the first week may escape serious risk during this interval. However, approximately 20% of these patients undergo all of their additional complications during this 3-week interval extending from day 7 to day 30. During this time, ischemic deficits, hydrocephalus, thrombophlebitis, pulmonary embolism, inappropriate secretion of antidiuretic hormone, and other signs of hypothalamic injury appear. Since this subgroup cannot be identified prior to operation, deterioration may appear after operation performed during the first week. Whether surgery can accelerate or convert asymptomatic vasospasm into the symptomatic variety has not been settled. When the clinical state deteriorates, the cause must be identified and appropriate therapy aimed at whatever pathological events are responsible.

Patients who arrive with decreased levels of consciousness (grades 3 and 4), have usually lost consciousness at the onset of their SAH for periods of half an hour or more. Motor activity may be increased, but the patient responds inappropriately and may be combative and belligerent. Vomiting may continue past the initial ictus. In this group, deep stupor, disorientation, and combativeness may continue although focal neurological deficits are usually not encountered. For patients who arrive in a stuporous state after major SAH, two clinical courses can be outlined. In one, there is gradual improvement in the level of consciousness and behavior. At the end of the first week, the patient may recover to grade 1 or grade 2 and be responsive. The second group deteriorates further, near the end of the first week, due to ischemic deficits and other complications. In the latter group, disorientation and stupor continue, and both focal and diffuse deficits appear. Deterioration during the second week is usually attributable to neurological causes but somatic factors including pulmonary function, deep vein thrombosis, and electrolyte disturbance may be the factor causing worsening. Ischemic deficits, brain edema, increased intracranial pressure (ICP), herniation, and subsequent brain stem compression cause neurological progression.

If vasospasm involves the A_1 portion, the small perforators that feed the septum and anterior hypothalamus may be affected. Rebleeding in this area is also particularly devastating. Blood tends to dissect along low-resistance pathways. When the aneurysm has been attached to the optic chiasm or nerve, it may cause sudden visual loss. Likewise, the aneurysm may be attached to the thin lamina terminalis and rupture directly into the hypothalamus and third ventricle. Motor and sensory disturbances involving the lower extremity may occur. With delayed ischemic deficits or vasospasm, there may also be aberrations with speech pattern and thought content.

Cerebro-Subarachnoid Hemorrhage

The course of these patients may be entirely different from those with primary subarachnoid hemorrhage. More patients are in poor neurological condition. The hematoma creates increased ICP interfering with cortical and brain stem function further. Axial dislocations predominate as a cause of neurological deterioration and death. If the hematoma occupies the medial basal frontal lobes, a diencephalic catabolic syndrome may ensue. This condition is characterized by temperature elevation, tachycardia, lethargy, and hypertension. Korsakoff's amnestic confabulatory syndrome may be present due to the involvement of the periventricular gray matter. Hematomas in the corpus callosum also lead to severe mental and behavioral problems and disconnection syndromes. Hematomas erupting into the ventricular system may obstruct the foramen of Monro or aqueduct of Sylvius, rapidly resulting in acute hydrocephalus. Asymmetrical hydrocephalus also may be encountered in which one ventricle expands at the expense of the other. In the second week, deterioration due to ischemic deficits and vasospasm also occurs. Hydrocephalus is more often a complication in patients harboring intraventricular hematomas.

ICP measurement is helpful in prognosticating outcome after SAH from an AComA complex aneurysm. Patients with good outcomes have significantly lower baseline ICP, and the height of plateau waves and

B-waves, unrelated to the location of the aneurysm, are less. Plateau waves are marginally higher in patients with aneurysms of the AComA complex.

The computed tomography (CT) scan is useful in predicting the site of hemorrhage from an aneurysm. Silver et al.[16] found that the scan correctly predicted the site in 77% of cases. Subarachnoid blood can be detected in as many as 95% if it is performed within 5 days of the hemorrhage. Cisternal blood is found in most patients with AComA aneurysms. Features associated with AComA aneurysms include involvement of the anterior interhemispheric fissure and a "typical" septal hematoma in a minority of cases. There may be infarction in the ACA distribution, and meningeal hyperemia may be seen on postcontrast scans. Punctate lesions in the hypothalamus and in the periventricular areas of the third ventricular are also commonly seen on CT scans. Intracerebral hematomas usually occupy the medial portion of one frontal lobe but may occur in the interhemispheric fissure. However, it is not uncommon to encounter hemorrhages in the subdural space alone or in combination with intracerebral hemorrhage. Hematomas dissect into the ventricular system, usually from the medial frontal lobes rather than through the lamina terminalis. However, rarely, the hemorrhage may dissect into the third ventricle directly or inferiorly into the optic chiasm and nerves. The clinical course of the disease in patients with AComA aneurysm rupture depends upon the extent and rapidity of onset as well as the direction that the aneurysm points and ultimately the dissection path that the blood takes through the brain.

Intraocular hemorrhage (Terson's syndrome) occurs in approximately one-fourth of all patients with SAH, and, of these, those bleeding from AComA aneurysms are the most likely candidates. Commonly, this occurs in the subhyaloid space but vitreous hemorrhages can also be found in three-fourths of those who have hemorrhages. They may obscure the optic disc and vascular pattern of the fundus. Most patients recover visual function within 6 months.

Congestive heart failure also occurs more commonly in patients bleeding from ACA aneurysms. The reason is not clear but perhaps derives from the close association of the dissecting blood and the sympathetic nuclei and tracts of the hypothalamus.

Surgical Options

In a prior era, A_1 and AComA aneurysms were considered appropriate only for direct intracranial clipping. The aneurysms, arising from small, difficult to access arteries, were considered inappropriate for endovascular catheters. Within the past five years, however, the introduction of high-resolution imaging and fine catheters such as the tracker catheter has permitted the catheterization of these vessels for endovascular repair of aneurysms. Both reconstructive and deconstructive alternatives may be applied to aneurysms arising from the A_1, AComA, or A_2 branches. Several factors dictate whether an endovascular or a direct surgical operation is preferred. The location of the aneurysm, the patient's condition, and the blood supply to the territory in question are the most important. For the endovascular approach, the first question to be answered is whether a deconstructive or reconstructive procedure will be applicable. In some aneurysms arising on this system, trapping may be appropriate, but only after test occlusion has been carried out safely. When deconstructive operations or trapping procedures must be used, the most appropriate method is clearly an endovascular one, sparing the patient an operative craniotomy. Reconstructive endovascular procedures are also applicable throughout the anterior cerebral system. Originally, only giant and unclippable aneurysms were considered for this form of therapy, but now even small and well-placed aneurysms are treated.

Direct methods are also widely applicable to aneurysms

TABLE 10.1. Operative alternatives for surgical management of ACA–AComA aneurysms

Type of aneurysm	Direct operation	Endovascular operation	Test occlusion	Combined operation
A_1 AComA				
<5 mm	+	−	−	−
>5 mm	+	+	+	−
>5 mm wide neck	+	−	−	+
>10 mm	+	+	+	+
A_2 aneurysm				
<5 mm	+	−	−	−
>5 mm	+	+	+	−
>5 mm wide neck	+	−	+	+
>10 mm	+	+	+	+

of the A_1, AComA, and A_2 segments. The most difficult lesions for direct craniotomy are those that are considered giant and would require extensive dissection for isolation of the neck and clipping. The success of the direct operation depends to a large extent upon the approach that is chosen. Whereas the pterional approach has become popular during recent years, the orbitocranial variation allows a wider and more anterior view of the lesion that projects superiorly and posteriorly. The latter approach provides additional working room for hands and instruments and less retraction for the large and giant lesion. As much working space as achievable should be planned when deciding the appropriate approach to the aneurysm from which thrombus or atheroma must be removed and microvascular surgery carried out. During the hemorrhagic period (within the first 2–3 weeks after aneurysm rupture), the direct approach is favored by most neurosurgeons. The direct operation facilitates removal of clot from the environs of the aneurysm, the subarachnoid space, and the ventricles, terminated with clipping of the aneurysm at the same sitting. The endovascular operation is indicated during the hemorrhagic period only in patients in low clinical grade and in those without evidence of cerebral vasospasm. The presence of vasospasm requires treatment using medical measures or with balloon angioplasty. Only after the patient's condition has stabilized should the endovascular approach then be reconsidered (Table 10.1).

Direct Approaches

Pterional Approach

The pterional exposure is used to approach many aneurysms of the basal arteries. The general techniques of this operation have been described in Chapter 6. Only those features peculiar to aneurysms of the A_1, A_2, and AComA will be described in this chapter.

Initially, the dura is opened in the upper edges of the bony exposure and the curve with the bony opening. It should be based directly over the sphenoid wing, held back, and sutured to the surrounding pericranium. The base of the frontal lobe and the sylvian fissure are then exposed as indicated. The connecting veins running between the middle cerebral vein and the sphenoparietal and cavernous sinus should be coagulated and divided only if tearing appears imminent. Self-retaining retractors are positioned and the microscope brought into place. The surgeon proceeds along the floor of the frontal fossa until the optic nerve and carotid artery can be identified. The carotid artery is dissected of its arachnoid covering and the ACA followed to the anterior communicating branch. The olfactory tract is usually visible. Since routine removal of the gyrus rectus is not carried out, the A_1 segment should be exposed and followed along its course. This provides a good road map for localizing the AComA and aneurysm. This vessel is identified by dissecting the arachnoid covering from the

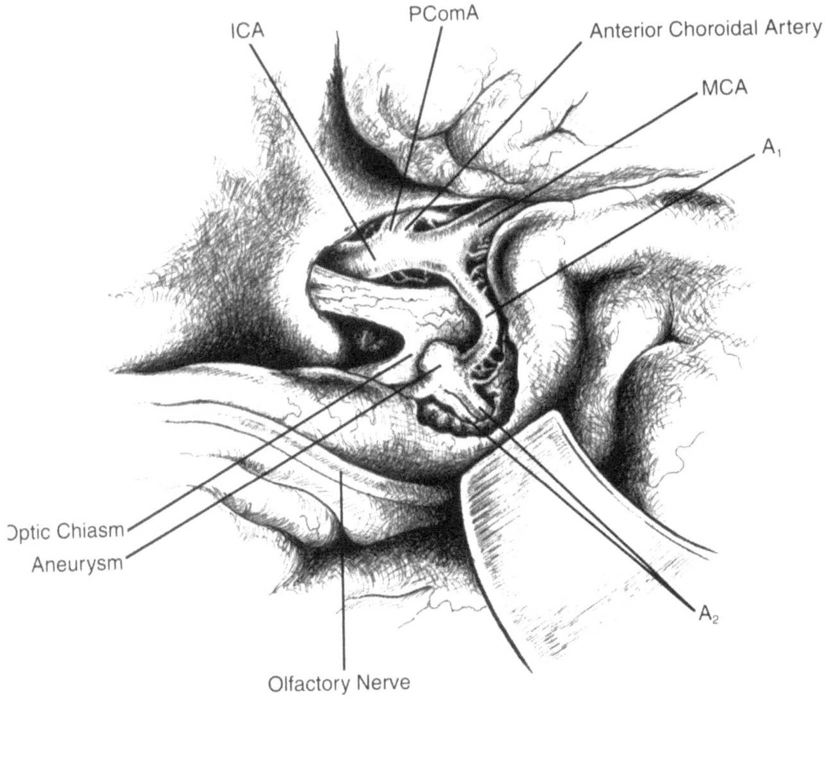

FIGURE 10.3. Right pterional approach to the anterior communicating artery aneurysm. In this case, the A_1 branches are demonstrated passing into the interhemispheric fissure. The gyrus rectus immediately overlying the optic chiasm has been resected to demonstrate the A_2 branches and the aneurysm. PComA, posterior communicating artery.

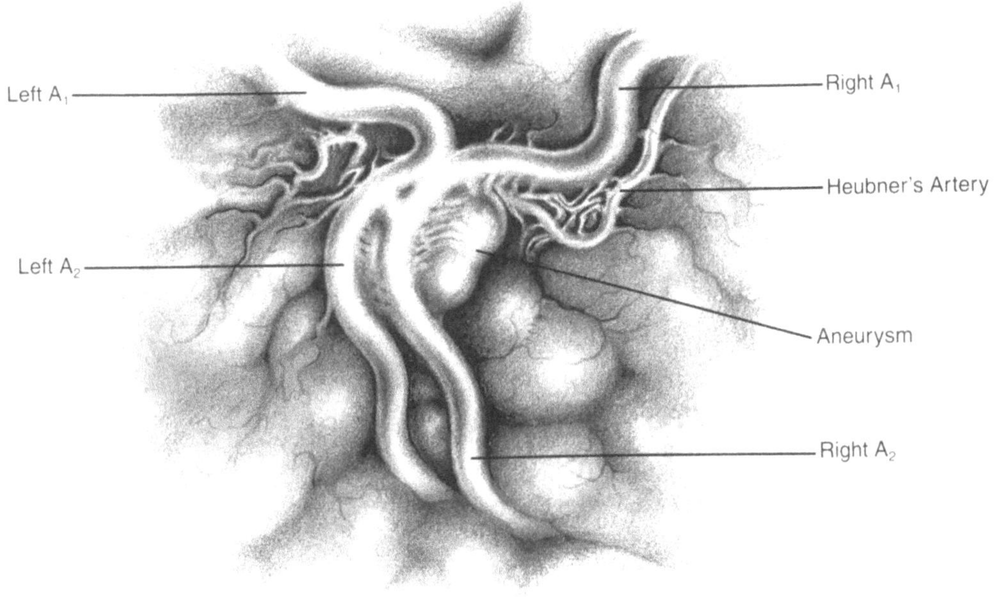

A

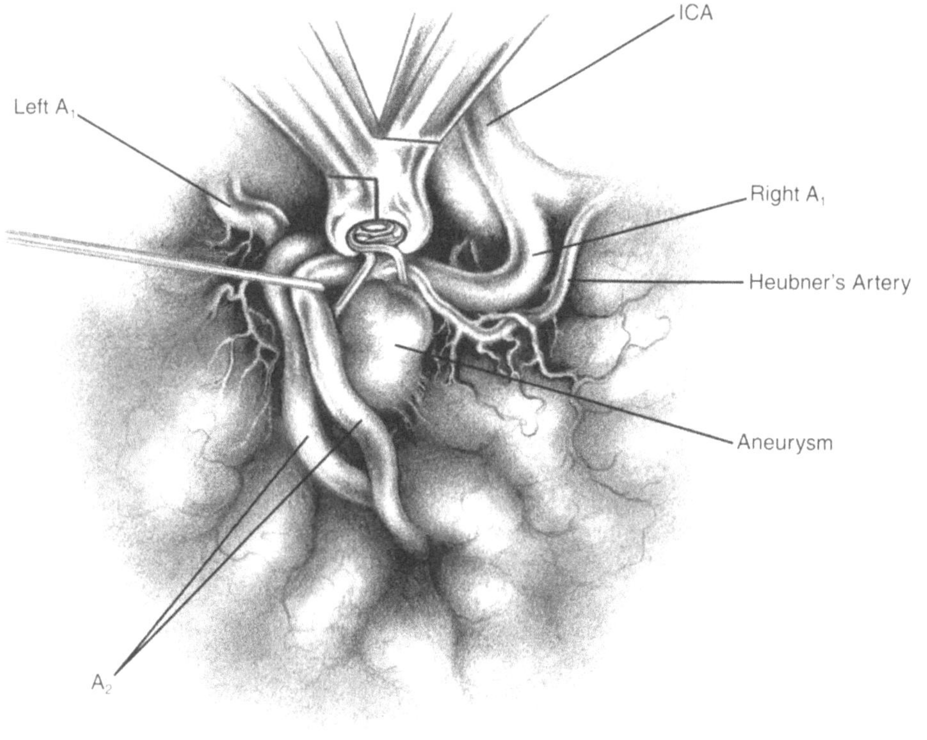

B

FIGURE 10.4. (A) An anterior communicating artery aneurysm projects posteriorly, a less common variant. From this position, important perforators encase the posterior fundus of the aneurysm. (B) For posterior projecting aneurysms, the A_2 branch on the side of approach should be elevated to apply the clip safely. The aneurysm must be depressed in order to visualize the opposite A_2 to assure that is not included in the clip.

carotid artery along its medial course. Further opening of the fissure inferiorly may be required. If the takeoff of the aneurysm from its origin is not clearly seen, however, a gyrus rectus incision must be performed.

A 2-cm incision is made into the gyrus rectus, beginning anterior to the optic chiasm and extending posteriorly until the posterior aspects of the chiasm can be seen (Fig. 10.3). Most aneurysms are found just superior and posterior to the optic chiasm. After cauterizing the gyrus rectus and making the incision, this is followed inward using coagulation and suction until the arachnoid membrane is seen marking the lateral wall in the interhemispheric fissure. The fissure is then opened exposing the two ACAs distal to the anterior communicating branch. If the aneurysm is pointing forward, the AComA should be identified first and followed anteriorly along its course until the aneurysm neck can be exposed.

Aneurysms that project posteriorly, between the A_2 segments, should be approached somewhat more anteriorly. In this case, A_1 becomes the reference point. This artery is followed toward the longitudinal fissure throughout its course. As it joins the AComA, the A_2 and Heubner's arteries are identified. These may adhere to the aneurysm and require both sharp and blunt microsurgical dissection to separate adhesions and arachnoid. The opposite A_1 should also be identified and its relationship to the A_2 and the anterior communicator established. Then the dissection proceeds along the AComA until the neck of the aneurysm has been isolated. Often, the neck will involve branches of the A_1, the A_2, or Heubner's artery. A temporary clip should be employed if rupture of the aneurysm seems likely. This clip should be applied close to the AComA itself if the aneurysm is confined to this vessel. Short arteries, whether they arise from the A_1, A_2, or AComA, should be excluded when possible. From here, the dissection is carried to the neck of the aneurysm, which is clipped separately (Fig. 10.4). The AComA clip may then be removed. After clipping, the most important step is to identify all significant branches and make certain that they have not been included in the clip or that they have not been compromised by clip torsion. In addition, the fundus of the aneurysm should be inspected to make sure that it is collapsed and not pulsatile. For AComA aneurysms, deliberate rupture of the fundus is not necessary. If no pulsations occur or no swirling blood can be detected, exclusion from the circulation can be expected. Figure 10.5 demonstrates the results of direct intracranial clipping of a small AComA aneurysm.

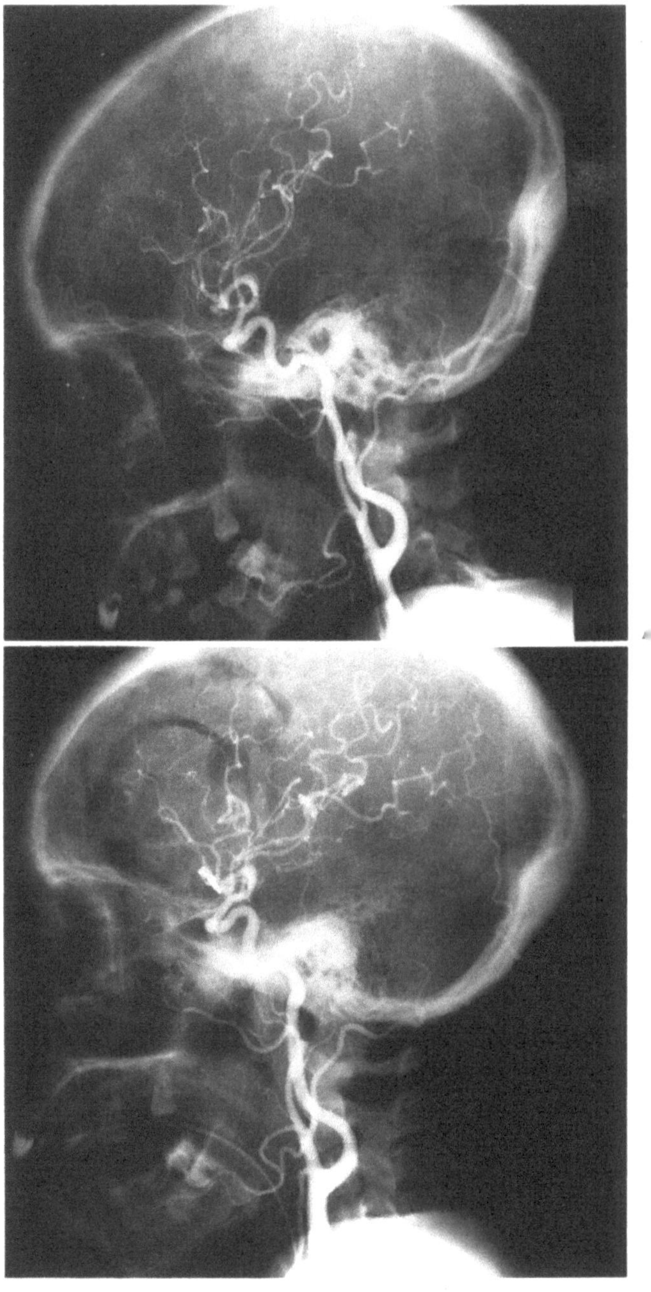

FIGURE 10.5. (A) Small aneurysm of the AcomA that has produced subarachnoid hemorrhage. (B) After clipping using a pterional approach.

Orbitocranial Approach

The orbitocranial approach is used for AComA aneurysms that require more anterior visualization. Aneurysms that project between the A_2 segments and adhere to these vessels are especially suited to this approach. Aneurysms that project forward are also well visualized using this approach. The operation provides the most direct and shortest route to the lesion. Just as it is sometimes necessary to view an AComA aneurysm through the orbit on the angiogram, this approach opens the overlying A_1 and A_2 segments and projects the anterior communicating region more clearly. The pterional approach provides a somewhat more lateral and posterior visualization of aneurysms that project posteriorly and the perforating arteries. The orbitocranial operation provides excellent cosmesis, although occasionally enophthalmos occurs, especially if the orbital contents are entered. The pterional operation is almost always associated with some atrophy in the temporal area and some flattening. The orbitocranial approach may be performed through an eyebrow incision, thus hiding the operative scar in the eyebrow and providing excellent cosmesis, especially for the patient with a receding hairline. However, division of the frontalis branch of the seventh nerve is almost always necessary as the eyebrow incision must be extended along its inferior base. Since most patients recover frontalis muscle function within 6 months, this rarely causes permanent loss. The orbitocranial approach sometimes obviates the need for gyrus rectus incisions. Unless the aneurysm projects inferiorly or forward, a gyrus rectus incision is usually needed when a pterional incision is used.

Using an orbitocranial approach, the surgeon may substitute the traditional scalp incision with an incision extending through the eyebrow and into the temporal area to the zygoma (Fig. 10.6). At this point, the incision should be directed somewhat more posteriorly to within 2 cm of the tragus. The incision is opened to the fascia and attempts are made to retract the frontalis nerve if it has not been severed. This should swing forward with the anterior portion of the incision. The temporalis muscle is dissected free of the temporal bone and reflected posteriorly. An opening is made at the pterion, in the most inferior portions of the squamosal suture as it approaches the zygomatic arch, and just above the supraorbital foramen. This opening may enter the frontal sinus, which must be dissected free of its mucosa. Then, using a small dissecting tool on the air drill, a small opening is made in the posterior wall of the frontal sinus.

The orbital fascia is identified under the supraorbital rim and dissected free with a Penfield dissector, exposing

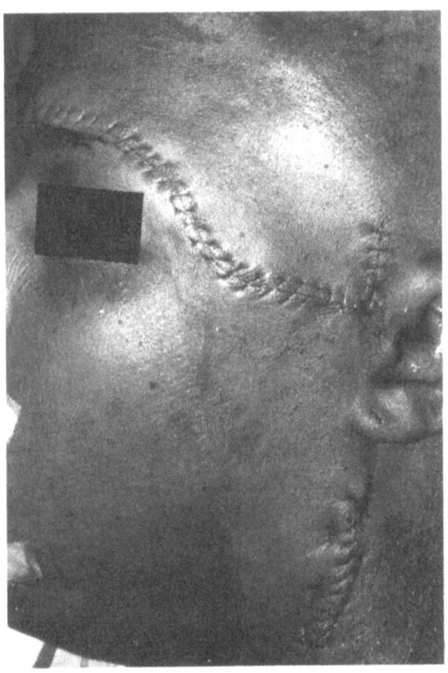

FIGURE 10.6. Eyebrow incision for the orbitocranial approach. The incision must extend to the tragus and superiorly in order to obtain exposure necessary for visualizing the anterior cerebral circulation. In this case, proximal control of the internal carotid artery was necessary because of the low origin of the aneurysm in the cavernous sinus.

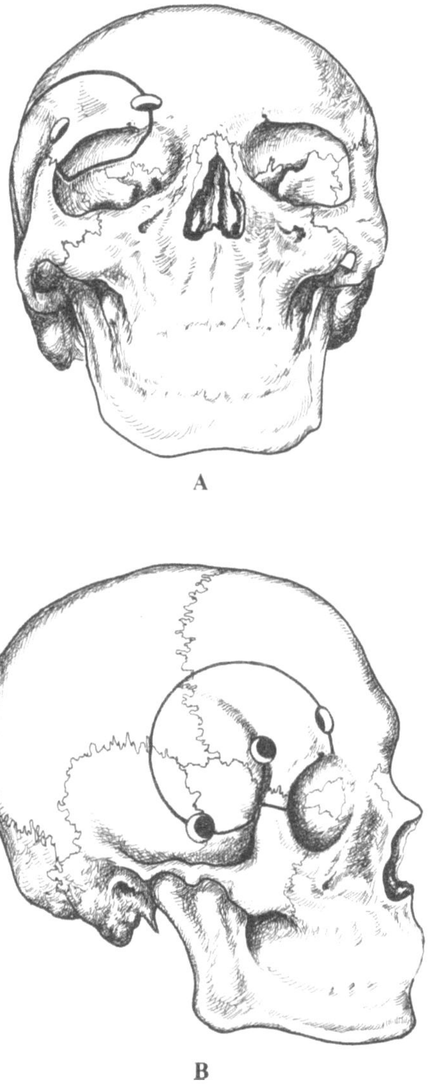

FIGURE 10.7. (A) The orbitocranial approach for aneurysms of the anterior circulation. One burr hole is placed over the supraorbital foramen, one at the pterion, one at the inferior extent of the squamosal suture, and others as needed. These are connected and a cut made at the zygomaticofrontal suture. Scoring the orbital roof facilitates fracture. (B) Lateral view of the orbitocranial approach. This exposure provides both pterional and frontal views of the lesion.

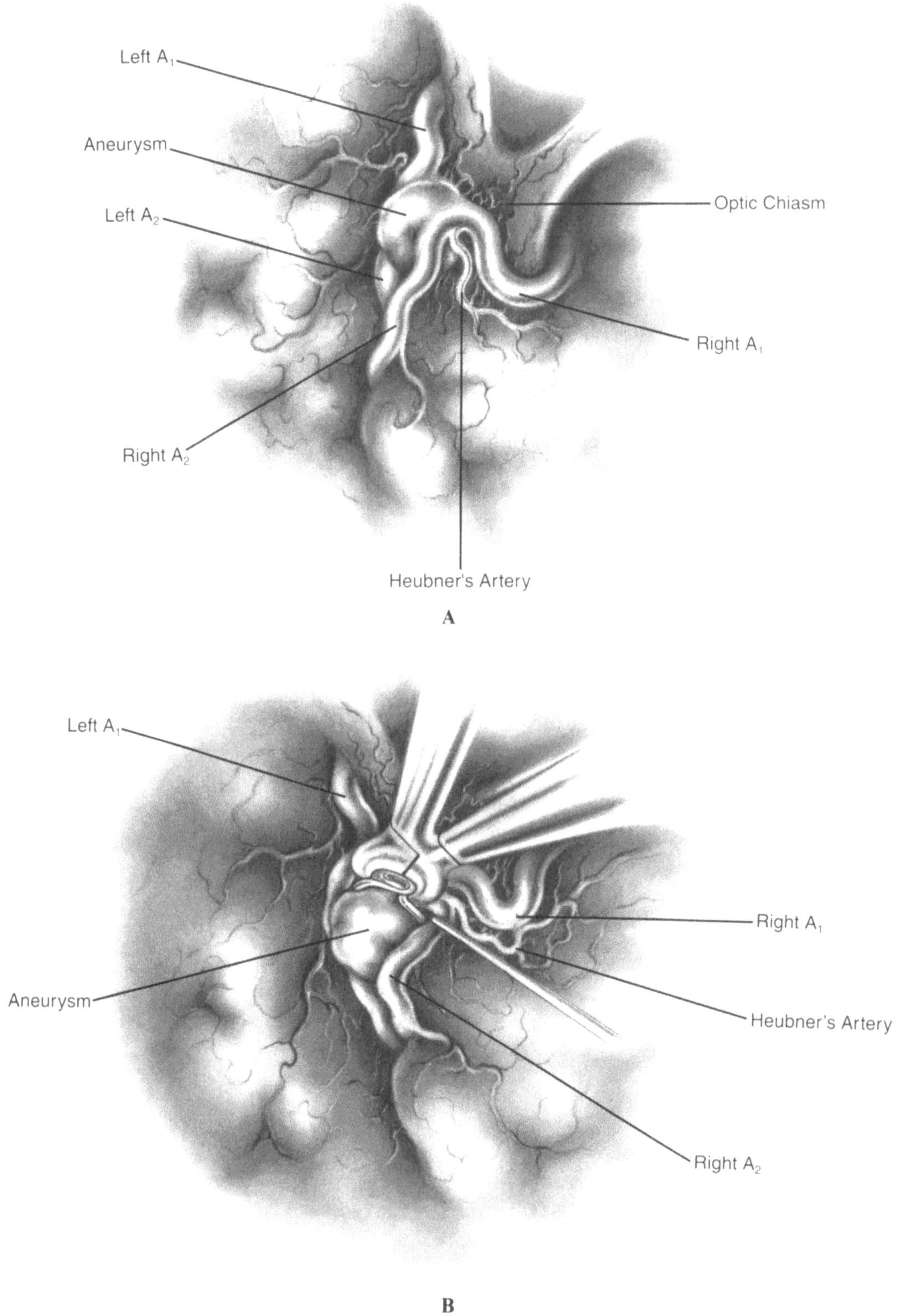

FIGURE 10.8. (A) An anterior communicating artery aneurysm projects anteriorly and superiorly. This view is from a right orbitocranial approach, which provides good visualization of both A_1 and A_2 branches. (B) Clipping of the aneurysm shown in A. The perforating arteries are not well seen but both A_2 branches are separated well from the A_1 branches.

the orbital roof approximately 2.5 cm from the glabella. Using a small dissecting drill, the surgeon scores the orbital roof along its course from the supraorbital foramen to the lateral orbital rim. Using the craniotome attachment, the zygomaticofrontal suture is used as a reference point to open the lateral orbital rim. The remainder of the openings are then connected. The bone will be fractured along the orbital roof. If the bone does not fracture easily, a Gigli saw blade should be passed through the openings and the orbital roof cut through or thinned enough to fracture easily (Fig. 10.7). In our experience, the orbital roof usually fractures smoothly approximately 2 cm from the glabella. If it is not scored sufficiently, however, it may fracture into the superior orbital fissure, causing damage to intimate structures. As the free bone flap is removed, any tears in the orbital fascia should be closed immediately because the escaping orbital fat may undergo necrosis even if it did not interfere with exposure. At this point, the dura mater should be opened along the posterior aspects of the cranial opening and allowed to cover the orbital contents. This exposes the frontal and temporal lobes. It also permits entry into the sylvian fissure. The veins are coagulated and a self-retraining retractor is placed between temporal and frontal lobes. A second retractor is usually placed directly under the frontal lobe, over the orbital roof, thus providing both a frontal and pterional projection. Usually, the frontal view is preferred for AComA aneurysms. This retractor is extended to the interhemispheric fissure, identifying the optic nerve and carotid artery en route. The interhemispheric fissure may be opened and the A_1 portion of the artery is usually visible at this point. The junction of the A_1 and AComA is identified on the right side, and this vessel is followed and dissected until the aneurysm neck can be visualized and clipped (Fig. 10.8).

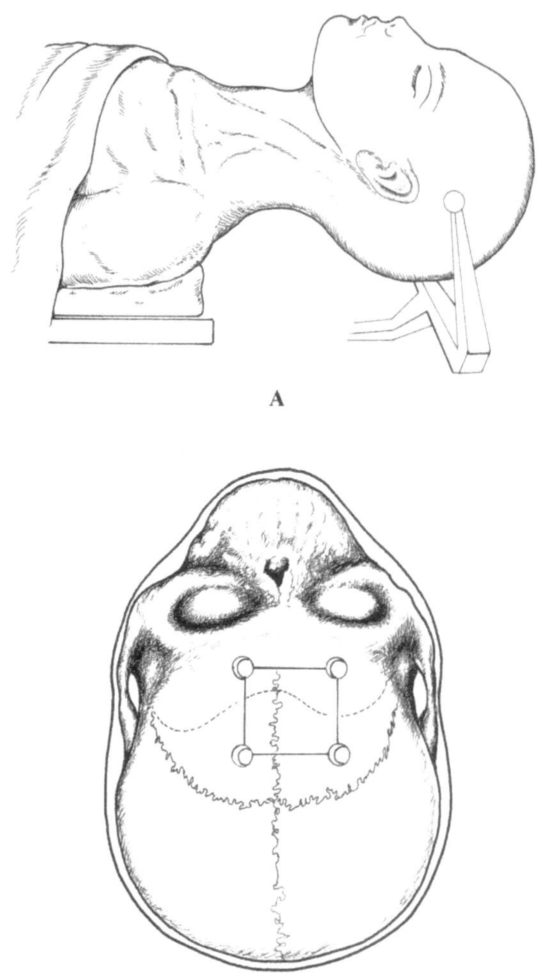

A

B

FIGURE 10.9. (A) Position for distal ACA aneurysms. The head is slightly extended in the head holder. (B) The bone flap is placed predominantly to the right of the midline and approximately 2 cm anterior to the coronal sutures.

Approach to Distal ACA Aneurysms

Aneurysms that arise distal to the AComA are located in the interhemispheric fissure. They should be approached via the midline, usually placing the craniotomy predominantly over the patient's right frontal lobe, which will be retracted away from the midline. For aneurysms arising on the distal callosomarginal or frontopolar arteries, transfalcine approaches have been offered; but the surgeons options are more limited and proximal, and distal control may not be easily achieved (Fig. 10.9).

For lesions that arise from the A_2 branch at the frontopolar or callosomarginal artery, the bone flap should be placed low, about 1 cm above the supraorbital ridge, to allow identification of the main A_2 segments as they pass from beneath the genu of the corpus callosum. The orbital artery exits the A_2 beneath the genu to supply the orbital surface and gyrus rectus. The frontopolar artery exits at the genu and supplies the medial part of the superior frontal gyrus. The callosomarginal artery also supplies the medial superior frontal gyrus along with part of the corpus callosum, the cingulate gyrus, and the anterior central gyrus. This artery arises superior to and approximately 15 mm distal to the anterior genu in most patients.

A scalp incision placed in the hairline usually permits enough bone exposure. Because the scalp is reflected anteriorly, the periosteum overlying the frontal bone should be preserved. This will be used to cover the posterior wall of the frontal sinus if it should be entered; therefore, as much as possible should be carefully dissected free of the bone posteriorly and left attached anteriorly. Later, this fascia will be sutured to the anterior aspects of the dura mater to separate the craniotomy site from the frontal sinus. There is no advantage to obliterating the sinus with fat or muscle if it is closed along its posterior surface.

The craniotomy should be placed across the midline so that the sagittal sinus may be divided if necessary. Ordinarily, a unilateral exposure is adequate because the A_2 lies close to the corpus callosum, and, except for large, upward projecting aneurysms, the falx will not interfere. Occasionally, the dome of an aneurysm may become adhered to the falx or inferior sagittal sinus. The A_2 branches intertwine and the aneurysm may be attached by adhesions to one or both. Only careful dissection along the A_2 segments provides the solution as to which is the origin and which is the secondary attachment. Temporary clips allow the dissection to proceed with lowered risk of premature rupture. There is still debate about whether the clips should be removed periodically to perfuse ischemic tissue. However, this technique has been applied to other tissues with success and should offer some protection for the ischemic brain as well. The A_2 branch may be occluded for periods of up to 40 min if the patient is anticoagulated. The nonanticoagulated safe occlusion times are unknown for this vessel (Fig. 10.10).

Right-angled microvascular clips are often required to occlude the neck without compromising flow in the respective A_2. The distal branches anastomose freely with branches from both the MCA and the PCA; therefore, sacrifice of this vessel is theoretically possible. However, A_2 preservation is the goal. In the case of fusiform aneurysms that have ruptured, several modifications in technique are feasible. If the lesion is short and the proximal and distal segments will reach after excision of the lesion, then end-to-end anastomosis is the best alternative (Fig. 10.11). Some lengthening is achievable by cutting the arachnoid strands along the A_2 branch. If the A_2 hugs the corpus callosum tightly and there is no redundancy in the vessel, a new lumen must be developed by the application of clips along the axis of the aneurysm. The primary complication bearing upon this method relates to the presence of thrombus, which invariably occupies the wall of fusiform aneurysms. Distal occlusion and embolization is thus the major complication.

Endovascular Technique

The endovascular operation, like the direct operation is best applied to patients in good neurological condition. The size and configuration of the aneurysm is also most important with aneurysms of the AComA and A_1 segments. With direct clipping, surgical results are best when aneurysms are less than 2 cm in size. Endovascular operations may be better for larger aneurysms and less suitable for smaller lesions measuring less than 1 cm. The endovascular approach is not only useful for aneurysm occlusion but is also useful diagnostically. Balloon occlusion of parent arteries indicates to the surgeon whether a vessel can be safely occluded temporarily or permanently.

Historically, aneurysms of the AComA complex have been the most difficult ones for endovascular methods. The first reports of an AComA aneurysm managed using endovascular techniques appeared in 1973.[17] In this case, an arteriovenous malformation (AVM) fed by both ACAs was associated with an aneurysm involving the AComA. The AVM occupied the posterior frontal lobes bilaterally in the interhemispheric fissure. The patient already had two previous hemorrhages, from either the aneurysm or the AVM. A small latex balloon, introduced into the carotid artery, passed rapidly into the A_1 segments intracranially, aided by the abnormal flow patterns. Then the balloon was manipulated into the AComA and into the aneurysm where it was inflated and detached. The aneurysm was thus occluded, sparing feeders to the AVM that were subsequently embolized using polysterol. Since 1973, endovascular techniques have flourished. Victor Shcheglov in Kiev has now accumulated perhaps the largest series of patients with lesions of the ACA numbering in the hundreds.[18]

Several problems had to be overcome in order to pass a catheter into the A_1 segment consistently. Many types of arterial balloons and catheters were developed and tested in order to negotiate the sharp turns encountered at the takeoff of the A_1 from the ICA. The microballoons that can be passed through these small vessels may still be of insufficient size to occlude large aneurysms of the AComA complex, the lesion regarded as most applicable for this technique.

Before deciding upon any endovascular approach, complete studies of both carotid arterial circulations, including oblique views of the anterior cerebral–anterior communicating artery complex are necessary. Oblique projections through the orbit provide good visualization of the AComA and allow the surgeon to make decisions concerning the neck of the aneurysm in relation to the parent artery. The ICA from which the aneurysm fills best is preferred for initial catheterization. If the aneurysm is fed equally from the right or the left ICA, the nondominant carotid artery should be almost always chosen for the entry site. Configuration of the takeoff of the A_1 from the ICA is important. An A_1 that leaves the ICA with an obtuse angle of more than 90o is more easily entered than those that take an inferior course or leave the artery at angles of 90° or less (Fig. 10.12). Contralateral occlusion of the carotid artery in the neck with simple compressive techniques may be helpful in changing flow pattern so that the catheter can be introduced into the A_1 segment. Otherwise, a balloon may be placed

FIGURE 10.10. (A) Right paramedian approach along the falx to an aneurysm arising from the pericallosal artery. Typical relationship of the A_2 vessels to the aneurysm is shown. (B) The neck of the aneurysm has been identified after microdissection and a right angled fenestrated clip applied, preserving flow in the right pericallosal artery.

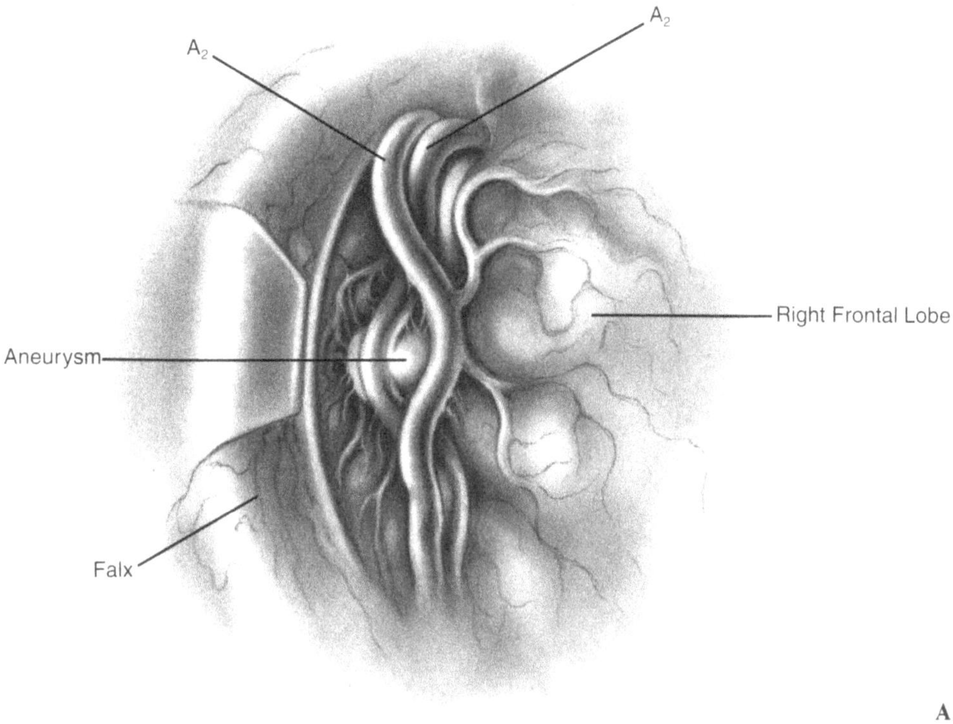

A

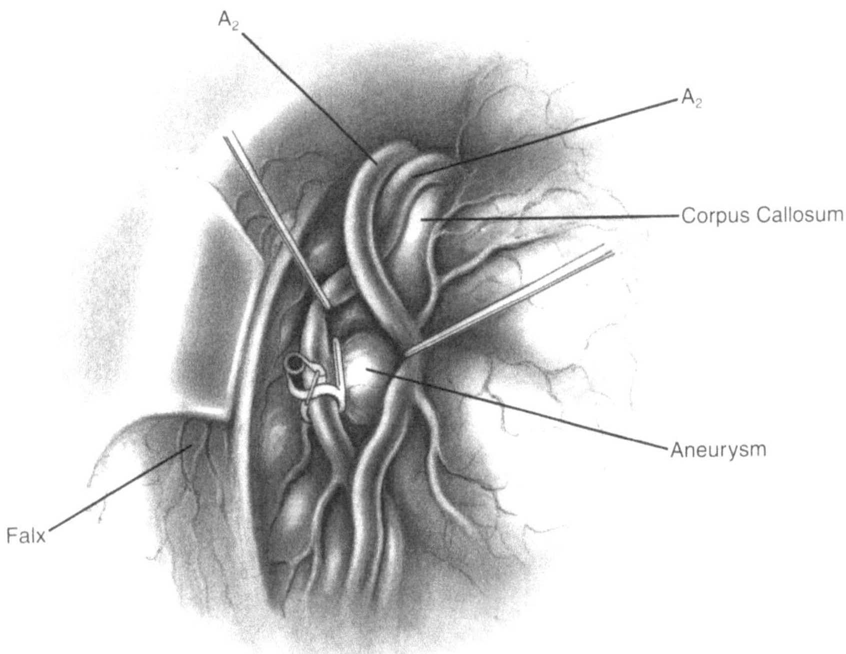

B

into the ipsilateral MCA and inflated to direct flow into the ipsilateral A_1 for manipulation of the balloon catheter. The aim of endovascular surgery for this aneurysm is to maintain flow in the AComA as well as in both A_1 and A_2 segments. It is perhaps easier to introduce balloons into those aneurysms that point anteriorly because contrast material that fills the balloon is somewhat lighter than blood and tends to migrate upward when the patient is placed in the supine position on the operating table. Deconstructive operations (wherein the parent artery is sacrificed) must sometimes be carried out in those cases in which the aneurysm occupies all of the AComA. In these cases, occluding the AComA is almost universal with balloon inflation. This effectively sepa-

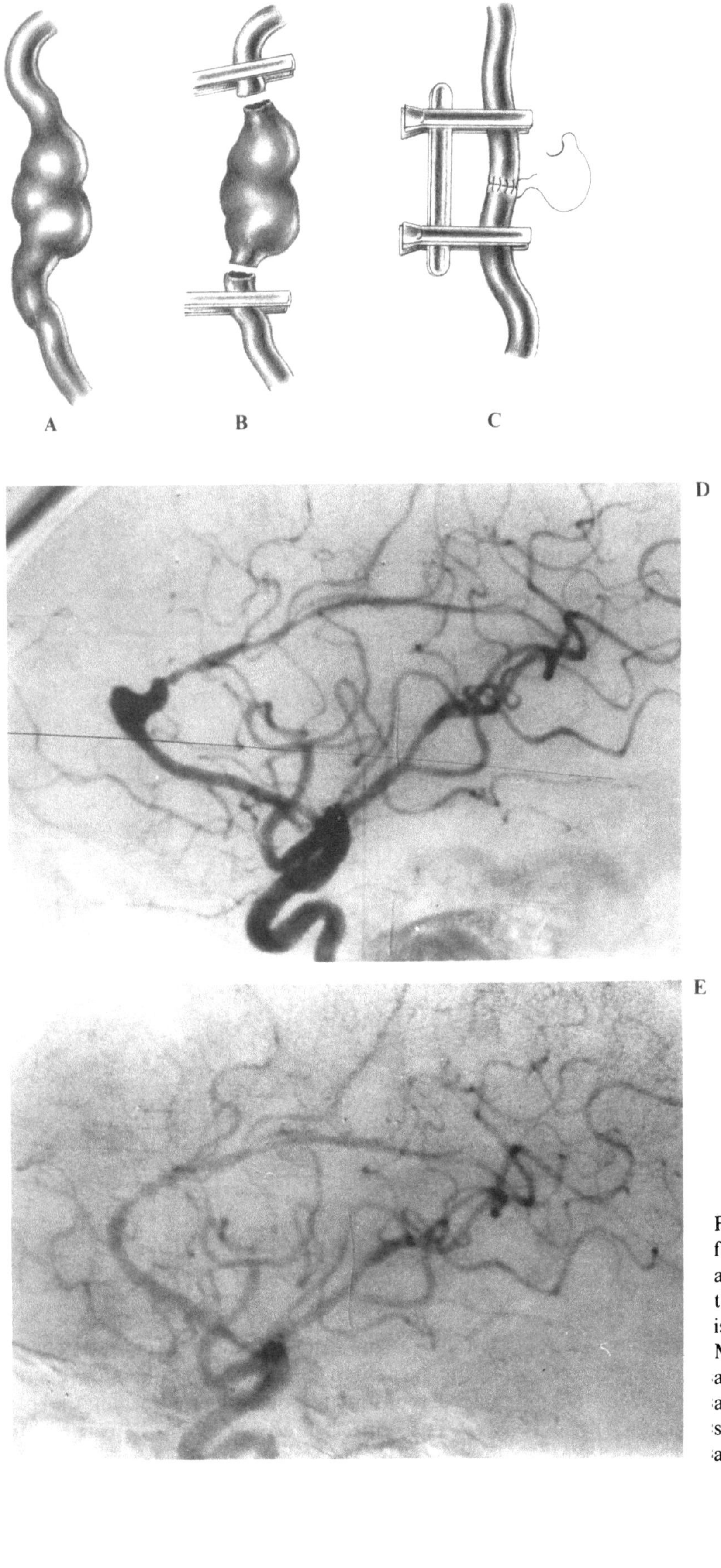

FIGURE 10.11. (A–C) Large and unclippable fusiform aneurysms may be managed by excision and end-to-end anastomosis when they involve the A_2 branches. In these cases, some dissection is needed proximally and distally to gain length. Multiple fine sutures are needed to secure the anastomosis. (D) Partially thrombosed giant aneurysm of the anterior cerebral artery causing subarachnoid hemorrhage. (E) After excision and end-to-end anastomosis.

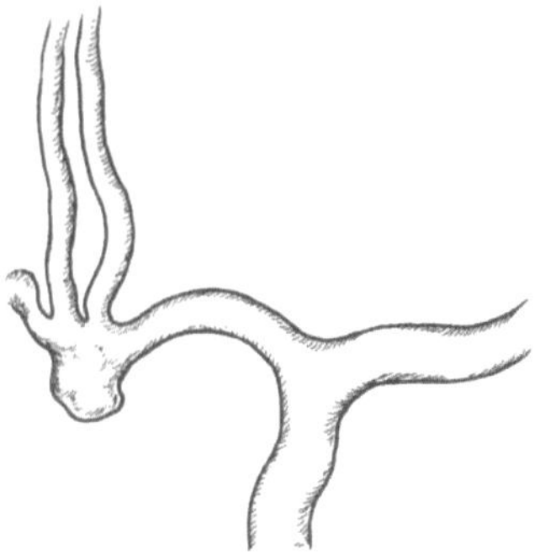

A

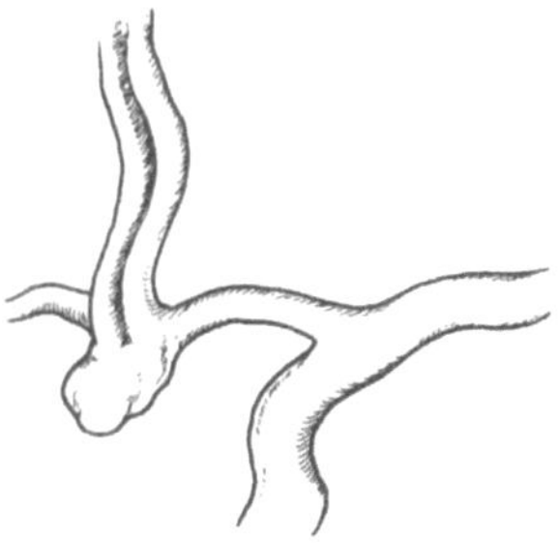

B

FIGURE 10.12. (A) The anterior cerebral artery takes off at an obtuse angle facilitating the passage of a balloon catheter. (B) The anterior cerebral artery exits at an acute angle making passage of the balloon catheter difficult.

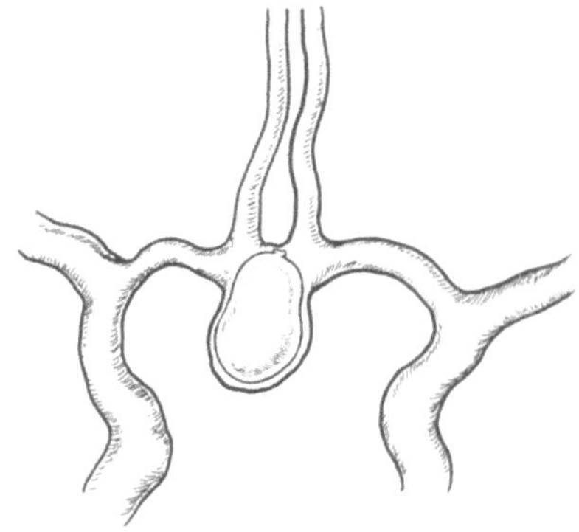

FIGURE 10.13. Deconstructive procedure for an AComA aneurysm. The balloon has been placed in the aneurysm separating the left and right anterior cerebral circulation.

rates the two anterior circulations but is usually well tolerated (Fig. 10.13). Test occlusions are employed with the patient awake to identify those patients dependent upon cross-flow through the AComA branch.

The second endovascular procedure found useful is occlusion of the dominant A_1 that feeds the aneurysm. The size of the balloon to be used and its position within the A_1 segment are important for this procedure. Since the perforating arteries from A_1 feed the medial basal forebrain, internal capsule, and caudate nucleus, the balloon must be short and well placed distally in the segment, as close to the aneurysm as possible. After A_1 occlusion, the angiogram should be repeated to see if the aneurysm fills from the opposite side. If it does, other procedures may be needed to effectively exclude this lesion from the arterial circulation. Test occlusions must

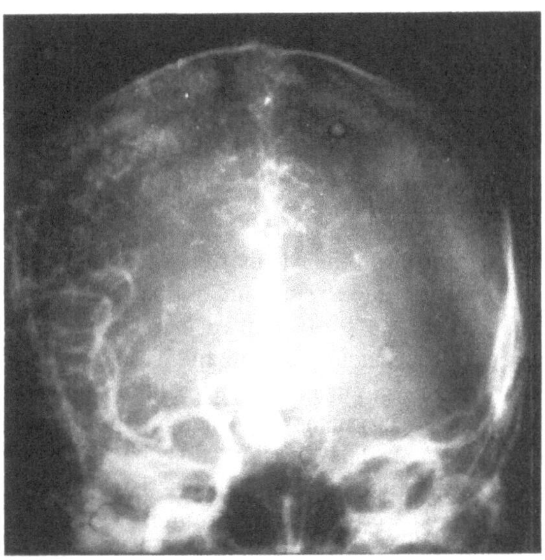

A

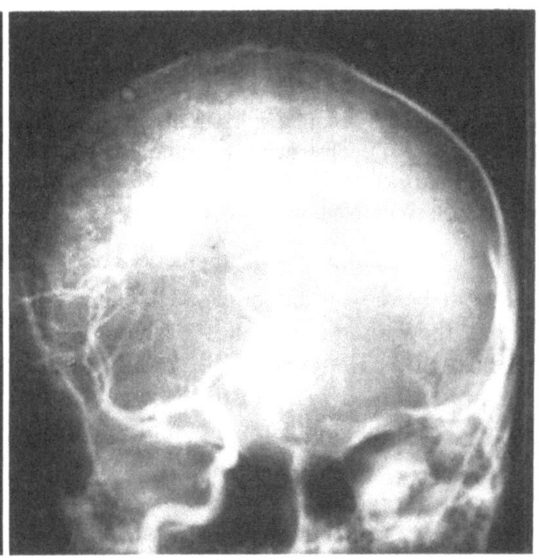

B

FIGURE 10.14. (A and B) A giant aneurysm of the anterior communicating artery before and after a balloon has been placed directly in the aneurysm cavity, excluding it from the circulation. Both A_2 branches fill.

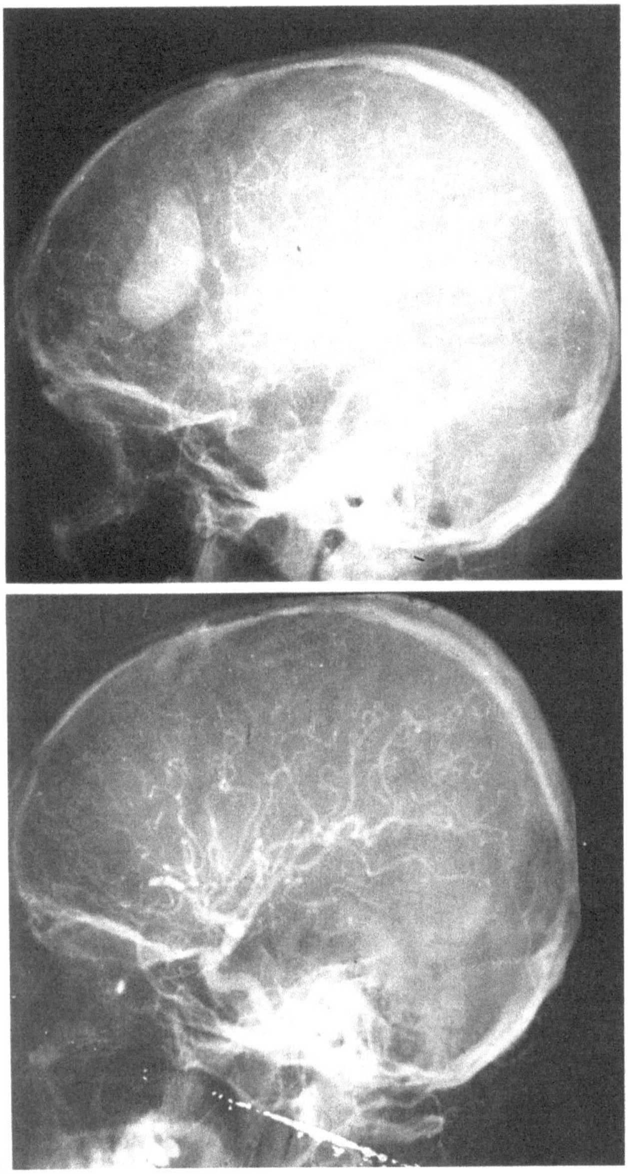

A

B

FIGURE 10.15. (A and B) Giant aneurysm of the distal anterior cerebral artery (A_2). Deconstructive operation with a balloon in the distal anterior cerebral artery proximal to the aneurysm orifice at the callosomarginal orifice.

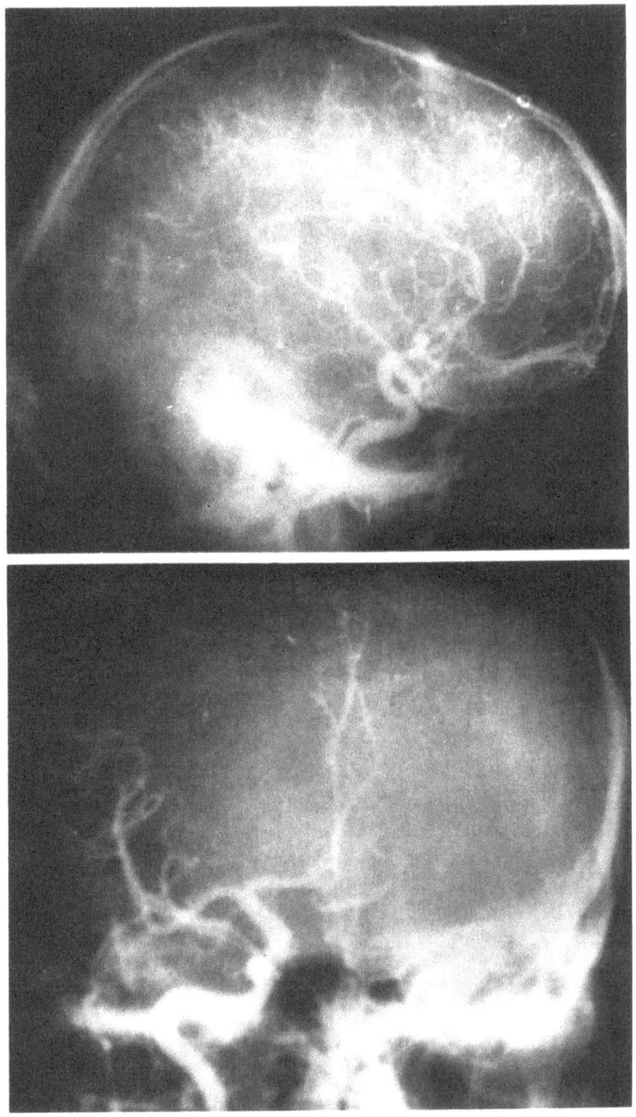

FIGURE 10.16. (A) Small superior projecting aneurysm of the anterior communicating artery. (B) The balloon is in the cavity of the aneurysm.

be carried out before the balloon is detached to make certain that the balloon does not occlude important perforators such as Heubner's artery prior to detachment. Figures 10.14–10.16 illustrate some results of endovascular occlusion of AComA complex aneurysms.

Conclusions

The decision about whether to use a direct intracranial operation versus an endovascular approach must take into account many factors. Among these are the experience of the surgeon, the facilities available, the patient's condition, the peculiarities in configuration and location of the aneurysm, and the patient's desires and wishes. Only the surgeon who has experience with the direct intracranial operation and clipping and with endovascular technique employing balloons and coils should make the decision as to which method is best for a given patient. The decision must be based upon answers to questions such as (1) Has the aneurysm recently ruptured? or (2) Is it unruptured? The size of the aneurysm is as important as its location in relation to the parent vessel and its orifice size.

In patients with recent rupture, these decisions must be made carefully. The risk of rupturing, causing rebleeding in this individual, are substantially greater than in the patient with a "cold" aneurysm. When the decision is reached that an aneurysm should be treated using an endovascular method, precautions must be taken. Preliminary plans should have been made to perform an emergency craniotomy, with all of the advance planning requisite for this procedure. If the endovascular surgeon is skilled and fortunate, bleeding may be arrested with a balloon placed in the parent artery at the aneurysm orifice. Only a short period of time, depending on many factors including the reserve energy state of the arterial territory in question, is available in which to make necessary decisions and to carry out the operation. This operation can succeed only if a skilled aneurysm surgeon is involved in the care of the patient.

References

1. Yasargil MG. *Microneurosurgery*. Georg Thieme, Verlag, Stuttgart; 1984;I.
2. Nathal E, Yasui N, Sampel T, Suzuki A. Intraoperative anatomical studies in patients with aneurysms of the anterior communicating artery complex. *J Neurosurg*. 1992; 76:629–634.
3. Padget DH. The development of the cranial arteries in the human embryo. *Contrib Embryol*. 1948;32:205–261.
4. Fischer E. Die Lageabweichungen der vorderen Hirnarterie in Gefassbild. *Zentralbl Neurochir*. 1938;3:300–312.
5. Maurer J, Maurer E, Perneczky A. Surgically verified variation in the A_1 segment of the anterior cerebral artery. *J Neurosurgery*. 1991;75:950–953.
6. Riggs HE, Rupp C. Variation in form of circle of Willis. *Arch Neurol*. 1963;8:8–14.
7. Wilson G, Riggs HE, Rupp C. The pathologic anatomy of ruptured cerebral aneurysms. *J Neurosurg*. 1954;11:128–134.
8. Von Mitterwallner F. Variationstatistische unter Suchungen an den basalen Hirngefassen. *Acta Anat*. 1955;24:51–88.
9. Perlmutter D, Rhoton AL. Microsurgical anatomy of the anterior cerebral anterior communicating recurrent artery complex. *J Neurosurg*. 1976;45:259–271.
10. Gomes FB, Dujovny M, Umansky F, Berman SK, Diaz FG, Ausman J, Mirchandani HG, Ray WJ. Microanatomy of the anterior cerebral artery. *Surg Neurol*. 1986;26:129–41.
11. Vincentelli F, Lehman G. Extracerebral course of the perforating branches of the anterior communicating artery microsurgical anatomical study. *Surg Neurol*. 1991;35:98–104.
12. Perlmutter D, Rhoton AL. Microsurgical anatomy of the distal anterior cerebral artery. *J Neurosurgery*. 1978;49: 204–228.
13. Gomes FB, Dujovny M, Umansky F, Ausman JI, Diaz FG, Ray WJ, Mirchandani HG. Microsurgical anatomy of the recurrent artery of Heubner. *J Neurosurgery*. 1984;60: 130–139.
14. Pieris J, Russel R. Giant Aneurysms of the carotid system presenting as visual field defect. *J Neurol Neurosurg Psychiatry*. 1980;43:1053–1064.
15. Zubkov YN. *Treatment of Patients with Intracranial Arterial Aneurysms in the Hemorrhagic Period*. Moscow; 1990. Thesis.
16. Silver AJ, Pederson ME Jr, Ganti SR, Hilal SK, Michelson W. CT of subarachnoid hemorrhage due to ruptures aneurysm. *Am J Nucl Radiol*. 1981;2:13–22.
17. Zubkov YN. Catheterization of brain vessels. *Ann Polenov Neurosurgical Institute* (Leningrad). 1973;5:218–227.
18. Fox AJ. Highlights of the First Congress of the World Federation of Interventional and Therapeutic Neuroradiology; October 11–13, 1991; Zurich, Switzerland. *AJNR*. 1992;13:1021–1024.

11
Middle Cerebral Artery Aneurysms

Middle cerebral artery (MCA) aneurysms make up approximately 30% of all intracranial aneurysms presenting with acute subarachnoid hemorrhage (SAH).[1] The incidence, however, varies from 21% in clinical series to 31% in autopsy series. Eighty to 85% are located at the bifurcation of the MCA at the junction of the M_1 and M_2. Ten percent, however, are found along the trunk of the M_1 at the lenticulostriate branches and the anterior temporal branch. Ten percent are found on the M_2 branches, distal to bifurcation.

Yasargil[2] classified MCA aneurysms into anterior temporal, lenticulostriate, bifurcation, second bifurcation, and distal, thus defining the aneurysm in relation to its nearest branch. Structurally, aneurysms of the bifurcation present the most difficult surgical problems because they commonly arise from a sessile base and the broad neck presents a problem for direct clipping. Unfortunately, this aneurysm makes up 80% of all of those of the MCA.

Eighty-five to 90% of all aneurysms of the MCA present with acute SAH. Unruptured aneurysms occasionally produce seizures, hemianopsia, hemiparesis, and speech disorders if they involve the dominant hemisphere. These unruptured aneurysms are usually of giant size, greater than 2 cm in diameter. They also present as a pulsatile mass. Of all giant intracranial aneurysms, those involving the MCA make up 16%.[3]

Microanatomy

During the third stage of Padget's embryologic classification (7–12 mm, 31- to 33-day embryo), the MCA extends from the primary internal carotid artery (ICA).[4]

The MCA is called the largest cerebral artery.[5] It originates from the ICA at the proximal end of the sylvian fissure, below the anterior perforated substance, posterior to the division of the olfactory tract into the medial and lateral olfactory striae and lateral to the optic chiasm. The diameter of the MCA at its origin is 2.4 to 4.6 mm, and, in 70% of cases, it is larger than the ipsilateral anterior cerebral artery (ACA).[2]

The MCA passes laterally below the anterior perforated substance, approximately 10 mm behind the sphenoid ridge, to the sylvian fissure (Fig. 11.1). The main trunk of the MCA courses within the sylvian fissure and divides into its secondary trunks (main division); then it turns posteriorly crossing over the limen of insula with a sharp angle that is called the genu and lies upon the surface of the insula. The branches of the MCA arising from its primary division, course between the insula medially and the opercula of the temporal, frontal, and parietal lobes laterally; then they pass around the opercular cleft and spread out over the lateral surface and part of the inferior surface of the cerebral hemisphere.

The MCA has few variations.[5–7] The most common anomalies are duplication and an accessory MCA. The duplicate MCA arises from the ICA close to the origin of the anterior choroidal artery. The accessory MCA most commonly arises from the lateral aspect of the ACA near the origin of the anterior communicating artery (AComA). The accessory MCA, like the recurrent artery of Heubner, passes laterally parallel to the proximal ACA; the recurrent artery of Heubner enters the anterior perforated substance but the accessory MCA passes the anterior perforated substance and the proximal portion of the MCA to enter the sylvian fissure.

The duplicate MCA and accessory MCA supply the cortical areas that are usually supplied by the MCA; they may give rise to the perforating arteries. MCA anomalies were reported in about 3% of cases.[6,8] Jain[6] reported the duplication in 0.7% and an accessory MCA in 2.7% of 300 cadavers.

Segmentation of the MCA

Gibo et al.[5] divided the MCA and its branches into four segments: the M_1 or sphenoidalis, the M_2 or insular segment, the M_3 or opercular segment, and the M_4 or cortical segment. The M_1 segment begins at the origin

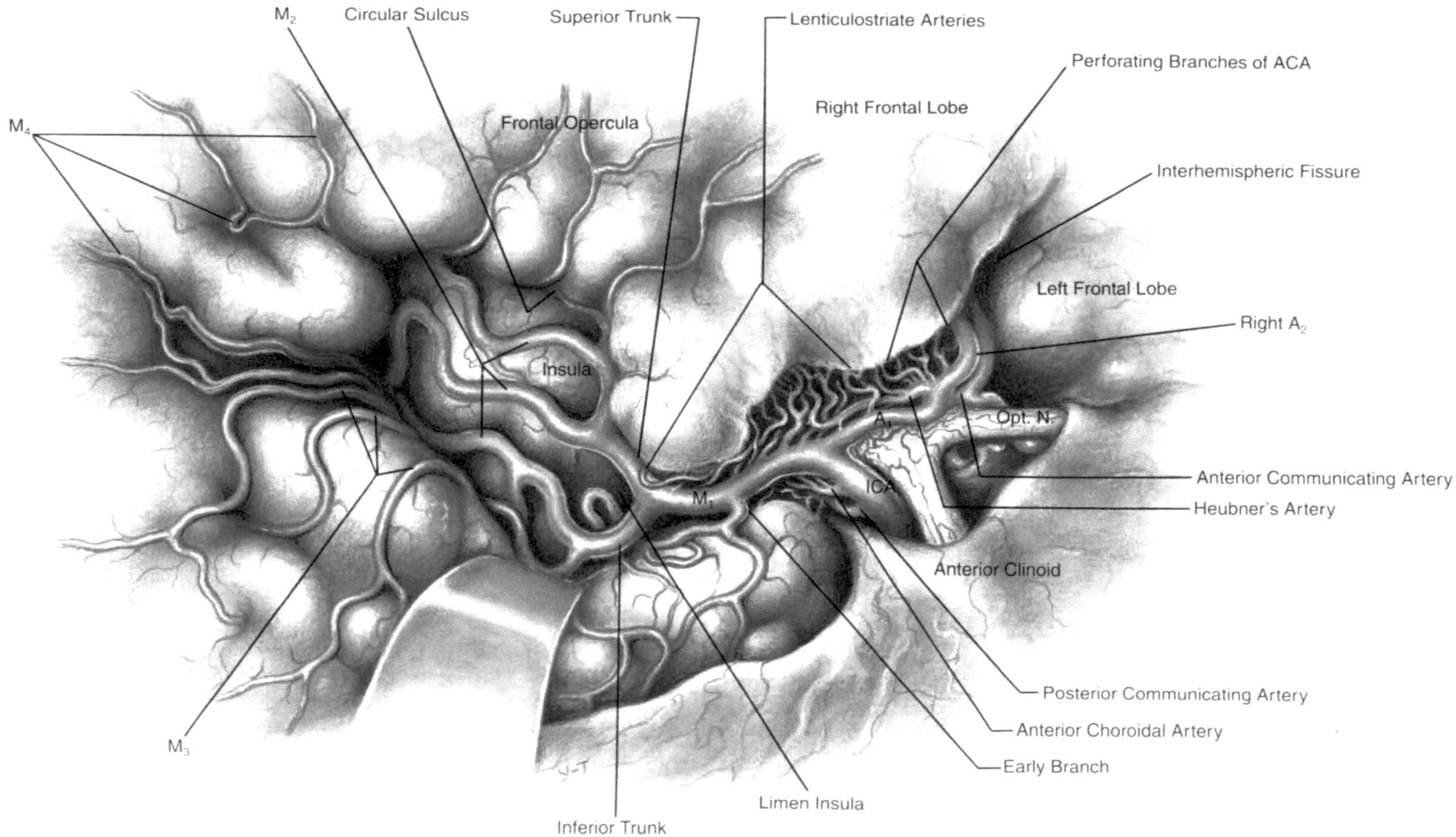

FIGURE 11.1. The deep branches of the right middle cerebral artery are shown from a right extended pterional approach. The superficial frontal cortex has been partially removed to demonstrate the penetrating arteries that originate on A_1 and M_1 and supply the deep nuclei. The right temporal lobe has been deflected inferiorly to show sylvian and insular branches of the middle cerebral artery.

of the artery and courses laterally in the depth of the sphenoidal portion of the sylvian fissure behind the sphenoidal ridge and then terminates at the site where the artery turns posterosuperiorly at about a 90° angle. This part of the artery is called the genu and is located at the junction of the sphenoidal and opercular compartment of the sylvian fissure and close to the limen of insula. The length of the M_1 segment, which is also called the horizontal segment, is about 14 to 16 mm long but may be as long as 30 mm.[2] The main division of the MCA is usually located proximal to or at the level of the limen insula. In one study, the main division occurred before the genu in 85% of the cases studied.[5] Most commonly, the artery divides into two trunks but it may divide into three or more secondary trunks. In the study conducted by Gibo et al.,[5] the MCA bifurcated into the superior and inferior trunks in 78% of the cases, trifurcated in 12%, and divided into multiple trunks in 10%. Umansky et al.[8] reported a bifurcation in 71%, a trifurcation in 20%, and multiple divisions in 9%. The early branches of the MCA arise from the main trunk of the artery before the main division.

The M_2 (or insular segment), including the secondary trunks of the MCA, begins at the genu, passes over the limen of insula, and then lies on the insular cortex. It terminates at the circular sulcus of the insula. The cortical branches originate from the secondary trunks at the insular area.

The outer diameter of the secondary trunks ranges from 1.4 to 2.3 mm and their length ranges between 12.1 and 14.9 mm.[3] When the MCA terminates into a bifurcation, the superior and inferior trunks may have unequal diameters. The larger trunk supplies more cortical areas than the smaller trunk.

Mobilizations of the insular compartment of the MCA are limited by several small, penetrating pial arteries. They may be lifted up 3 to 5 mm without stretching the small pial arteries. The M_3 or opercular segment of the MCA begins at the circular sulcus and consists of the branches originating from the secondary trunks. These branches divide into superior and inferior groups, reaching the circular sulcus. The superior group passes downward on the medial surface of the frontal and parietal opercula to reach the superficial part of the sylvian fissure, then passes over the lateral surface of the opercula in an upward direction to spread over the surface of the cerebral cortex. The inferior group, which irrigates the temporal lobe, turns upward and laterally, then courses around the temporal operculum, and, after passing the external surface of the sylvian fissure, turns downward to spread over the temporal cortex. The M_3 segment terminates at the superficial part of the sylvian fissure.

The M_4 segment of the MCA is made up of cortical branches that begin at the superficial part of the sylvian fissure and course over the frontal, parietal, temporal, and some parts of the occipital lobe to irrigate the cerebral cortex in these areas.

The Middle Cerebral Artery Branches

The MCA gives rise to perforating arteries and cortical branches. The small perforating arteries, also called the lenticulostriate arteries, originate from the superior surface of the proximal MCA and penetrate the anterior perforating substance. The number varies from 5 to 17.[9] Perforating arteries are called the end arteries, but some authors have reported the existence of extracerebral anastomosis among the perforating branches of the ACA, the recurrent artery of Heubner, and the perforating branches of the MCA.

Most commonly, the perforating arteries arise from the main trunk of the MCA, but they may also originate from the point of the main division, secondary trunks, and early branches of the MCA.[9,10] In 600 hemispheres studied by Jain,[6] 54% of the perforating arteries arose from the main trunk of the MCA, 26% from the first major division of the MCA, and 20% from a branch of the MCA distal to the main division. The perforating arteries have been divided into the medial and the lateral groups, but in some cases no clear anatomical distinction can be made between them.

The lateral lenticulostriate arteries originate distal to the medial group, create an acute angle (about 30°–85°) immediately after they originate,[6] and pursue a recurrent course in a posterosuperior and medial direction for 2 to 5 mm; they then follow a superior and lateral curve for a distance of 9 to 30 mm before entering the lateral two-thirds of the anterior perforated substance. In the cisternal course, they may bifurcate into the smaller branches.[3] After penetration of the anterior perforated substance, these branches course laterally around and through the putamen, then medially through the superior half of the internal capsule and caudate nucleus. From the lateral view, they spread out superiorly and anteroposteriorly in a fan-shaped pattern and supply the internal capsule.

The perforating arteries usually reach only the lateral edge of the putamen. The structures situated most laterally, including the claustrum and the external capsule, are irrigated by the cortical branches of the MCA. In one study,[10] the average length of the medial lenticulostriate arteries was 9.25 ± 0.9 mm and of the lateral group, 16.67 ± 1.4 mm. In some cases, the medial perforating arteries may be replaced by the perforating branches of the proximal ACA and the recurrent artery of Heubner. The average diameter of perforating arteries arising from the MCA is 0.5 to 1 mm. The smaller perforating arteries (less than 0.5 mm outer diameter) usually originate from the most proximal portions of the MCA, and the larger branches most frequently arise distally. Grand[9] described three patterns of perforating arteries arising from the MCA: in 14% of cases, the larger perforating branches were found in the proximal half of the main trunk of the MCA before its major division; in 39%, the larger perforating arteries arose from the distal half of the MCA before its major division; in 47%, the larger perforators originated from the branches of the MCA distal to the main division. Of the 508 perforating arteries observed by Umansky et al.,[10] one-half arose as single branches and the other half as branches of the stem perforating arteries. Each stem gave rise to 2 to 13 small branches. Anomalies of the perforating arteries include elongation, dilatation, tortuosity, and constriction. Microaneurysm in these arteries has been demonstrated by microangiography.[11]

The perforating arteries supply the substantia innominata, the lateral portion of the anterior commissure, the dorsal half of the internal capsule, the body and dorsal aspect of the head of the caudate nucleus, most of the putamen, and the lateral segment of the globus pallidus.

Cortical Branches of the MCA

The cortical branches usually originate from the stem arteries,[12] but they may arise directly from the main and secondary trunks of the MCA.[5]

In cases in which the MCA bifurcates, the orbitofrontal, prefrontal, precentral, and central arteries usually originate from the superior trunk; the temporopolar, anterior temporal, middle temporal, posterior temporal, temporooccipital, and angular arteries arise from the inferior trunk (Fig. 11.2).

The cortical branches arising from the main trunk proximal to the division are called early branches. Grand[9] found early branches in 61% of hemispheres. Seventy-seven percent supplied the temporal lobe and 23% were distributed to the frontal lobe. The early branches to the frontal lobe usually supply the orbitofrontal and prefrontal areas; those terminating on the temporal lobe supply the anterior and lateral part of the temporal lobe.

The MCA supplies the lateral surface of the cerebral hemisphere, all the insular and opercular surface, the lateral half of the orbital surface of the frontal lobe, the temporal pole, the lateral part of the inferior surface of the temporal lobe, uncus, and parts of the parahippocampal gyrus. The cortical branches that supply the parietal and temporal lobes overlap onto the lateral occipital gyri.

Recently, Zwan and associates[13] demonstrated variations in the territory of the MCA; in 32% of hemispheres the cortical branches reached the interhemispheric fissure for variable distances between the precentral sulcus and the occipital pole.

Michotey et al.[14] divided the distribution area of the MCA into 12 territories: the orbitofrontal, prefrontal, precentral, central, anterior parietal, posterior parietal, angular, temporooccipital, posterior, middle and anterior temporal, and the temporopolar. Most commonly, one cortical branch, and less frequently, two or more, irrigates each of these cortical territories.

In several studies, the angular and temporooccipital arteries were the largest cortical branches of the MCA; the orbitofrontal and temporopolar arteries were found to be the smallest.[5,8] The area around the posterior end of the sylvian fissure is the site of the largest cortical branches of the MCA. According to Gibo et al.,[5] the average distance between the external auditory canal and the posterior end of the sylvian fissure is about 6.6 cm in adults. Chater et al.[15] found the cortical branch with a diameter more than 1.0 mm in the angular area in 100% of hemispheres, in the area around the temporal pole in 70% of hemispheres, and in the frontal convexity area in only 52% of hemispheres.

The orbitofrontal branch supplies the orbital portions of the middle and inferior frontal gyri and the inferior part of the pars orbitalis. The prefrontal artery irrigates most of the middle frontal gyrus, the anterior part of the pars opercularis, the pars triangularis, and the superior portion of the pars orbitalis. The precentral branch supplies the posterior pars opercularis, middle frontal gyrus, and the inferior and middle portions of the precentral gyrus. The central branch supplies the superior part of the precentral gyrus and the inferior half of the postcentral gyrus.

The anterior parietal artery goes to the superior postcentral gyrus, the upper central sulcus, the anterior part of the inferior parietal lobule, and the anteroinferior region of the superior parietal lobule. The posterior parietal branch supplies the posterior aspect of the superior and inferior parietal lobules as well as the supramarginal gyrus. The angular branch irrigates the posterior portion of the superior temporal gyrus, some parts of the supramarginal and angular gyri, and the superior portion of the lateral occipital gyri.

The temporooccipital branch supplies the posterior one-half of the superior temporal gyrus, the most posterior segment of the middle and inferior temporal gyri, and the inferior portion of the lateral occipital gyri. The posterior temporal artery goes to the posterior two-thirds of the superior temporal gyrus, the posterior one-third of the middle temporal gyrus, and the posterior end of the inferior temporal gyrus.

The middle temporal artery irrigates the superior temporal gyrus beyond the pars triangularis and pars opercularis, the middle portion of the middle temporal gyrus, and the posterior two-thirds of the inferior temporal gyrus.

The anterior temporal branch usually supplies the

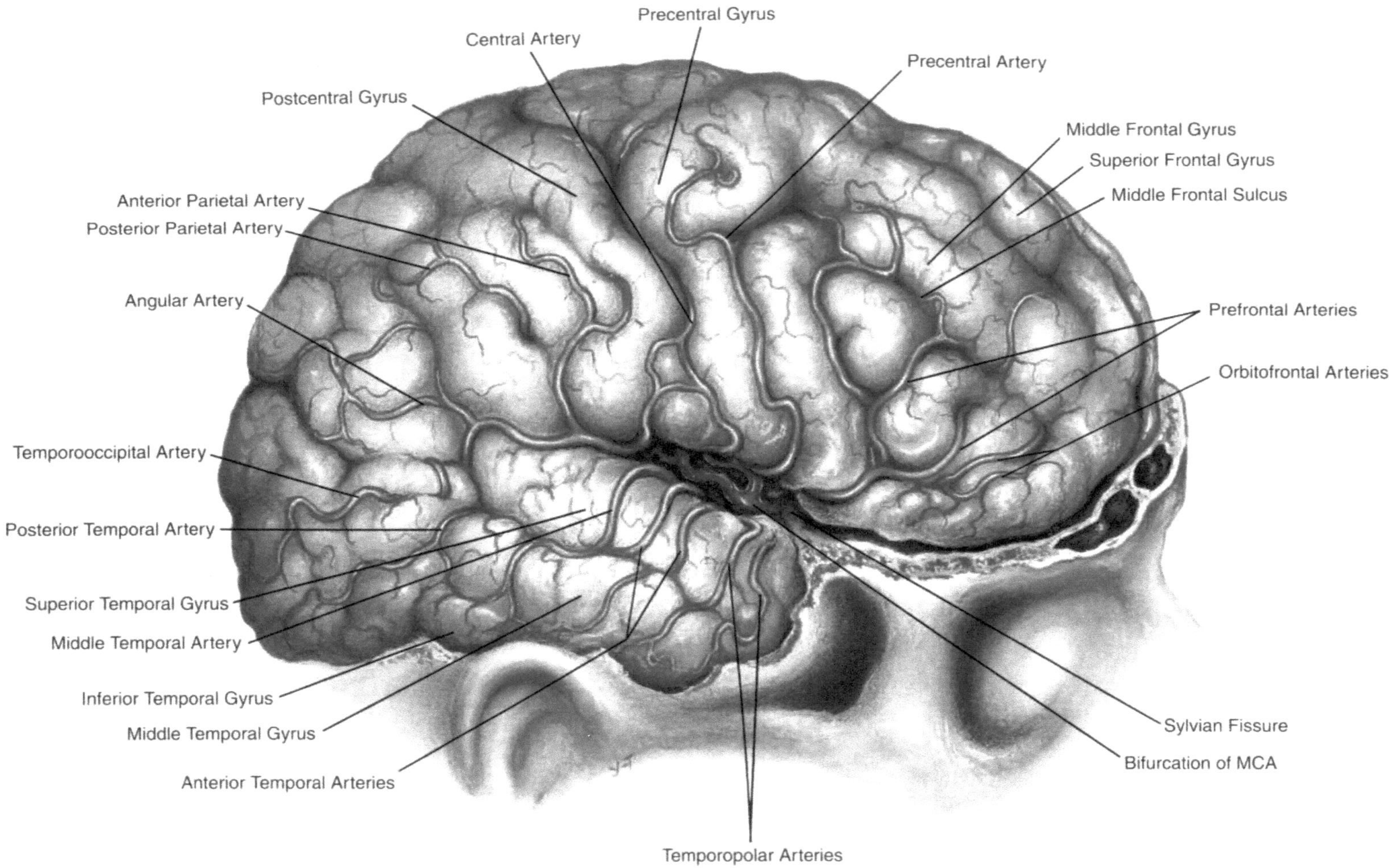

FIGURE 11.2. Right anterolateral view of the cerebral cortex with slight opening of the sylvian fissure to demonstrate the superficial branches of the middle cerebral artery and their distribution on the cortical surface.

anterior portion of the superior, middle, and inferior temporal gyri. The temporopolar artery irrigates the anterior pole of the superior, middle, and inferior temporal gyri; this artery was absent in 30% of hemispheres studied by Umansky et al.,[8] and its territory was irrigated by collateral branches of the anterior temporal artery. The temporopolar artery was frequently the first cortical branch of the MCA seen when the sylvian fissure was separated.

Clinical Features

The clinical features, associated with acute aneurysmal hemorrhage, depend upon the size of the aneurysm, the size of the hematoma, the location of the hematoma, the presence of increased intracranial pressure (ICP), and the presence of vasospasm. In approximately 50%, the signs are related to acute SAH. In the other 50%, symptoms are caused by cerebro-SAH. Of all the intracranial aneurysms, the MCA aneurysm is most likely to lead to a localized intracerebral hematoma. Pasqualin et al.[16] described 197 patients with MCA aneurysm, 108 (55%) of whom had intracranial hematomas. Eighty-three percent of these were located in the temporal lobe, 9% were in the subdural space, 8% were intraventricular, 7% were in the frontal lobe, and 4% were in less typical locations. The patient with an MCA aneurysm was most likely to deteriorate rapidly.

The clinical course of the patient following acute SAH depends not only on the rate of bleeding from the aneurysm but also on the size of the hemorrhage and the location. Blood clots develop asymmetrically in the subarachnoid pathways, occurring predominantly, however, in the sylvian fissure containing the aneurysm. For this reason, vasospasm may develop asymmetrically with predominating signs related to the vessels involved in the subarachnoid clot.

In patients with a small SAH [one in which less than 1 mm of blood is found in the subarachnoid space on initial computed tomography (CT)], the clinical features attributable to the SAH may be surprisingly mild. Meningeal signs may be minimal, headache may be mild, and there are few focal or general neurological symptoms. The patient is generally awake and alert. Near the end of the first week, generalized symptoms may appear. Local signs attributable to the MCA hematoma, however, may be more pronounced than in those with aneurysms in other locations in which generalized signs predominate. This is because ischemia develops in the territory of the penetrating and distal branches of the MCA. When SAH is severe, the patient is always in higher clinical grade. A sharp rise in ICP with associated herniation syndromes may be expected in this group, even early in the course. Major complications that may be seen result from increased ICP and hydrocephalus along with ischemic deficits.

Patients with severe SAH experience a high rate of complications during this intermediate phase. Because the vast supply of the MCA includes the cerebral cortex, subcortex, and brain stem, severe SAH may be associated with massive neurological involvement. Hemiparesis, hemianopsia, hemisensory deficits, and disorders of the sensorium may be encountered.

In patients harboring parenchymal hematomas, the clinical course is always more complicated. In those with small hematomas, the condition may rarely compensate in grade 1 or 2. Large hematomas occupying the cerebral substance or ventricles are associated with higher grades. Mortality varies from 78% for those with large intraparenchymal hematomas to 97% in patients with massive intraventricular hematomas. The first role of the neurosurgeon is to treat intracranial hypertension. With intracranial hematomas, vasospasm is also a more common feature. Perhaps this is because clots accumulate in the sylvian fissure, surrounding the MCA but also in the subarachnoid pathways elsewhere.

Treatment Options

The basis for treatment of aneurysms in this location is no different from aneurysms elsewhere except that the structural peculiarities of aneurysms that arise in this location must be given due consideration. The greatest number of these aneurysms is located at the bifurcation of M_1 to M_2. Usually, the neck is not well defined, and the aneurysm may have a sessile base. In addition, important vessels may arise from the dome of the aneurysm. Microneurosurgery with anastomosis, reimplantation, or a multiple clip application, may be needed to occlude the most difficult lesions. Sometimes, only portions of the aneurysm may be clipped, the remaining portion being invested with muslin or muscle. Perforating major branches may exit the wall of the aneurysm, calling for special techniques to spare these important vessels. Because short penetrating arteries may be compromised during dissection or by the use of either temporary or badly placed permanent clips, ischemic lesions occur postoperatively. Vasospasm may also involve the short branches, leading to focal neurological deficits.

Several factors must be considered prior to clipping. Among these, the neurological condition of the patient is paramount. If the patient's condition is unstable, the factors responsible for his decompensated state must be managed appropriately so that direct operation can be applied safely. Intracranial hematomas complicate half of all ruptured aneurysms in this location. Therefore, the decision to evacuate the clot must be made early. Removal of the hematoma may improve clinical grade. In these cases, clipping of the aneurysm should accompany removal of the hematoma because the rebleeding frequency in this group of patients in whom the hematoma has been evacuated is extremely high. In those entering this phase with hematoma and in poor neurological condition, mortality is high, with extreme morbidity among the survivors.[16]

Because of structural peculiarities, the choice of a procedure, either direct or endovascular, is an extremely complex problem. The best endovascular surgical candidate is one in whom the aneurysm is greater than 5 mm in diameter at its greatest dimension; the aneurysm should have a generous orifice for introduction of the balloon, and there must be no major branches exiting from the fundus. Before placement of a temporary balloon, test occlusion should be carried out to ensure that blood flow to the hemisphere and to the deep structures has not been compromised. In this test, the vessel or aneurysm is occluded with the test balloon for a period of 30 min. Monitoring of neurological and physiological parameters are carried out continuously during test occlusion. Endovascular therapy can be applied more appropriately to patients with large and giant aneurysms than in those with small aneurysms. During the hemorrhagic period (the first 6 weeks after onset), the endovascular procedure should be done only in patients who are compensated (grade 1). It should be applied only after vasospasm (if it is present) has been treated with angioplasty or has abated as determined by angiography or TCD. In this time period, the coagulogram should be normal or there should be a tendency toward hypocoagulability. Table 11.1 compares the method of treatment for MCA aneurysms using endovascular procedures, direct operations, test occlusion, and combined approaches.

Direct Surgery for MCA Aneurysms

Varying approaches have been used to clip aneurysms arising from the MCA. Among these, the frontal approach, frontal lateral approach, and a temporal approach have been popularized. Recently, the frontolateral or pterional approach with varying modifications has been more popular with microsurgeons. The basic pterional operation has been illustrated in Chapter 6. The following points should also be considered for aneurysms that arise on the MCA.

1. After the craniotomy, the ICA cisterns may be opened for cerebrospinal fluid drainage.
2. Opening the terminal aspects of this cistern allows safe retraction of the frontal lobes.
3. Any intracerebral hematomas should next be removed with suction.
4. The sylvian cistern along the base should be opened, exposing the M_1 for proximal control.
5. The sylvian fissure is opened distally to provide good exposure of the branchings of the MCA.
6. The dissection is carried along the anterior aspect of the MCA separating the branches of the M_2 from the aneurysm dome and origin.
7. The lenticulostriate arteries are isolated and identified.
8. The aneurysm is excluded from the circulation with a clip.
9. Remaining hematoma is removed from the sylvian fissure.
10. Papaverine may be applied to the cerebral vasculature in the region.

This approach is satisfactory for aneurysms that take-off from the M_1 or even for those arising from the anterior temporal branch (Fig. 11.3). Most MCA aneurysms arise at the branchings of the M_1 and M_2. The transsylvian approach has many advantages, including less retraction, and dissection is favored by many neurosurgeons. After identification of the sylvian fissure laterally, the arachnoid is opened near the sylvian vein. The sylvian vein may be retracted to either the frontal or the temporal side but usually more easily toward the temporal lobe. This permits entry into the sylvian fissure, exposing the branches of the M_2 and the aneurysm. Proximal control can then be achieved by dissecting proximally along the M_1 segment (Fig. 11.4). Tönnis and Walter[17] have introduced an approach through the

TABLE 11.1. Operative alternatives for surgical management of MCA aneurysms

Type of aneurysm	Direct operation	Endovascular operation	Test occlusion	Combined operation
Aneurysm < 5 mm	+	–	–	–
Aneurysm > 5 mm with good neck	+	+	+	+
Aneurysm > 5 mm with wide neck	+	–	–	+
Aneurysm < 10 mm large and giant	+	+	+	+

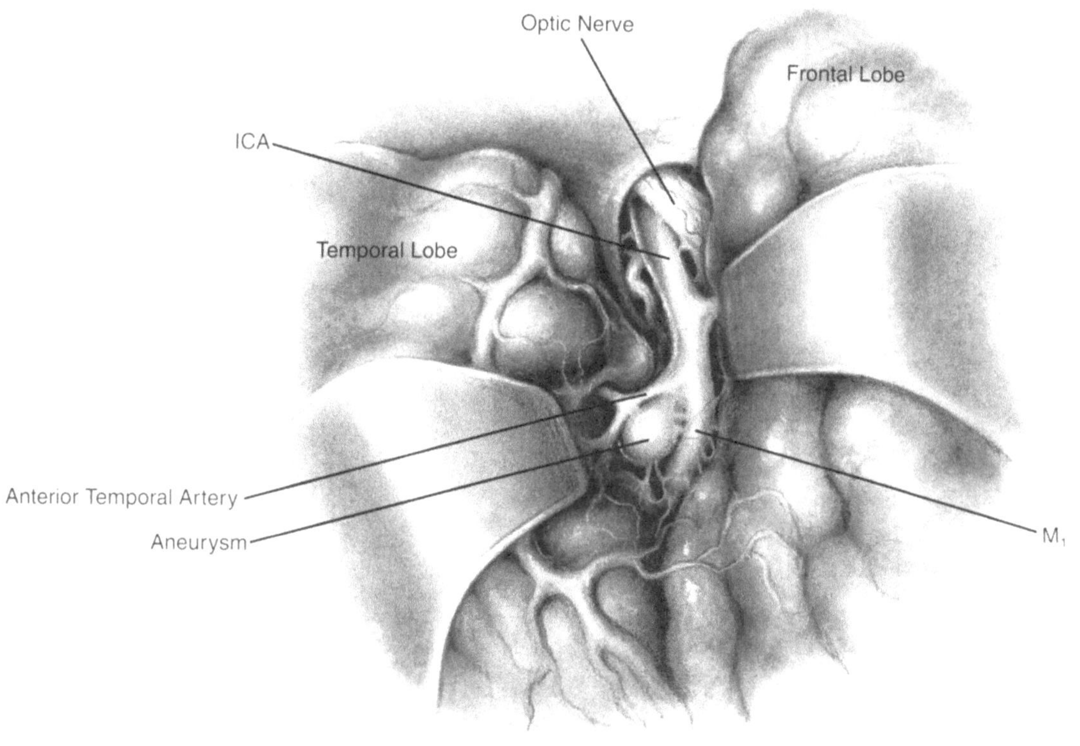

FIGURE 11.3. Left pterional approach to a proximal aneurysm of the left middle cerebral artery arising at the anterior temporal branch, projecting inferiorly. This aneurysm usually originates from the M_1 or bifurcation but may arise from the anterior temporal branch. ICA, internal carotid artery.

superior temporal gyrus. This approach has also been advocated by Heros et al.[18] This is useful when large hematomas can be seen within the temporal lobe.

Any manipulation of the MCA or its branches may precipitate ischemic complications.

Measurement of sensory evoked potentials may be useful in the surgery of MCA aneurysms. Friedman and co-workers[19] defined the changes of significance to be expected with clip application. In type 1 there was no change in potential. In type 2, there was rapid return to baseline. In type 3, significant change was seen that did not return to baseline. Type 4 patterns showed complete loss of potential. Types 3 and 4 had new neurological defects after clip application. Four of five patients with type 2 changes had no new deficits and recovered after prompt removal of temporary clips or by adjustment of the permanent clip.

The detailed anatomical relationship between the MCA aneurysm and the vessels that surround is important for microdissection. After determining this relationship, a method to exclude the aneurysm from the arterial circulation can then be selected. Among the surgical options are clipping of the neck of the aneurysm, clipping or partial clipping of the fundus of the aneurysm, or investment. Reimplantation of major branches into the main trunk of the MCA after excision of the aneurysm or extracranial–intracranial (EC-IC) bypass may be required to preserve flow in distal branches. Some aneurysms must be approached aggressively. After temporary clips have been applied to the M_1 and M_2 branches, aneurysm excision may be the only option. The clips should be applied distal to the lenticulostriate perforators. Occlusion of the MCA may be tolerated for periods of 40 to 50 min or perhaps longer if the penetrating branches are not included in the clips. Heparinization is also useful during this interval, and arterial pressure must be elevated.

Other methods may be required for large and giant aneurysms filled with atheroma and/or thrombus. After removal of the thrombus and atheroma, the ostium can usually be identified and clips applied so as to preserve nearby vessels (Fig. 11.5). In large thick-walled aneurysms, aneurysmectomy may be required and reconstruction after removal of the major portion of the mass-producing fundus. Purse-string sutures or encircling ligatures may also be used to obliterate aneurysms of the MCA. However, the tension necessary is critical. Excessive tension may force atheroma or thrombus back into the main trunk of the MCA or inadequate tension may allow filling of the aneurysm. Intraoperative angiography is useful.

Intracerebral hematoma occurs disproportionately in

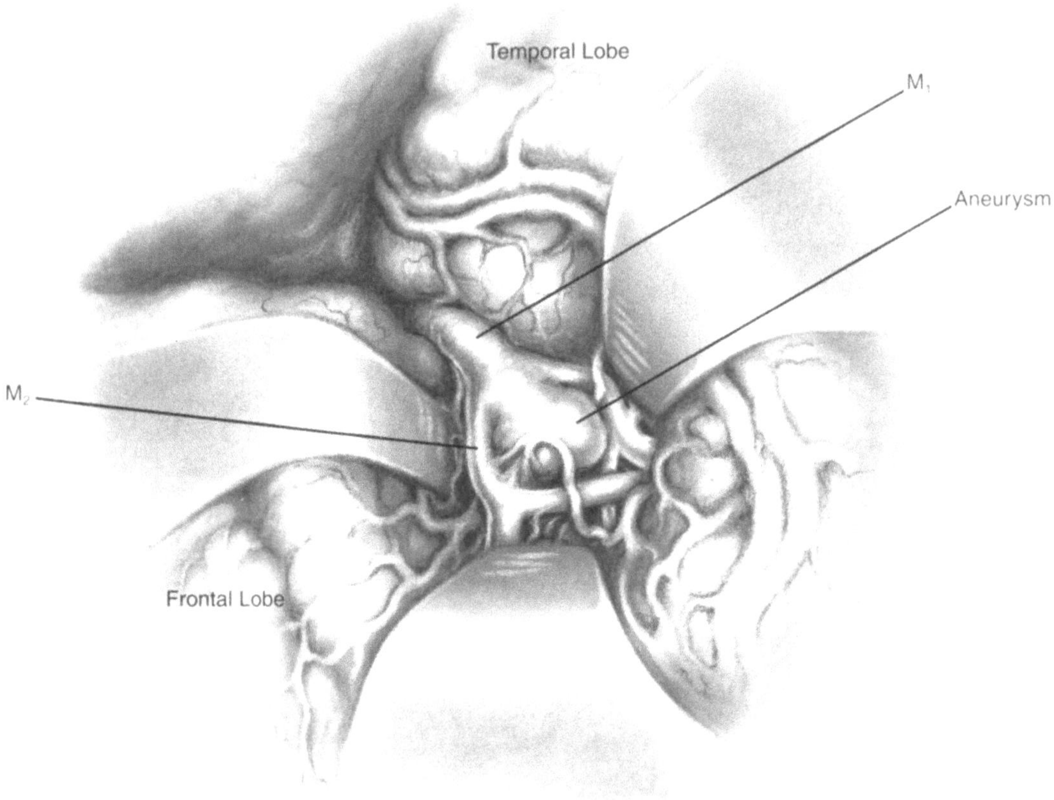

A

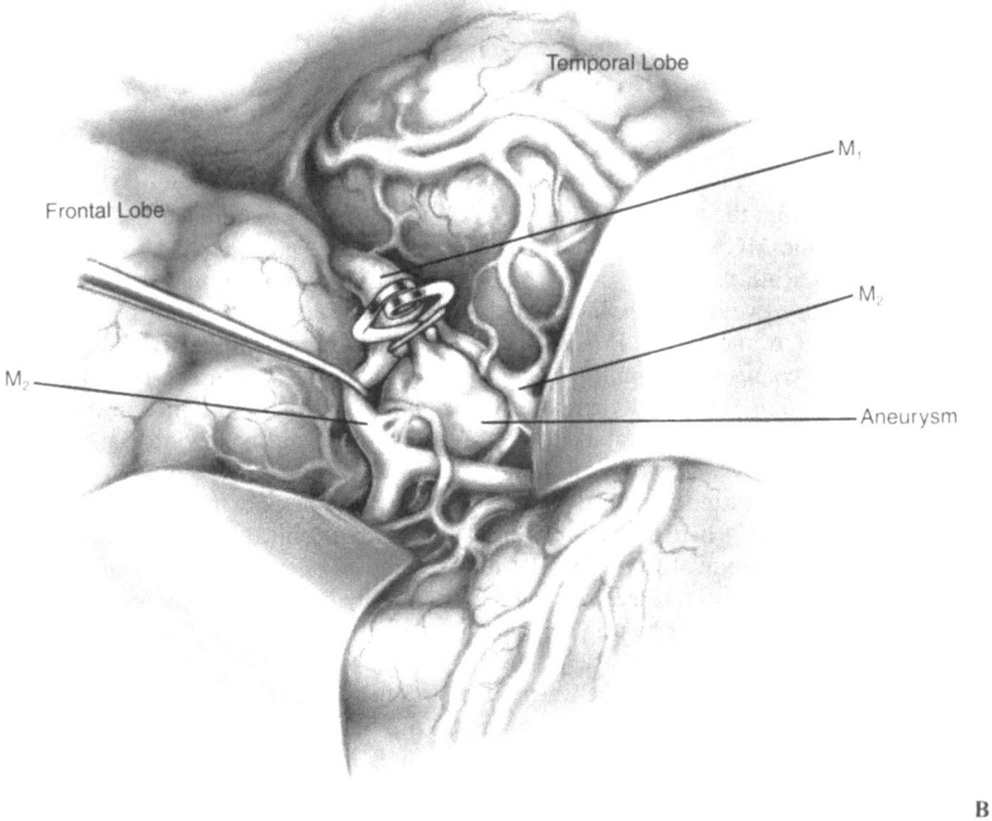

B

FIGURE 11.4. (A) Right transsylvian approach to a multilobulated aneurysm of the middle cerebral artery bifurcation. Penetrating arteries to the frontal and temporal lobes cross the aneurysm fundus. The sylvian veins have been retracted temporally. (B) This aneurysm may be managed by using temporary clips on the M_1 branch. The major and minor branches have been dissected free so that the permanent clip can be applied at the aneurysm orifice.

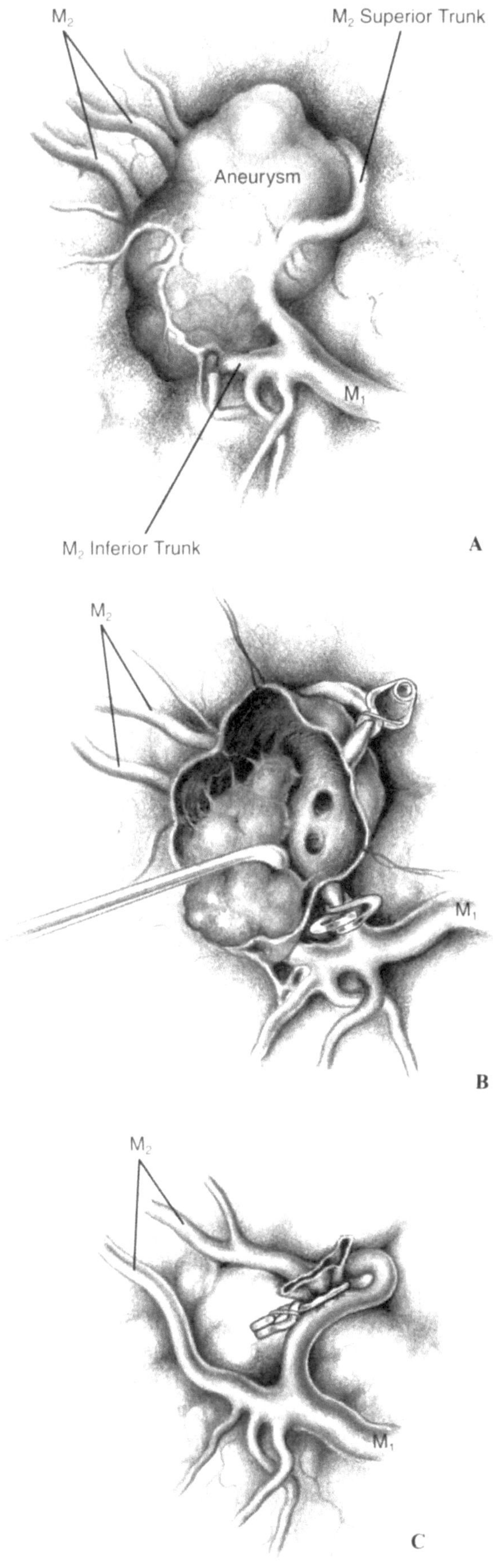

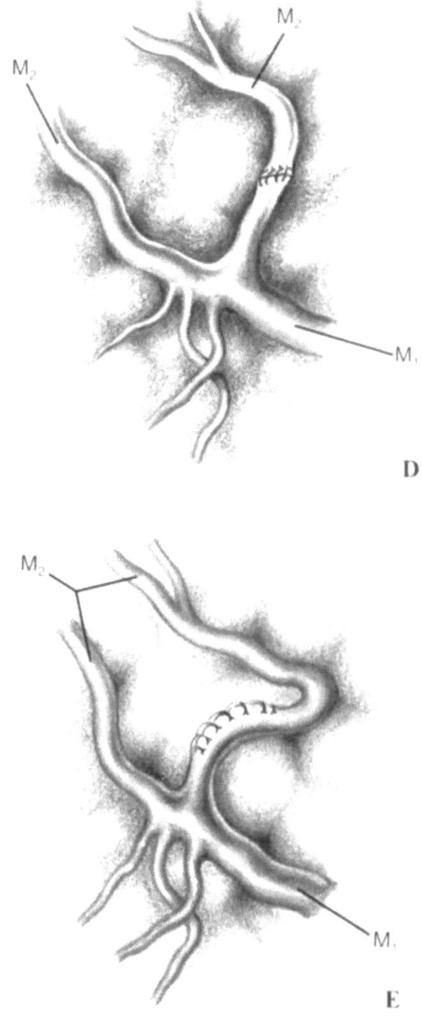

FIGURE 11.5. (A) The aneurysm arises from M_2 and important branches enter and exit the aneurysm. In addition, it is filled with atheroma and thrombus, precluding routine clipping. (B) The aneurysm has been opened and the atheroma and thrombus dissected away, exposing the ostia of the important entering and exiting vessels. (C) The vessel has been remade using a clip. (D) The aneurysm has been excised and an end-to-end anastomosis of the proximal and distal branch is carried out. (E) The aneurysm has been excised and repaired using microvascular suture.

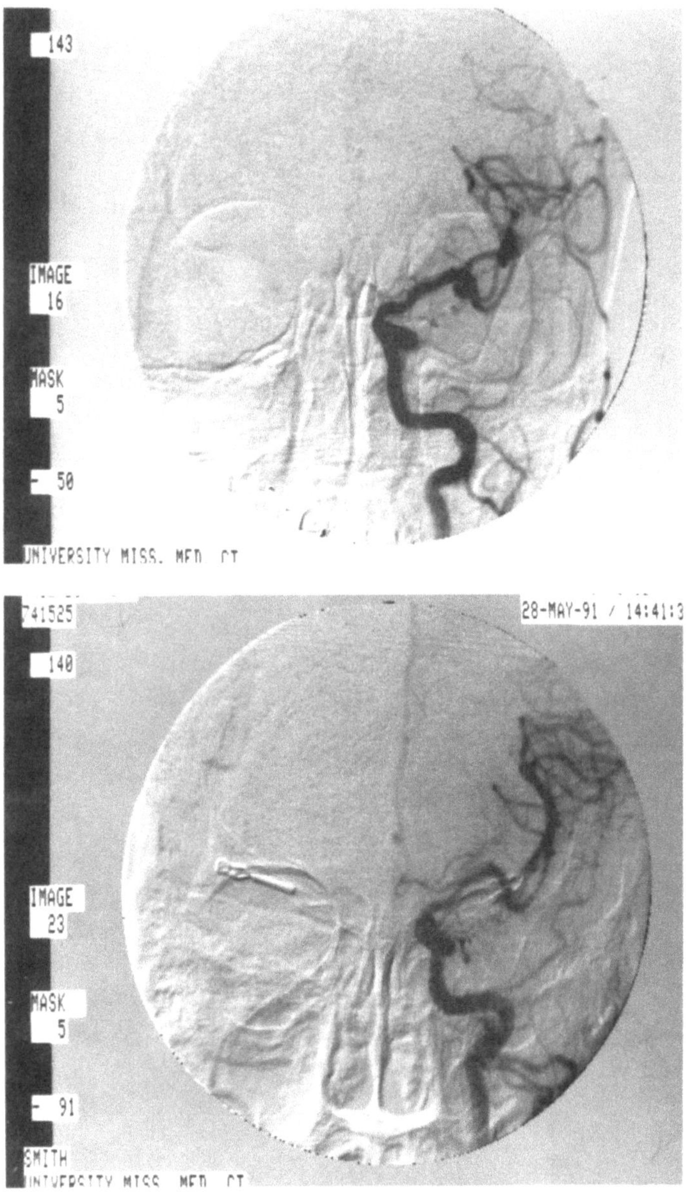

A

B

FIGURE 11.6. (A) Middle cerebral artery aneurysm with elevation of the middle cerebral artery. (B) After clipping of the aneurysm. There was a mirror aneurysm at the opposite middle cerebral artery bifurcation.

patients with MCA aneurysms. The aim of therapy should be complete removal of the hematoma with clipping of the aneurysm at the same operation. Intravenous mannitol and controlled hypotension and/or temporary clips may be required to gain exposure in some patients. The aneurysm usually lies deep to the hematoma, and evacuation may allow entry to the aneurysm for clipping. Brain edema is also a constant feature in the patient with intracerebral hematoma. Most patients arrive in higher clinical grades, and mortality overall exceeds 50% irrespective of the treatment given.[16] However, in those not operated, the mortality is higher, and most of the deaths are attributed to rebleeding of the aneurysm. Figure 11.6 demonstrates the results of direct intracranial clipping of a MCA bifurcation aneurysm.

Endovascular Approaches

Deconstructive procedures are those in which the main arterial trunk is sacrificed, the distal territory of which must be nourished by collateral channels. These procedures are rarely applicable to the MCA. The main trunk of the MCA must be preserved if neurological deficits are to be avoided. Overall, however, endovascular approaches to these aneurysms are gaining in utility and feasibility. Because of the importance of the MCA to perfusion of the hemisphere, temporary test occlusion with the balloon in the aneurysm is essential for a safe endovascular approach. Procedures for test occlusion are similar to those used with other aneurysms. The detachable balloon is placed in the aneurysm and inflated to its permanent size and configuration. Afterward, the patient is evaluated neurologically and with physiological methods to assess flow in the MCA. In addition, angiography is carried out after the balloon has been inflated to its maximum permanent size. After 30 min, if the patient's neurological condition remains stable and if there is no retardation of flow, consideration is given to permanent detachment. If signs (such as hemiparesis, hemisensory, speech disturbances, or visual impairment) appear during this 30-min interval, the balloon must be deflated and the procedure terminated. Test occlusion also serves a useful purpose for the surgeon who is planning a direct clipping because the test demonstrates which vessels are important. Those arising from the fundus of the aneurysm may be critically assessed and surgical planning finalized. If the patient develops ischemic symptoms during the 30-min occlusion testing period, if velocity falls 50% or greater in the MCA, or if there is an inadequate flow pattern on the angiogram, further deterioration is likely after permanent occlusion. In the patient who fails the first balloon occlusion test, a second balloon occlusion test may be carried out with a more successful result. This usually requires modification of systemic arterial pressure and anticoagulation. Thus, a single failure of temporary test occlusion may not always negate the endovascular option for permanent occlusion.

Complex aneurysms of the middle cerebral bifurcation may bear a complex relationship to the M_1 or M_2 branches, with preservation unlikely using clipping. An EC-IC bypass may be considered as a preliminary procedure. Thereafter, a second test occlusion may be carried out, recognizing that sacrifice of major vessels may still be needed but perhaps better tolerated. Permitting the EC-IC bypass to mature for 3 to 4 months is advisable. During this time, blood flow through the bypass may increase significantly. Occasionally, however, the EC-IC bypass will not remain open due to high flow and pressure within the MCA. The function of the extracranial bypass should be evaluated both with Doppler and with angiography prior to a second endovascular testing procedure.

Two possibilities for endovascular treatment arise after a successful bypass. In one of these, the endovascular surgeon may perform a deconstructive procedure in which the M_1 or M_2 branches are sacrificed. In the other, the balloon is again detached in the main body of the aneurysm, sparing these vessels. Sacrifice of the M_1 should always be carried out with trepidation, realizing the importance of this artery to the circulation of the hemisphere and the likelihood that deficits will follow, even with a successful EC-IC bypass. For permanent balloon occlusion of the MCA, the short branches must be spared and the balloon must be placed as close to the orifice of the aneurysm as feasible. On the M_2 side, the balloon must also be as close to the aneurysm as possible to spare the short branches that exit the M_2 branches and penetrate the operculum to supply deep structures.

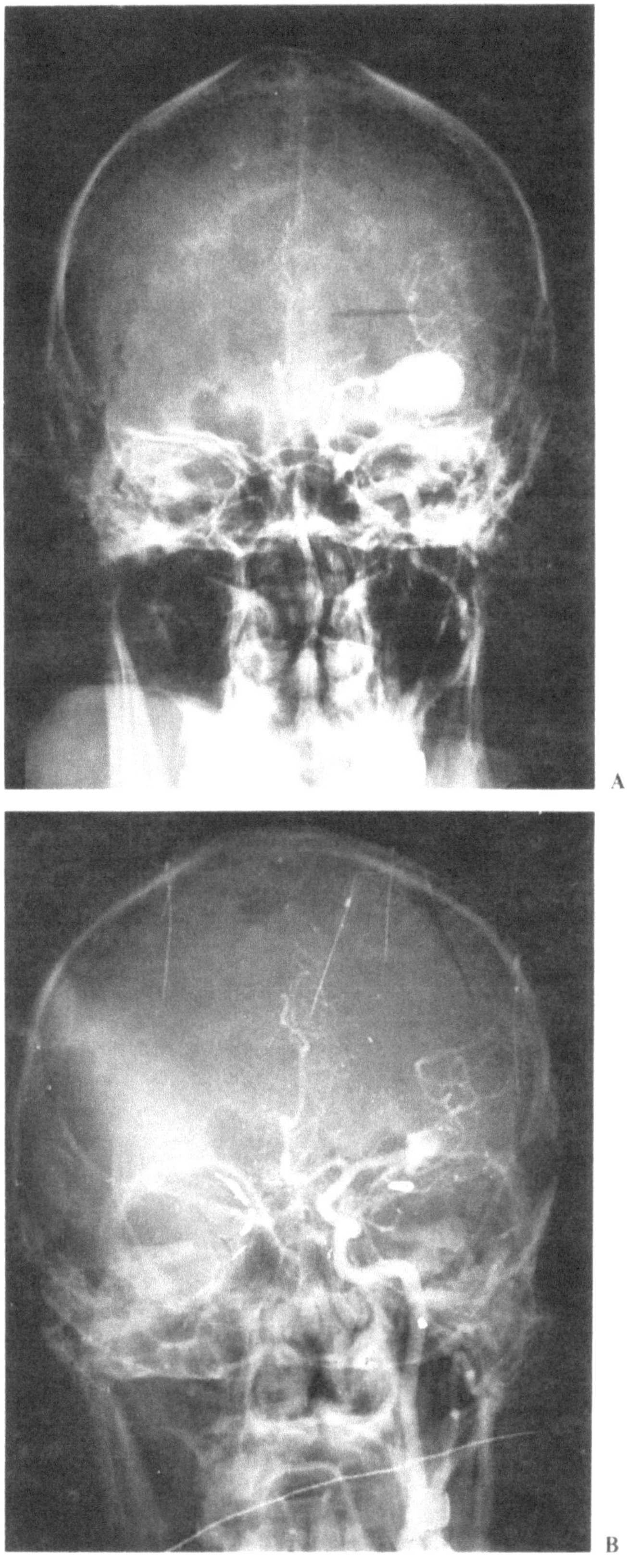

A

B

FIGURE 11.7. (A) Giant aneurysm of the MCA bifurcation. (B) After occlusion of the aneurysm with a balloon. Attempt had been made unsuccessfully to occlude this aneurysm with direct craniotomy. The electrodes have been placed in the scalp to record EEG during the endovascular operation.

Reconstructive operations are those in which the M_1 and M_2 branches are spared by placing the balloon or coil directly in the aneurysm sac. This is the preferred treatment course and is often feasible with MCA aneurysms. If neurologic deficits do not appear within 30 min of test occlusion, velocity is not significantly reduced and the angiogram shows good filling of the distal branches, then permanent occlusion may be carried out safely. Both liquid and hard material are useful for producing the final permanent balloon inflation. For large and giant aneurysms, liquid contrast material is preferred because, as weeks go by, leakage from the balloon allows thrombosis and shrinkage of the aneurysmal mass. For smaller aneurysms, those 1 cm or less, the use of hard material is preferred because immediate protection is provided, and late thrombosis in this aneurysm is less likely to occur due to its flow characteristics.

In detaching the balloon, once it has been permanently inflated with either hard material or with liquid, the use of a helper balloon is preferred. The helper balloon is placed in the parent artery adjacent to the orifice to occlude the aneurysm. The catheter onto which the balloon is attached inside the aneurysm is held against the wall of the aneurysm by the inflated helper balloon. Upon detachment, the helper balloon places tension against the orifice of the aneurysm, keeping the detachable balloon in place and preserving the parent artery. The balloon also allows some protection against bleeding should it occur during detachment. The introduction of the balloon into the aneurysm is perhaps easiest when dealing with middle cerebral bifurcation aneurysms because the aneurysm often arises in a direct line with the M_1 segment through which the balloon passes.

Aneurysms that arise from the M_1 segment usually exit at an acute angle from the M_1 pointing anteriorly and inferiorly. Placing a detachable balloon in this particular

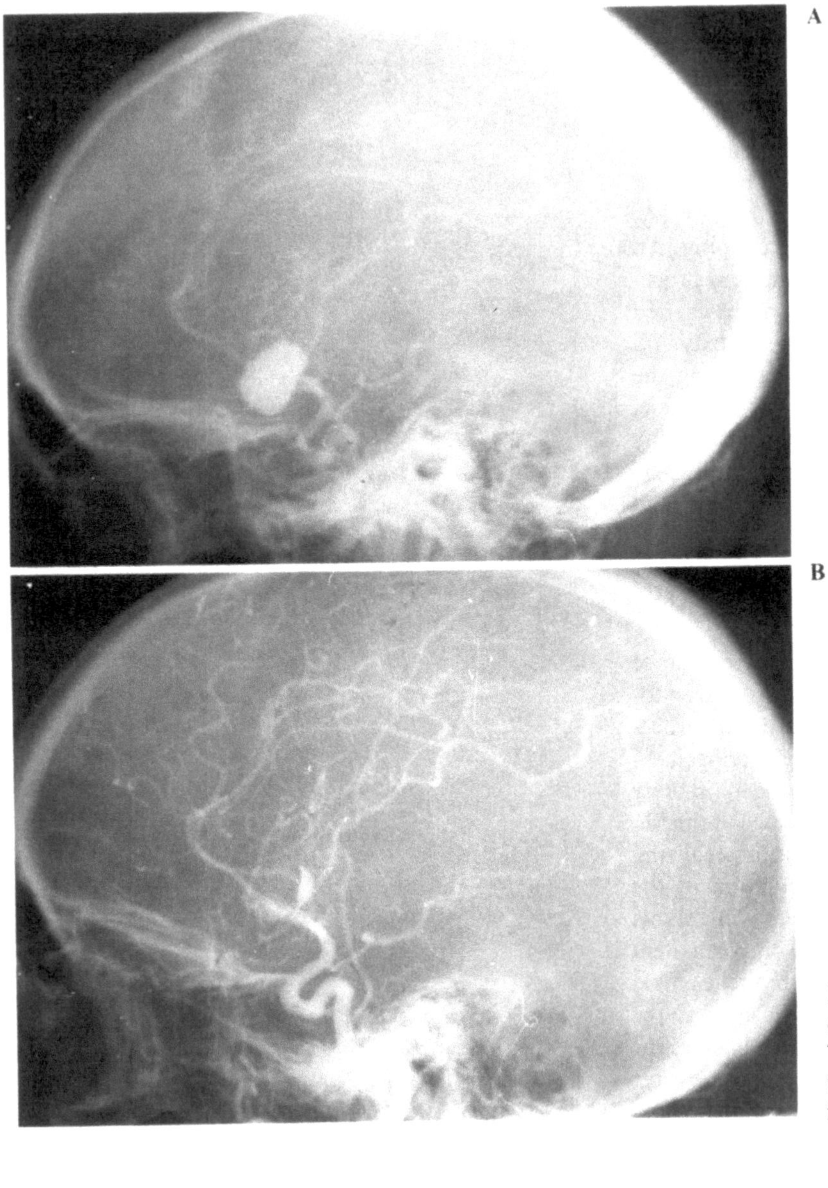

FIGURE 11.8. (A) MCA bifurcation aneurysm. (B) Aneurysm occluded with a latex balloon. The contrast material shown is in the apex of the balloon. The remainder of the balloon is filled with polymer.

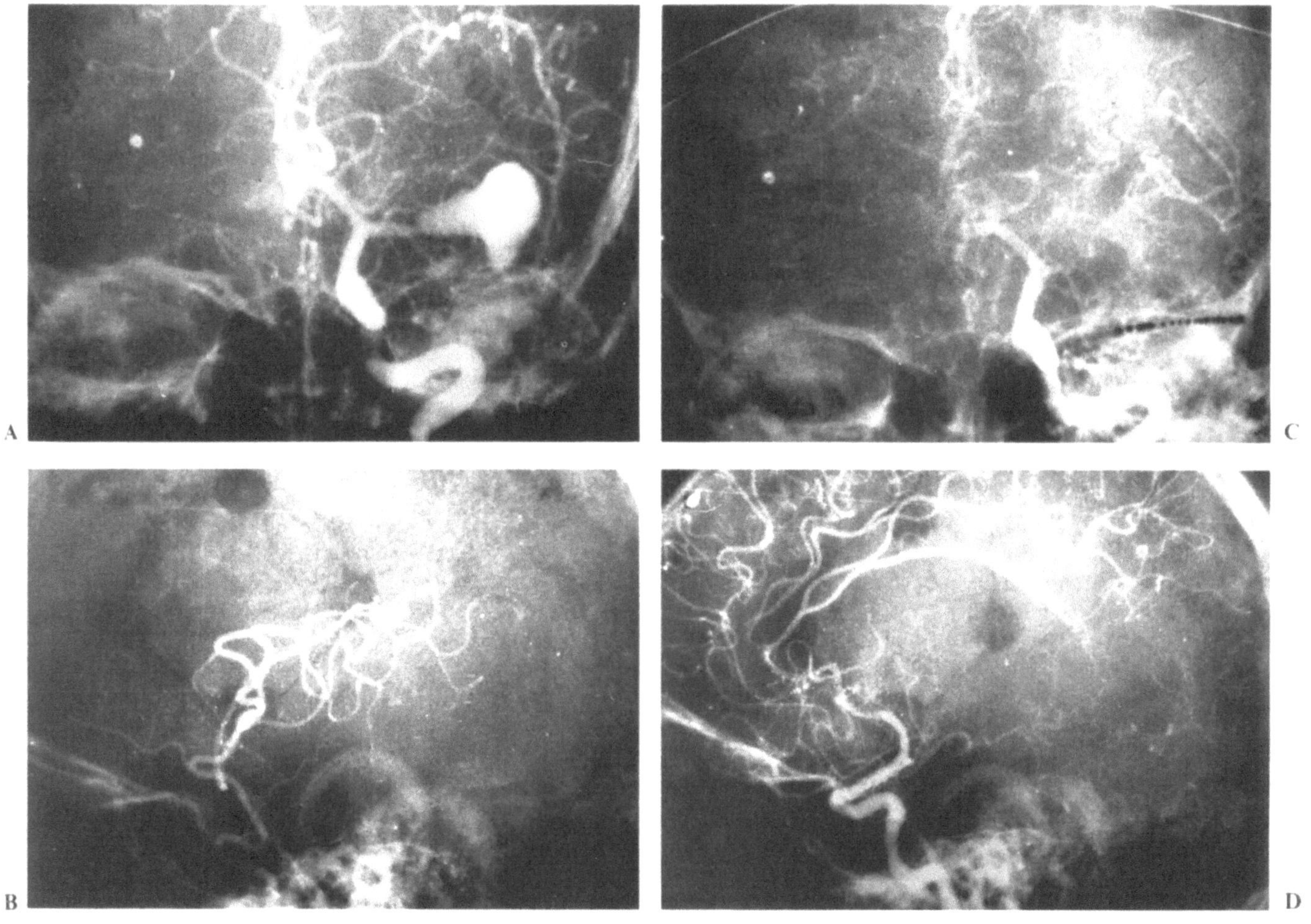

FIGURE 11.9. (A) Giant aneurysm of the MCA bifurcation. (B) Following superficial temporal to cortical branch bypass. (C) Occlusion of the MCA with good filling of the distal MCA branches and nonfilling of the aneurysm. (D) Lateral angiogram shows occlusion of the MCA with nonfilling of the aneurysm following a STA/MCA bypass.

aneurysm may require all of the techniques available. Changing the patient's head position in relation to the balloon may be necessary, but, always, a helper balloon is placed near the orifice in order to reduce flow in the MCA and to serve as a deflector for the primary balloon.

Postoperatively, maintaining homeostasis in the circulatory system is important. The blood pressure should not be allowed to fall greatly, and coagulation should be reduced with aspirin or heparin. After 24 hours of observation, it is unlikely that deficits will appear if they have not done so during this interval and the patient may be discharged home. Figures 11.7–11.9 show some results of endovascular operations for MCA aneurysms.

Conclusions

Gains have been recently made in the technical management of MCA aneurysms by both the direct and endovascular surgeon. Many MCA aneurysms are associated with mass lesions due to hematomas. Therefore, direct evacuation of the hematoma with concurrent clipping of the aneurysm is the preferred management method. While reconstructive endovascular techniques have a role, deconstructive methods in which the main trunk or secondary branches are occluded should not be used if other alternatives are available. Occlusion of major branches or perforating arteries can lead to extensive neurological sequelae.

References

1. Ebina K, Shimizu T, Sohma M, Iwabuchi T. Clinicostatistical study on morphological risk factors of middle cerebral artery aneurysms. *Acta Neurochir (Wien)*. 1990; 106:153–159.
2. Yasargil MG. *Microsurgical Anatomy of the Basal Cisterns and Vessels of the Brain, Diagnostic Studies, General Operative Techniques and Pathological Considerations of the Intracranial Aneurysms. Microneurosurgery*. New York:

Thieme Stratton Inc.; Stuttgart and New York: Georg Thieme Verlag; 1984:I:72–84.
3. Weir B. *Aneurysms Affecting the Nervous System*. Baltimore, MD: William & Wilkins; 1987:325–328.
4. Padget DH. The development of the cranial arteries in the human embryo. *Contrib Embryol*. 1948;32:205–261.
5. Gibo H, Carver CC, Rhoton AL Jr, Lenkey C, Mitchell RJ. Microsurgical anatomy of the middle cerebral artery. *J Neurosurg*. 1981;54:151–169.
6. Jain KK. Some observations on the anatomy of the middle cerebral artery. *Can J Surg*. 1964;7:134–139.
7. Truemper E, Fischer AQ. Cerebrovascular embryology and anatomic variation. In: Newell D, Ward R, eds. *Transcranial Doppler*. New York: Raven Press; 1992:231–282.
8. Umansky F, Juarez SM, Dujovny M, Ausman JI, Diaz FG, Gomes F, Mirchandani HG, Ray WJ. Microsurgical anatomy of the proximal segments of the middle cerebral artery. *J Neurosurg*. 1984;61:458–467.
9. Grand W. Microsurgical anatomy of the proximal middle cerebral artery and the internal carotid artery bifurcation. *Neurosurgery*. 1980;7:215–218.
10. Umansky F, Gomes FB, Dujovny M, Diaz FG, Ausman JI, Mirchandani HG, Berman SK. The perforating branches of the middle cerebral artery, microanatomical study. *J Neurosurg*. 1985;62:261–268.
11. Leeds NE, Goldberg HI. Lenticulostriate artery abnormalities. Value of direct serial magnifications. *Radiology*. 1970;97:377–383.
12. Carpenter MB. *Context of Neuroanatomy*. Baltimore, MD: Williams & Wilkins, 1991:438–461.
13. Zwan AV, Hillen B, Tulleken CA, Dujovny M, Dragovic L. Variability of the territories of the major cerebral arteries. *J Neurosurg*. 1992;77:927–940.
14. Michotey P, Moscow NB, Salamon G. Sect. II, Anatomy of the cortical branches of the middle cerebral artery. In: Newton TH, Potts DG, eds. *Radiology of the Skull and Brain. Angiography*. St. Louis, MO: CV Mosby; 1974: 1471–1478.
15. Chater N, Spetzler R, Tonnemacher K, Wilson CB. Microvascular bypass surgery. Part I: anatomical studies. *J Neurosurg*. 1976;44:712–714.
16. Pasqualin A, Bazzan A, Cavazzani P, Scienza R, Licata C, Da Pian R. Intracranial hematomas following aneurysmal rupture: experience with 309 cases. *Surg Neurol*. 1986;25:6–17.
17. Tönnis W, Walter W. Ein neuer operativer Zugang zu den sackfrmigen Aneurysmen der basalen Hirngefsse. *Wien Med Wochenschr*. 1960;110:145–147.
18. Heros RC, Ojemann RG, Crowell RM. Superior temporal gyrus approach to middle cerebral artery aneurysms. Technique and results. *Neurosurgery*. 1982;10:308–31.
19. Friedman WA, Kaplan BL, Day AL, Sypert GW, Curran MT. Evoked potential monitoring during aneurysm operation: Observation after fifty cases. *Neurosurgery*. 1987;20: 678–687.

12
Aneurysms of the Vertebrobasilar System

According to Stehbens,[1] these aneurysms account for 4.9% of all those presenting to clinicians. From postmortem anatomical studies, aneurysms in this location make up 11.7%. In reviewing the Cooperative Study series, Sahs et al.[2] found them to make up 4% of all aneurysms in all locations. The true incidence of vertebrobasilar aneurysms must depend, in part, on the persistence of the clinician in identifying the sources of subarachnoid hemorrhage (SAH). In older literature, the angiogram may not have adequately covered the vertebrobasilar system.

Both the origin of the aneurysm from the nearest parent artery and the branch nearest to which the aneurysm arises has been used to classify these aneurysms.[3-6] The discussion that follows attempts to conform to traditional views, and aneurysms of the basilar artery (BA) apex, the basilar artery trunk, and those that arise from the vertebral arteries themselves are given special consideration. Aneurysms that actually arise from the posterior cerebral artery (PCA), the superior cerebellar artery (SCA), the posterior inferior cerebellar artery (PICA), and the anterior inferior cerebellar artery (AICA) will also be discussed separately.

Any consideration of aneurysms of the posterior circulation must include the anatomical relationships since, in this location more so than others, the adjacent structures determine to a great extent the results and complications to be expected. The vertebrobasilar system is well known for the large and giant aneurysms that arise from it. Perhaps one-fourth of all giant aneurysms arise from the vertebrobasilar system. Fusiform aneurysms also occur predominantly on the posterior cranial circulation.

The anatomy of this arterial system is well known and many articles have appeared, describing both gross and microsurgical dissections.

Microanatomy of the Posterior Circulation

The microscopic anatomy of the vertebrobasilar arterial system has been reported in detail.[7-12]

According to Padget's[13] classification, the posterior circulation appears during the first embryologic stage (4–5 mm, 28- to 30-day-old embryo) in the form of paired longitudinal neural arteries that lie ventrolateral to the midline of the hindbrain. During the same stage the upper intersegmental arteries extend from the embryo's aorta to the seven cervical segments of each side. By the second stage (5–6 mm, 28- to 30-day-old embryo), both longitudinal neural arteries join together and form the primary BA. The distal portion of the seven cervical intersegmental arteries form perpendicular branches in the cephalic and caudal direction, and these branches anastomose together and form the primary vertebral artery (VA) on each side. Embryologically, the longitudinal neural arteries are the continuum of the primary VAs. By the third stage (7–12 mm, 31- to 33-day-old embryo), the intersegmental arteries lose their proximal connection to the aorta, but the connection of the seventh intersegmental artery to the aorta persists and creates the future subclavian artery on each side. During the fourth stage (12–14 mm, 34- to 36-day-old embryo), the posterior circulation begins to receive blood from both VAs.

The Vertebral Artery

After giving rise to the muscular and radicular branches, the VA leaves the foramen transversum of the first cervical vertebra and passes posteriorly around the superior articular process of the atlas. Then it courses anteromedially and penetrates the atlantooccipital membrane and dura to enter the subarachnoid space of the posterior fossa through the foramen magnum; subsequently, it lies within the lateral cerebellomedullary cistern and courses superiorly, anteriorly, and medially to reach the anterior surface of the medulla and finally to the pontomedullary sulcus. At this point, the artery joins the opposite VA to form the BA.

The VA lies anterior to the first dentate ligament and to the hypoglossal, accessory, vagus, and glossopharyngeal nerve rootlets. The hypoglossal rootlets, which emerge from the preolivary sulcus and extend to the hypoglossal canal, are close and immediately posterior to the VA. In some cases the VA is tortuous and elongated, and it may stretch and push these rootlets posteriorly, close to the accessory, vagus, and glossopharyngeal nerves (Fig. 12.1).

The two VAs join together at the level of the pontomedullary junction, against the lower border of the clivus, but their union site may be located a few millimeters above to 15 mm below this point. The caliber of the VA varies tremendously and there may be differences between the two. The left VA is usually larger than the right.[14–16] In elderly patients, the artery may be elongated and tortuous.

Anomalies of the VA, including hypoplasia, aplasia duplication, fenestration, and abnormal anastomosis with the internal carotid artery (ICA) have been reported.[6,14–17] In 0.2% of cases, it may terminate in the PICA, and, in such cases, the BA originates from the contralateral VA.[6] In one study, the VA was absent in 2% of the hemispheres.[10] Anomalies of the VA have frequently been associated with aneurysms and arteriovenous malformations (AVMs) of the posterior circulation.[18]

Branches of the Vertebral Artery

The posterior meningeal artery: This artery arises from the VA at the level of the foramen magnum, usually between the occipital bone and the dura. It supplies the bone, the diploe, and the dura of the posterior fossa including the falx cerebelli.

The posterior spinal artery: This artery most frequently

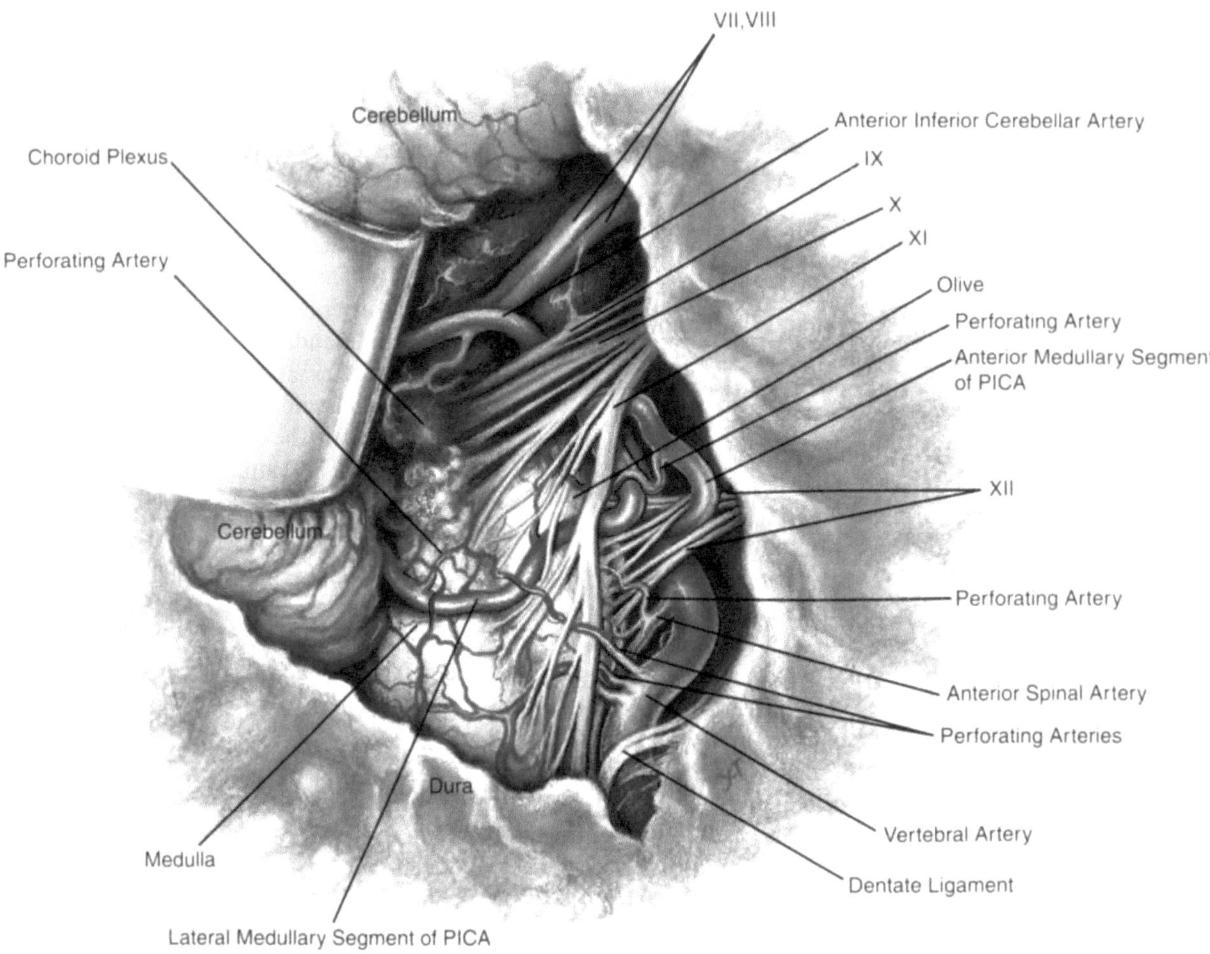

FIGURE 12.1. An anterolateral view of the right vertebral artery as seen from a suboccipital approach. The penetrating branches from the vertebral artery and posterior–inferior cerebellar artery (PICA) are seen entering the lateral medulla. The normal course of the PICA is shown in its relation to the cranial nerves, olive and lateral medulla.

originates from the PICA, but it may arise from the VA. It descends along the posterior surface of the lower portion of the medulla and spinal cord, usually as two main branches anterior and posterior to the dorsal roots of the spinal nerves. Some small branches of the posterior spinal artery (PSA) anastomose with branches of the PICA on the posterolateral sulci of the medulla. The PSA supplies the posteroinferior portion of the inferior cerebellar peduncle, gracile, cuneate fasciculi, and their nuclei, and some parts of the vagus and solitary tract nuclei.[7,19]

Anterior spinal artery: The anterior spinal artery (ASA) originates from the distal portion of the VA and descends on the anterior surface of the medulla to join with its counterpart within the premedullary cistern at the pyramidal decussation or midmedullary level to create the single trunk of the ASA, which courses downward on the ventral midline sulcus of the spinal cord. Various anomalies of this artery have been reported and are common.[15]

Some branches terminating in the medulla originate in the ASA, and these branches usually penetrate the anterior medial sulcus of the medulla. The upper end of the anterior medial sulcus of the medulla is called the ventromedial pontomedullary perforated zone, which is bounded by the lower border of the pons and two pyramids of the medulla. The foramen caecum is located in the rostral part of this area. Several perforating arteries originate from the rami, and the upper portion of the single trunk of the ASA, distal VAs, and the proximal BA enter this area to supply the lower half of the anterior surface of the medulla.

The ASA supplies the pyramids, the medial longitudinal fascicles, the dorsal motor nucleus of the vagus nerve, the medial lemniscus, the hypoglossal nucleus, the caudal part of the solitary nucleus, and the medial accessory olive. Occlusion of one ASA may cause a medullary lesion with inferior alternating hemiplegia (ipsilateral tongue paralysis with contralateral hemiplegia).[19]

Medullary perforating branches: Several small branches originate from the VA as direct and circumflex perforating arteries and penetrate the medulla at the ventromedial pontomedullary and preolivary perforated areas as well as at the posterior surface of the medulla. They supply the anterolateral, lateral, and posterolateral medulla. Their irrigation areas are the medullary pyramids, the inferior olivary complex, the cephalic part of the hypoglossal nucleus, the dorsal motor nucleus of the vagus nerve, some parts of the solitary nucleus, and the reticular formation.

The perforating arteries arise all along the VA. These arteries and those arising from the ASA divide into short perforating and long medullary perforating branches that may extend to the floor of the fourth ventricle. In some cases, small branches arise from the VA, distal to the origin of the PICA, and supply the choroid plexus protruding from the foramen of Luschka.[10]

Posterior Inferior Cerebellar Artery

The posterior inferior cerebellar artery (PICA) has the largest caliber among the branches derived from the VA. The PICA encircles the lower brain stem (medulla) and supplies the medulla, the cerebellar suboccipital surface, the cerebellar tonsil, the vermis, the tela choroidea, the inferior medullary velum, and the choroid plexus of the fourth ventricle. The origin of the PICA, though variable, is usually 14.0 to 26.0 mm above the foramen magnum. Commonly, the PICA arises 13 to 16 mm below the junction of the VAs. The diameter of the PICA at its origin is 0.5 to 3.4 mm (average 2.0 mm), about half the diameter of the VA at the origin of the PICA. Hypoplasia of the PICA occurs in 5% to 16% of cerebellar hemispheres.[20,21]

The PICA has a single trunk in 90% of the cases and duplicated in 2% to 6%, absent in 4% to 26%, and bilaterally absent in 2%.[20–22]

The PICA may arise from the BA, or it may have a common origin with the AICA. It commonly arises from the posterolateral surface of the VA within the anterior medullary cistern, anterior or lateral to the olivary protrusion; it then courses mostly posteriorly, laterally, and superiorly, and passes around the body or lower border of the olive within the lateral cerebellomedullary cistern. The artery has a variable relationship to adjacent cranial nerves (see Fig. 12.1). The hypoglossal nerve arises as a line of rootlets from the preolivary sulcus, which is situated between the olive and the medullary pyramids and extends to the hypoglossal canal. The hypoglossal rootlets are usually posterior to the VA. Most frequently, the PICA originates from the VA at the level of the hypoglossal rootlets (66%), but it may arise rostral or caudal to the nerve. The PICA usually passes posteriorly above, below, or between the hypoglossal rootlets; in some cases it loops before or after passing the hypoglossal nerve.

Posterior to the hypoglossal rootlets, the PICA courses from the lateral to the posterior surface of the medulla while it passes between the rootlets of cranial nerves IX, X, and XI, but most frequently between the lower rootlets. The PICA passes above the glossopharyngeal rootlets in 5% of the cases, between the glossopharyngeal nerve and vagus rootlets in 2%, between the vagus rootlets in 24%, between the vagus and accessory nerves in 31%, and between the accessory rootlets in 38%.

The proximal portion of the PICA usually courses below the origin of the facial and vestibulocochlear nerves, but in some cases the artery loops between the hypoglossal nerve anteriorly and among the glossopharyngeal, vagus, and accessory nerves posteriorly.

This loop may form superiorly; thus, it will lie close to cranial nerves VII and VIII and may compress these nerves. The PICA bifurcates into a medial and lateral trunk in 88% of the cases.[10]

The medial trunk of the PICA passes rostrally in the fissure between the vermis and the cerebellar hemisphere (verohemispheric fissure) and supplies the vermis and adjacent portion of the cerebellar hemisphere. The lateral trunk courses laterally and leaves the telovelotonsillar fissure to supply the surface of the tonsil and the cerebellar hemisphere (Fig. 12.2).

Lister et al.[10] divided the PICA into five segments in relation to the medulla and cerebellum: the anterior medullary, the lateral medullary, the tonsillomedullary, the telovelotonsillar, and the cortical segments. The anterior medullary segment is located between the origin of the PICA and the most prominent portion of the inferior olive and is 1.0 to 15.0 mm long. In some cases, the PICA originates lateral to the medulla; thus, this segment will be absent.

The second segment of the PICA is situated between the olive and the origin of cranial nerves IX, X, and XI. The length of the artery in this segment depends on the direction of its course; it may pass directly or may create a loop in various directions. The length of this segment ranges from 5.0 to 32.0 mm.

The tonsillomedullary segment passes the origin of cranial nerves IX, X, and XI, courses posteromedially between the lower border of the tonsil and the medulla, creates a loop that is called the caudal or inferotonsillar loop, and ends at the medial surface of the tonsil. The length of this segment measures 10 to 43 mm. The lower limit of the caudal loop of the PICA is above the foramen magnum in 60% of the cases, at the level of the foramen magnum in 5%, and below the foramen magnum in 35%.[23] Thus, the low situation of the caudal loop cannot serve as evidence of the tonsillar herniation in angiographic studies.

The fourth segment of the PICA, the telovelotonsillar segment begins at the midportion of the medial surface of the tonsil, ascends toward the roof of the fourth ventricle, and makes a loop with the superior convexity that is called the cranial or supratonsillar loop. The fourth segment exits the fissure between the tonsil, the vermis, and the cerebellar hemisphere to reach the surface of the cerebellar hemisphere. The cranial loop usually lies below the fastigium of the fourth ventricle. The arterial branches that supply the choroid plexus of the fourth ventricle most commonly arise from this segment of the PICA.

The cortical segment of the PICA begins where the PICA leaves the fissure between the vermis, the hemisphere, and the tonsil; it ends at its terminal branches.

The main trunk or the branches of the PICA usually pass to the surface of the hemisphere from the superior and lateral border of the tonsil.

Branches of the PICA

Three groups of arteries originate from the PICA and its main divisions:

The perforating arteries: Several small perforating branches arise from the PICA, especially from its first three segments, and supply the anterior, lateral, and posterior medulla. These arteries anastomose and overlap the perforating branches of the VA on the surface of the medulla. They most frequently arise from the tonsillomedullary segment of the PICA.[10] The perforating arteries originating from the PICA may dip to the brain stem immediately after origination (direct perforation), but they may also be short or long circumflex types that course a distance around the medulla before penetration.

The choroidal branches: The choroidal arteries most commonly arise from the tonsillomedullary and telovelotonsillar segments of the PICA, but they may arise from the lateral medullary segment. Their average number is six, and they supply the tela and the choroid plexus at the midline and paramedian portion of the roof of the fourth ventricle.

The cortical branches: The cortical branches of the PICA usually distribute and supply most portions of the suboccipital surface of the cerebellar hemisphere, the cerebellar tonsil, and half of the vermis on the ipsilateral side. In some cases, cortical branches are distributed to a larger surface and overlap the superior or tentorial surface in the same side and the same part of the contralateral hemisphere. The PICA is rarely so small that its cortical branches supply only the ipsilateral tonsil. The cortical branches of the PICA divide to the hemispheric, vermian, and tonsillar arteries.

The hemispheric arteries arise from the cortical segment or the lateral trunk of the PICA and pass laterally above the tonsil and distribute on the suboccipital surface of the cerebellar hemisphere. Most commonly, the hemispheric arteries consist of the medial, intermedial, and lateral branches, which supply the medial to lateral surface of the hemisphere.[10] They overlap the cortical branches of the SCA and the AICA adjacent to the tentorial and the lateral or petrosal surface of the cerebellum. They anastomose medially with the vermian arteries.

The vermian arteries: Most frequently, one or two small branches arise from the medial trunk of the PICA in the fissure between the vermis and the ipsilateral hemisphere and supply the vermis.

The tonsillar arteries of the PICA originate from the main or lateral trunk of the PICA and supply the ipsilateral cerebellar tonsil.

Occlusion of the PICA or the medullary branches of the VA produces the lateral medullary syndrome due to ischemia of the dorsolateral part of the medulla. The PICA also supplies the lateral medullary region rostral to

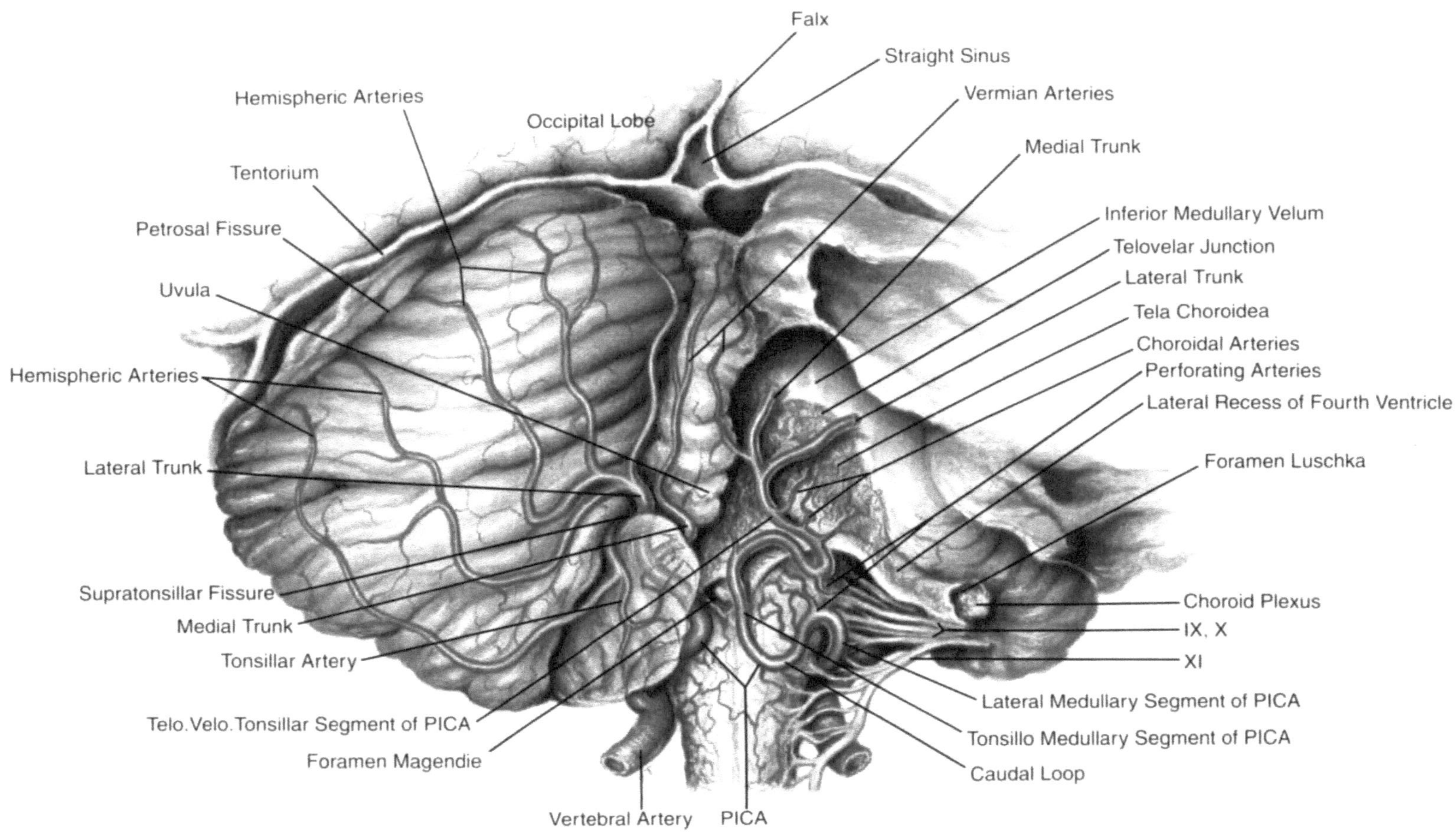

FIGURE 12.2. A midline suboccipital view of the vertebral artery and PICA. The right cerebellum has been removed to show the course of the lateral medullary segment of PICA and its deep distribution. Perforating and choroidal branches are shown. The left PICA has been shown transparently beneath the left cerebellar tonsil.

the area supplied by the direct medullary branches of the VA.

The Basilar Artery

The two VAs join to form the BA at the pontomedullary sulcus (Fig. 12.3). From this point, the BA extends upward on the shallow groove at the midline of the anterior surface of the pons between the two abducent nerves and behind the clivus within the prepontine cistern. The distal portion of the BA enters the interpeduncular cistern and ascends to the level of the dorsum sellae. At this region it separates a few millimeters from the anterior mesencephalon. The terminal portion of the BA may curve posteriorly between the two cerebral peduncles. The BA usually terminates at the level of the pontomesencephalic junction and bifurcates into both PCAs immediately distal to the oculomotor nerves. The BA bifurcates at the level of the pontomesencephalic junction, opposite the interpeduncular fossa in 88% of cases, but it may divide below the junction or as far rostrally as the level of the mamillary bodies. The distance between the bifurcation and mamillary bodies is 0 to 14 mm.[12] The BA ends at the level of the dorsum sella in 51% of patients, superiorly in 30%, and below the dorsum sella in 19%.[24] In one angiographic study, the distance between the tip of the BA and the dorsum sella was 6.8 $\pm$ 2.8 mm in the adult cases.[23]

Krayenbuhl and Yasargil[24] pointed out that the distance between the basilar apex and the dorsum sella measured 1 to 5 mm in 39% of their cases, 5 to 9 mm in 48%, and more than 9 mm in 18%.

The length of the BA varies from 25 to 39 mm and the diameter measures 2.7 to 4.3 mm. Saeki and Rhoton[12] found some dilatation of the artery at the bifurcation in 16% of the cases studied. The BA has a straight course in only 25%, but in aged persons the course of the BA becomes tortuous and elongated, deviates from the midline, and achieves an S-shaped configuration. In this situation the proximal portion of the artery has a concave curve toward the larger VA.

Regarding the embryologic data, several types of anomalies have been found in the BA. The BA may be formed by one VA while the other VA terminates in the PICA.[17,21] Localized fenestration of the artery has been reported in 1%.[6] An intraluminal septum is found in 0.3%, and a complete duplication or fetal type is extremely rare. The BA may anastomose abnormally with the ICA as discussed previously,[17,25] and these anomalies may be associated with aneurysms.[18]

Branches of the Basilar Artery

The following arteries arise from each side of the BA: the perforating arteries, the AICA, the SCA, and the PCA.

The perforating arteries originate from the BA and its

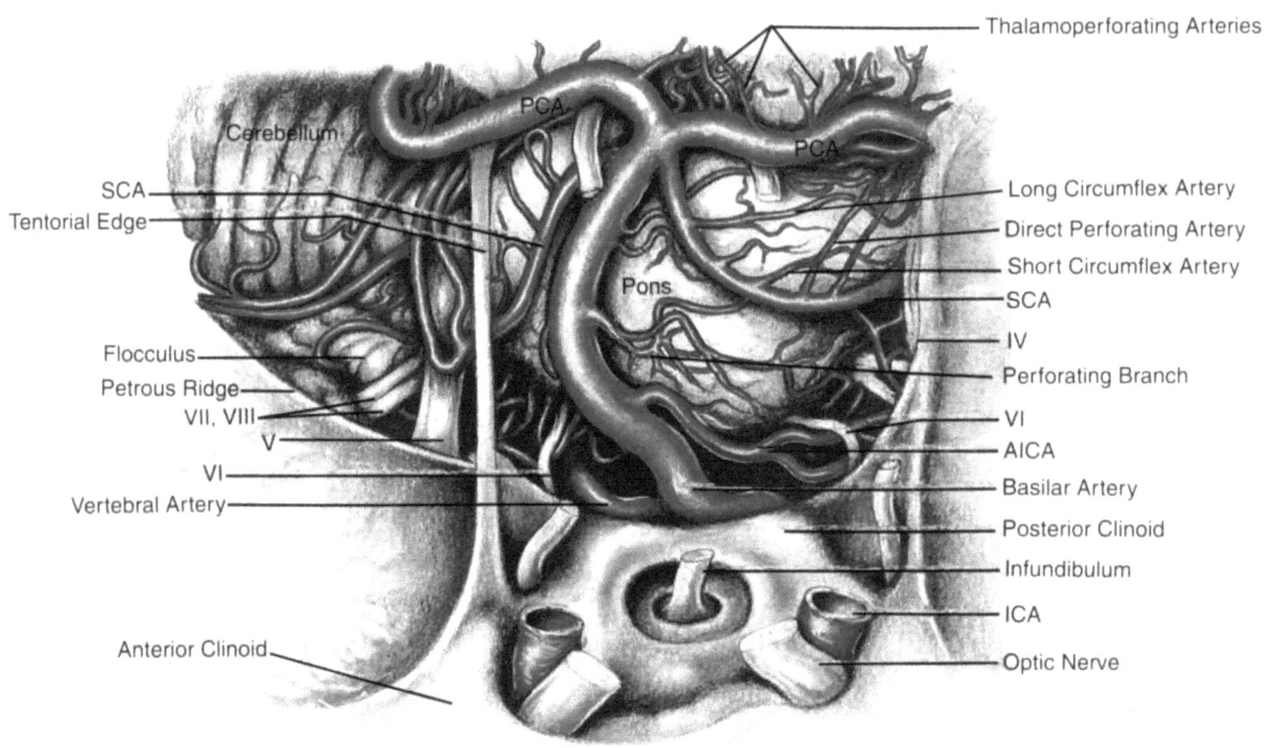

FIGURE 12.3. An anterior and basal view of the basilar artery and its branches and relationships of structures along the cranial base to cranial nerves. AICA, anterior inferior cerebellar artery; ICA, internal carotid artery; SCA, superior cerebellar artery.

major branches to supply the brain stem, the cranial nerves, and the cerebellar peduncles. Those branches arising directly from the BA consist of the paramedian perforating and the short and long circumflex arteries. Most of them originate from the rostral portion of the BA, but some, especially the surface pontine arteries, originate from the midportion or lower segment. A few small perforating arteries may arise from the most proximal BA and enter the ventromedial pontomedullary perforated area near the foramen caecum. The distal centimeter of the BA has the most perforating arteries, also referred to as the superior mesencephalic arteries. Their average number is 0 to 18.[8,12] These branches originate from the posterior surface of the BA in 50% of the cases and from each lateral surface in 25%. No perforating artery arises from the anterior surface of the BA, but Grand and Hopkins[8] found that a single artery with a 0.5 to 1.0 mm diameter arose from the anterior-superior basilar tip, which coursed posterosuperiorly to enter the interpeduncular fossa in two of 30 cadavers. The upper paramedian direct perforating arteries usually originate 2 to 3 mm below the basilar bifurcation. They intermingle with the perforating branches of the proximal posterior cerebral artery (P_1) and enter the interpeduncular fossa and the posterior perforating substance. Perforating branches arising from the upper segment of the BA supply the mesencephalon. The ventral surface of the pons is supplied by three groups of perforating arteries that originate directly from the posterior and lateral surface of the BA. Grand and Hopkins[8] found their highest origin 1 to 2 mm below the origin of the SCA, and their diameters ranged from 0.25 to 1.0 mm.

1. *The paramedian pontine arteries:* These perforating branches arise from each side of the BA as three to four small branches,[26] but in some cases, they may be absent. They usually wind and twist together and anastomose, or they overlap superiorly and inferiorly and finally penetrate the pons along the margin of the anterior pontine sulcus. These branches supply the midpontine region (including the pontine nuclei, corticospinal, corticopontine, and corticobulbar tracts), and some parts of the ventromedial pontine tegmentum.
2. *The short circumflex pontine arteries:* These branches, described by Stopford[15], originate from the BA and then course laterally to the paramedian group to supply the anterolateral surface of the pons.[7,23] Obstruction of these arteries produces cerebellar symptoms and impairment of contralateral sensory and autonomic functions.[7,23]
3. *The long circumflex pontine arteries:* The number of these arteries is one to four and in some cases they may be absent. The lateral surface of the pons is divided into three areas based on their relationship to the trigeminal nerve origin. These areas are anterior, inferior, and posterior to the trigeminal nerve. The long circumflex arteries course superiorly and inferiorly to the trigeminal nerve and distribute on the lateral surface of the pons. They also give branches to the trigeminal nerve. The SCA and the AICA also send branches to the superior and inferior portion of lateral surface of the pons. The long circumflex arteries supply the lateral surface and the tegmentum of the pons and the lateral part of the middle cerebral peduncle.

The Anterior Inferior Cerebellar Artery

The AICA arises most frequently from the lower third of the BA (73–75%), but it may originate from the middle third (16–21%) or from the most proximal few millimeters of the BA (6–9%).[27] In Stopford's[15] reports, the AICA arose at the same level on both sides in 85% of the cases, and caliber of the AICA was equal bilaterally in only 15%.

The AICA courses laterally within the prepontine cistern and crosses the abducent nerve ventrally in 66% of the cases and dorsally in 34%[23]; it then turns backward around the pons toward the cerebellopontine angle within the cerebellopontine cistern. At this point, the AICA has a close relationship to the facial and vestibulocochlear nerves and usually lies ventromedial to their roots. Within the cerebellopontine cistern, the AICA is located slightly inferior and close to the pons and usually gives rise to small branches that supply the lower two thirds of the lateral surface of the pons. Most frequently, the AICA bifurcates into two major trunks, the rostral (lateral) trunk and the caudal or inferomedial trunk, beside cranial nerves VII and VIII. The site of bifurcation occurs proximal to the VII and VIII cranial nerves in two thirds of the cases and after crossing them in one third of the cases.[28] The AICA may send small branches to the olive and the upper lateral surface of the medulla. The rostral trunk of the AICA most commonly passes laterally above the flocculus and runs toward the middle cerebellar peduncle; it then courses within the horizontal or petrosal fissure and supplies the surface of the cerebellum facing the petrous bone and the superior and inferior semilunar lobules. The distal hemispheric branches anastomose with the cortical branches of the SCA and the PICA.

The caudal trunk courses inferomedially toward the medial and anterior borders of the cerebellum and usually below the flocculus close to the brain stem. The caudal trunk supplies the biventral lobule, the inferomedial portion of the petrosal surface of the cerebellum, the middle cerebellar peduncle, and the pons.[23] The terminal branches of the caudal trunk often anastomose with branches of the PICA. The AICA arises from each side of the BA as a single artery in 72% to 73% of the cases, as a duplicate in 25% to 26%, and as a triplicate in 1% to 2%.[21,28]

Hypoplasia of the AICA is found in 20% of the cases and is usually associated with enlargement of the ipsilateral PICA; inversely, when the PICA becomes hypoplastic, the AICA supplies its territory.[22] In eight cases (six cases reported by Yasargil[6] and two reported by Stopford[15], the AICA penetrated the abducent nerve and ran between its fibers.

The AICA may be divided into three segments, in relation to cranial nerves VII and VIII and the internal auditory meatus: the premeatal, the meatal, and the postmeatal segments.[28] The premeatal segment lies between the origin of the AICA and the internal auditory meatus. This segment of the AICA usually consists of the main trunk of the AICA, although the artery may bifurcate in this segment.

The meatal segment is adjacent to the meatus, and usually one or both of its major trunks is nerve-related, creating a loop with lateral convexity before turning again toward the brain stem. This arterial loop may be located medial to the meatus, but, in half of the cases, it lies adjacent to the meatus or protrudes into the internal auditory canal. Sunderland[29] found the loop of the AICA at the level of the meatus or protruding into the canal in 64% of the specimens. In this segment, the artery usually lies anteroinferior or between the seventh and the eighth cranial nerve roots.

The postmeatal segment is located distal to the facial and vestibulocochlear roots. After passing these nerves, the AICA or its major trunks course medially and are normally situated posteroinferior to these nerves; but, they may lie superior or between cranial nerves VII and VIII. Finally, the AICA or its main divisions course medially, reach the brain stem and the petrosal surface of the cerebellum, and supply these structures.

The Branches of the Anterior Inferior Cerebellar Artery

The AICA gives rise to the perforating, the internal auditory, the subarcuate, and the cortical branches (Fig. 12.4).

The perforating arteries originate from the AICA or its major trunks, proximal or distal to cranial nerves VII and VIII, and supply the pons, particularly its lateral surface and the medulla. *The recurrent perforating arteries* are small branches that are found in over 80% of the cases.[28] They arise from the AICA beside cranial nerves VII and VIII, course toward and occasionally into the

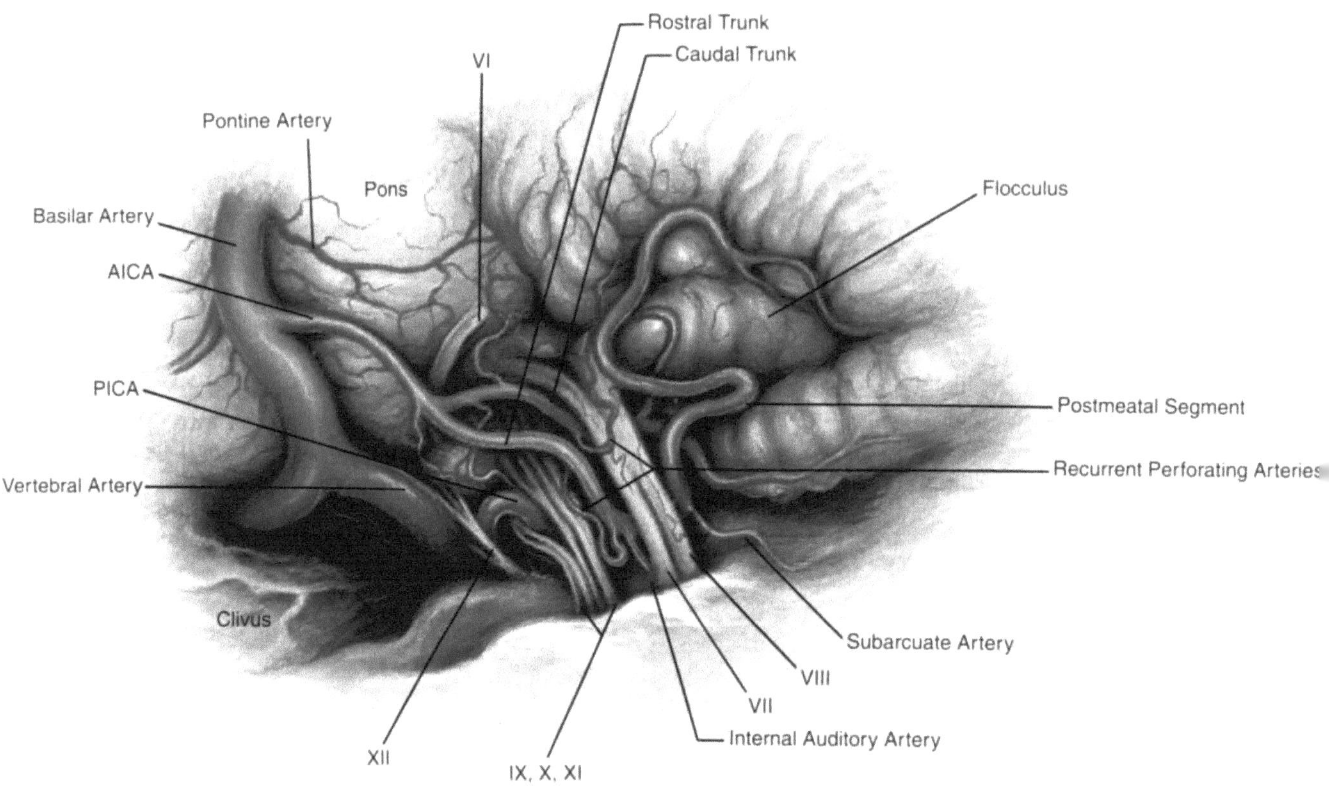

FIGURE 12.4. Left anterolateral view of the AICA and its branches. The relationship of the rostral and caudal trunk to the seventh and eighth nerves are shown. The perforating branches from AICA are demonstrated.

internal auditory meatus, and, after forming a loop, take a recurrent course along the roots of cranial nerves VII and VIII and reach the brain stem. These arteries supply the facial and vestibulocochlear roots and the brain stem around their entry points to the brain stem. They also supply the middle cerebellar peduncle, the pons (particularly around the trigeminal root entry zone), the superior part of the lateral surface of the medulla, the choroid plexus protruding to the cerebellopontine cistern and the lateral recess of the fourth ventricle, and the glossopharyngeal and vagus rootlets. The recurrent arteries lie between the facial and the vestibulocochlear roots in 65% of the cases, inferior to them in 34% of the cases studied, and superior in 1%.[23]

The *internal auditory artery* (IAA) originates from the AICA in 83% to 95% of the cases but may also arise from the BA.[23,29] The IAA usually arises from the premeatal and meatal segments of the AICA or its major trunks and most frequently arises from the apex of the loop, which is formed by the artery near the meatus. In one study, the artery originated from the AICA medial to the internal auditory meatus in 60% of the cases, at the level of the meatus in 8%, and within the internal auditory canal in 32%.[28]

Fisch[30] found the IAA as a single branch in 50% of the specimens and as a duplication in 50% of specimens. He also pointed out that the IAA enters the canal from the anterior inferior rim of the meatus. The IAA supplies the bone and dura covering the internal auditory canal, cranial nerves VII and VIII within the canal, and the vestibulocochlear sensory organs. Rarely, the artery originates from the other branches of the AICA. The subarcuate artery arises from the AICA beside cranial nerves VII and VIII, medial to the acoustic meatus. It runs laterally and penetrates the dura covering the subarcuate fossa. The subarcuate artery enters into the subarcuate canal and supplies the semicircular canals and the mastoid. The subarcuate fossa is located posterior to the acoustic meatus and lies inferior to the groove of the superior petrosal sinus on the upper portion of the posterior surface of petrous bone.[28]

The cortical branches of the AICA supply the petrosal surface of the cerebellum including the superior and the inferior semilunar lobules, which are separated by the horizontal fissure and the biventral lobule. The cortical branches of the AICA anastomose with the cortical branches of the SCA and the PICA.

The Superior Cerebellar Artery

The SCA is the most consistent in location and origin among the posterior circulation arteries (see Fig. 12.3). The artery arises near the basilar apex, immediately close and adjacent to the origin of the PCA in 84% of the cases, below this point in 14%, and from the most proximal portion of the PCA in 2%.[23] It normally arises as a single trunk but is duplicated in up to 28%.[21,31] Absence of the SCA is extremely rare. The average diameter of the SCA is 1.9 mm at its origin. It originates within the interpeduncular cistern and courses laterally below the oculomotor and trochlear nerves and above the trigeminal nerves (Fig. 12.5). It then encircles the brain stem in the groove between the pons and the mesencephalon. After forming a shallow loop with caudal convexity within the lateral ambient cistern, the SCA reaches the groove between the posterior surface of the midbrain and the anterosuperior border of the cerebellum. Distal to this point, the branches of the SCA distribute on the superior surface of the cerebellum.

Normally, the SCA bifurcates into two major trunks: a rostral or superior trunk and a caudal or inferior trunk. The SCA usually bifurcates on the lateral surface of the brain stem, but it may divide proximally or distally. Hardy and Rhoton[32] measured the bifurcation of the SCA 0.6 to 34 mm distal to its origin. It bifurcates anterior to the brain stem in 30% and on the lateral surface in 70%.[21] The terminal branches of the rostral trunk of the SCA supply the vermis and adjacent portion of the superior surface of the cerebellum. The caudal trunk terminates on the lateral portion of the superior surface.

The SCA and its major trunks have important anatomic relationships to the adjacent cranial nerves, arteries, and tentorium cerebelli. The SCA passes the oculomotor nerve inferiorly and, in most cases, contacts the nerve. In 36% of the cases that were most frequently associated with various types of abnormalities (such as duplication low origination of the SCA, and the fetal type of PCA), the SCA passed 0.7 to 5.2 mm away from the third cranial nerve.[9] The trochlear nerve exits the midbrain below the inferior colliculus and courses laterally within the cerebellomesencephalic groove and crosses the branches of the rostral and caudal trunks of the SCA. When the nerve reaches the lateral surface of the brain stem, it lies inferior to the tentorium and superior to the SCA. The trochlear nerve touches the SCA in this area in 92% of the cases.[9]

The SCA encircles the brain stem above the trigeminal nerve. The nerve exits the lateral portion of the pons in an anterosuperior direction and runs under the tentorial attachment to enter Meckel's cave. The artery or its major trunks may contact the trigeminal root, particularly when its loop projects most caudally. The SCA frequently touches the superior and superomedial surface of the trigeminal root, usually a few millimeters distal to the trigeminal root entry zone.[32] This occurred in 52% of the SCAs studied.

The posterior border of the tentorial incisura is located between the occipital lobe superiorly and the colliculi inferiorly. The proximal portion of the SCA usually lies

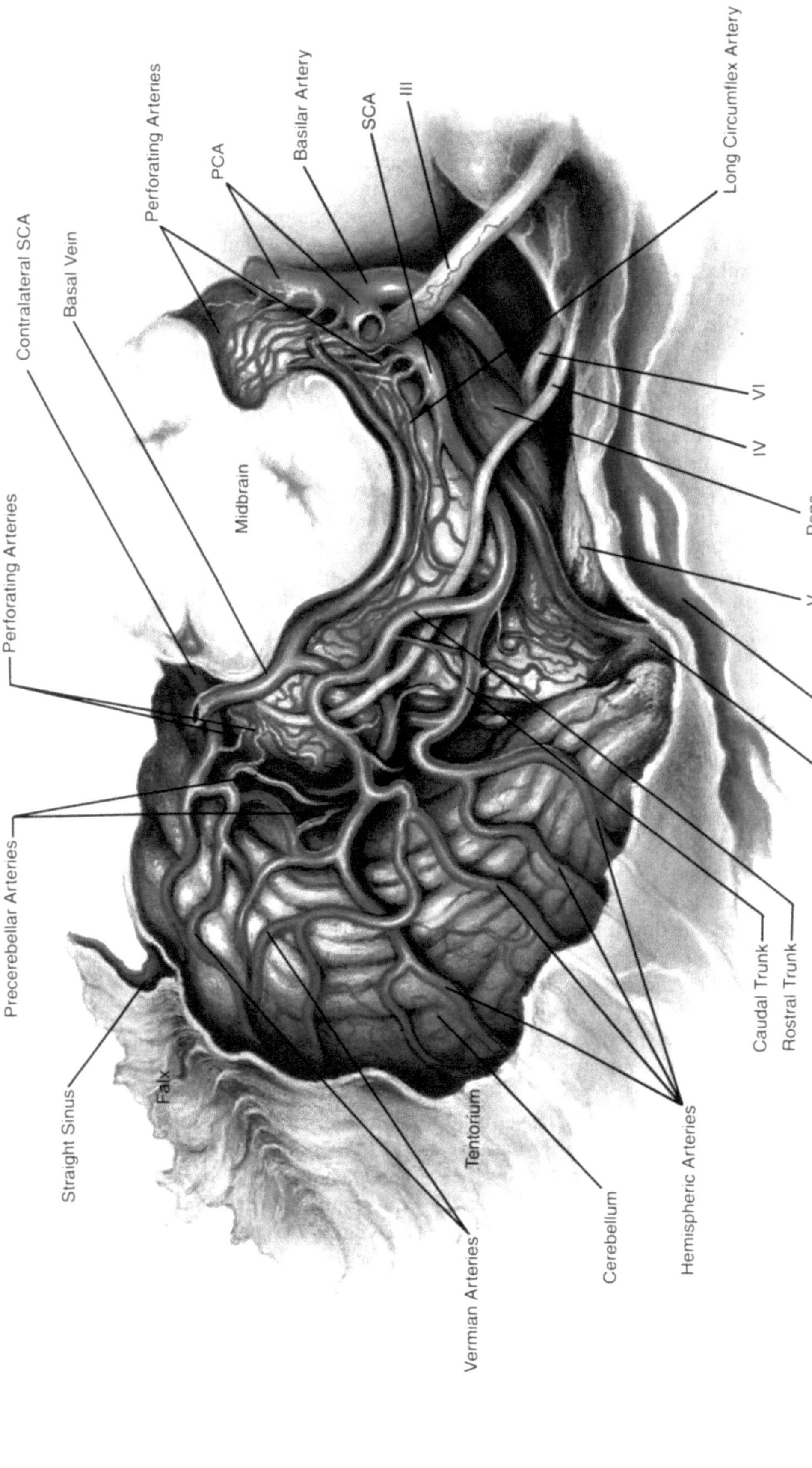

FIGURE 12.5. Right anterolateral view of the superior cerebellar artery and its branches. The precerebellar fissure has been opened to show the perforating arteries and the precerebellar arteries. The usual course of the fourth nerve in relation to the superior cerebellar artery branches has been depicted.

0 to 5.0 mm medial to the anterior third of the tentorial free edge. Distally, the SCA and its major trunks pass below the tentorium while it loops caudally. In the posterior portion of the incisura, some branches of the artery lie medial to the free edge of the tentorium and subsequently course beneath the tentorium. The SCA and its major trunks may be so close that they touch the free tentorial edge. In some cases, the artery may arise from a highly placed basilar apex. The origin of the SCA is then above the tentorial edge with distal segments passing below it.

The SCA may be divided into four segments: the anterior pontomesencephalic, the lateral pontomesencephalic, the cerebellomesencephalic, and the cortical segments.[9]

The anterior pontomesencephalic segment, also called the anterior pontine segment, is the part of the SCA lying between the origin of the SCA and the anterolateral margin of the brain stem.

The lateral pontomesencephalic (ambient) segment, which may be seen through the tentorial free edge, passes below to the tentorium and forms a loop caudally. The trochlear nerve courses above to the midportion of this segment. The basal vein of Rosenthal and the PCA pass parallel and above the SCA. This segment of the SCA terminates at the beginning of the cerebellomesencephalic groove. This groove is formed by the folia of the cerebellum posteriorly, the colliculi, the anterior medullar velum, and the superior cerebellar peduncle anteriorly. The groove is shallow laterally and is deepest in the medial portion. The superior part of the groove is situated within the quadrigeminal cistern. The third segment of the SCA, which is also called the quadrigeminal segment, and its branches loop into the groove, then course again superiorly, to reach the posterosuperior border of the groove and then pass over the cerebellum.

The cortical segment of the SCA consists of multiple branches that leave the cerebellomesencephalic groove and supply the superior surface of the cerebellum.

The Branches of the Superior Cerebellar Artery

The SCA gives rise to three groups of branches: The perforating, the precerebellar, and the cortical arteries.

Several perforating arteries originate from the SCA and penetrate the brain stem. They follow three patterns: (1) the direct perforating, (2) the short, and (3) the long circumflex arteries that wind around the brain stem before penetration. These branches arise from the main artery or its major trunks.

The majority of perforating arteries originating from the SCA terminate at the area between the superior and middle cerebellar peduncles and penetrate into the tegmentum (60–65%). Other perforating branches enter the quadrigeminal area to supply the colliculi; some branches also enter the cerebral peduncles and the interpeduncular fossa, which are mostly the direct perforating arteries.

The precerebellar arteries arise from the proximal portion of the cortical branches within the cerebellomesencephalic groove. The branches arising from the hemispheric cortical arteries penetrate the cerebellum and supply the deep cerebellar nuclei. Those branches arising from the vermian cortical arteries terminate in the inferior colliculi and the superior medullary velum.

The cortical branches: The SCA supplies the superior or tentorial surface and some parts of the petrosal surface of the cerebellum. The cortical branches of the SCA divide into the vermian and the hemispheric arteries. The vermian arteries usually originate from the rostral trunk of the SCA within the precerebellar as the cerebellomesencephalic groove and most frequently divide into median and paramedian vermian arteries.

The hemispheric arteries arise from the rostral and caudal trunk within the precerebellar groove and distribute on the tentorial surface of the cerebellum, lateral to the vermian arteries.

Usually, there are three hemispheric cortical arteries on each side: the medial hemispheric artery, which supplies approximately the medial one third of the superior surface of the cerebellar hemisphere; the intermediate hemispheric artery; and the lateral hemispheric artery. The latter two supply the middle and lateral third of the cerebellar hemisphere on the superior surface.

The marginal artery is a cortical branch that originates from the proximal SCA, and, when it exists, 50% to 60% course laterally to supply the cerebellum adjacent to the petrosal fissure.[9,21]

The Posterior Cerebral Artery

Two PCAs originate from the basilar apex within the interpeduncular cistern, usually 0.6 to 3.0 mm distal to the origin of the SCA. The PCA courses superior to the oculomotor nerve and passes around the cerebral peduncle and reaches the posterolateral surface of the mesencephalon; it then leaves the tentorial incisura and passes posteriorly over the tentorium to distribute its terminal branches (Fig. 12.6).

In the embryo, the artery is irrigated by the ICA, but, with development, the connection between the BA and the PCA becomes enlarged, and subsequently the carotid segment of the artery, which forms the posterior communicating artery (PComA), decreases in caliber. In the normal pattern, the PCA is larger than the PComA, and receives blood from the BA, but, in 15% to 40% of cases the PCA has a fetal-type configuration, and the proximal PCA (P_1) is smaller than the PComA. The PCA is then

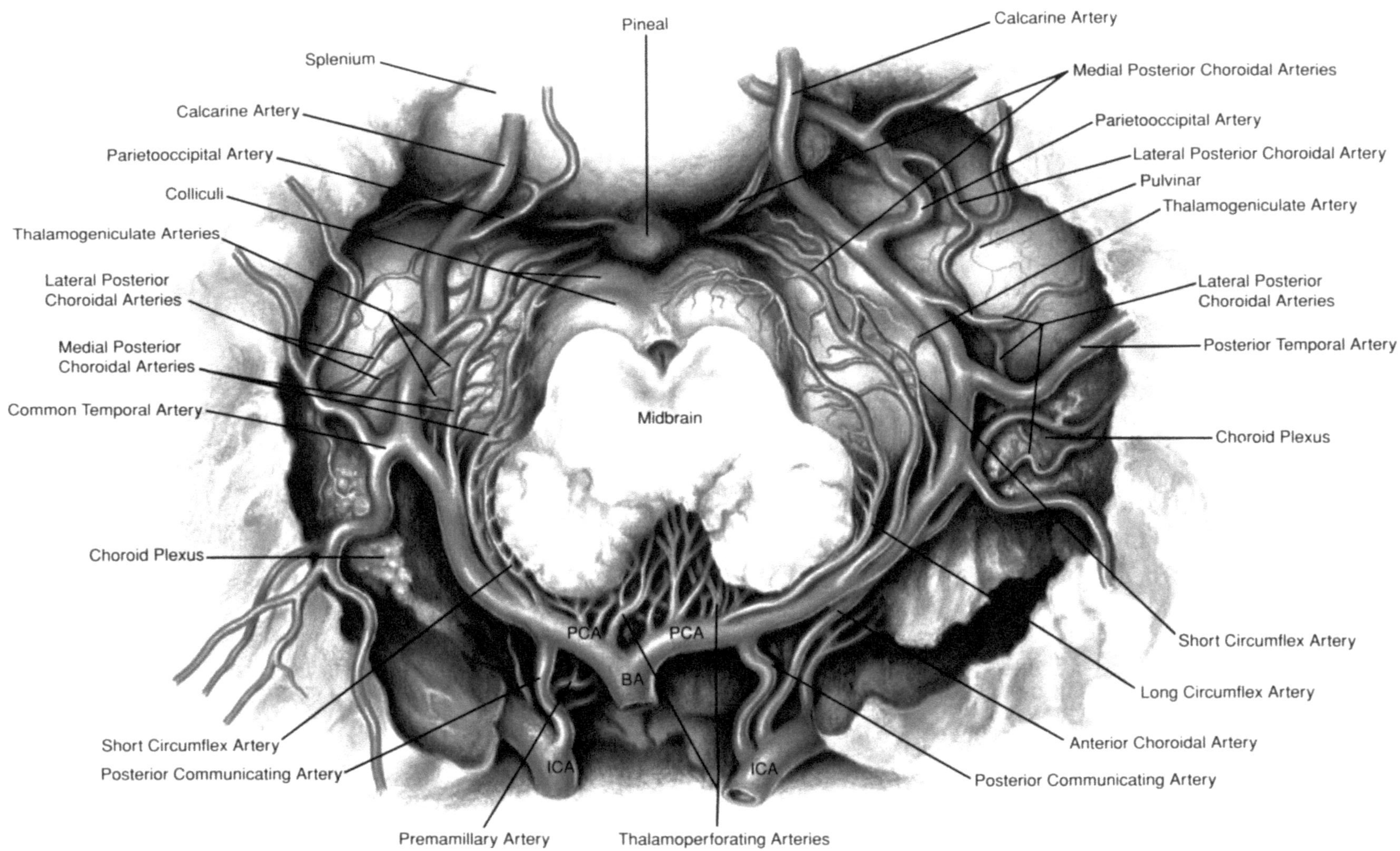

FIGURE 12.6. Basal or inferior view of both posterior cerbral arteries. The medial part of both temporal lobes have been removed. Both pulvinars are shown above the midbrain.

supplied mainly by the ICA. The PCA supplies the midbrain, the thalamus, the choroid plexus, the walls of the lateral and third ventricles, and the posterior portion of the cerebral hemisphere.

Krayenbuhl and Yasargil[24] divided the PCA into four segments, P_1 through P_4. The P_1 segment is also called the proximal, or precommunical segment, which is the portion of artery proximal to the PComA. The average diameter of the P_1 is 2.2 mm.[8]

The P_1 was larger than the PComA in 58% of the specimens studied, the intermediate type (the P_1 and the PComA had equal caliber) in 2%, and the fetal type (P_1 smaller than PComA) in 40%.[33]

In the fetal-type PCA, the oculomotor nerve may course inferomedially to the junction of the P_1 and the PComA. But in the normal pattern the nerve usually passes inferolaterally to this point.

The P_2 segment begins at the PComA and winds around the cerebral peduncle within the peduncular and ambient cisterns and terminates at the posterior margin of the midbrain. The P_2 segment may be subdivided into anterior (P_{2A}) and posterior (P_{2P}) compartments. The P_{2A} begins at the PComA and passes around the cerebral peduncle medial to the hippocampus, inferior to the optic tract and the basal vein of Rosenthal, and then enters the proximal portion of the ambient cistern.

The P_{2P} begins at the posterior border of the cerebral peduncle and courses along the posterolateral surface of the midbrain to the area inferolateral to the geniculate bodies and the pulvinar. The artery lies inferior and parallel to the optic tract and basal vein and superomedial to the tentorial edge and trochlear nerve.[33]

The P_3 segment is found between the posterior midbrain and the anterior limit of the calcarine fissure. This segment lies within the quadrigeminal cistern, and its average length is about 20 mm. At the area posterior to the colliculi, the two PCAs course medially; the average distance between them is 8.9 mm. The terminal branches of the PCA are the calcarine and the parietooccipital arteries, and they usually arise from the parent artery proximal to the calcarine fissure. The P_4 segment of the PCA consists of terminal branches that supply the posterior portions of the cerebral hemispheres.

The Branches of the Posterior Cerebral Artery

The PCA gives rise to direct perforating and to short and long circumflex arteries that supply the brain stem, to the medial and lateral posterior choroidal arteries, and to the cortical and splenial arteries.

The direct perforating arteries originate from the P_1 and P_2 segments and are constituted by the posterior thalamoperforating arteries that mostly arise from the P_1 segment, the thalamogeniculate arteries, and the peduncular branches that usually arise from the P_2 segment[33] (Figs. 12.6 and 12.7).

The posterior thalamoperforating (PTP) arteries are perforating branches that originate from the P_1 and the BA bifurcation. These have also been referred to as the arteries of Percheron.[34] The anterior thalamoperforating (ATP) arteries or polar arteries may arise from the PComA.[27] Peele[35] pointed out that the PTP arteries may also arise from the distal portion of the PComA. In two series reported by Rhoton and associates, the posterior thalamoperforating (PTP) arteries originated from the posterior and superior aspect of the P_1 segment.[12,33] The average number of PTP arteries arising from each P_1 segment is three, and their caliber varies from 0.2 to 1.0 mm.

The PTP arteries enter the interpeduncular fossa, the medial surface of the cerebral peduncles, and the posterior perforated substance. These arteries supply the base of the oculomotor nerve, the posterior thalamus, the periventricular and median nuclei of the thalamus, the substantia nigra, the red nucleus, the midline midbrain structures, and the rostromedian floor of the fourth ventricle. Some of the perforating arteries may originate from the proximal P_2 segment (the P_{2A}) and penetrate the cerebral peduncles to supply the corticospinal and corticobulbar tracts, the substantia nigra, the red nucleus, and a part of the tegmentum.

The thalamogeniculate arteries also arise from the P_2 segment, below the lateral thalamus, and within the ambient cistern. They usually terminate on the inferior surface of the lateral and medial geniculate bodies. Their caliber is about 0.2 to 0.6 mm, and the number of these arteries varies from one to seven in each hemisphere.[23]

The thalamogeniculate arteries supply the optic tract, the posterior limb of the internal capsule, and the posterior half of the lateral thalamus.[33]

The circumflex arteries most frequently arise from the P_1 and P_2 segments of the PCA (see Fig. 12.6).

The short circumflex arteries course around the cerebral peduncle, medial to the main trunk of the PCA, the long circumflex, and the choroidal arteries. They terminate on the posterolateral surface of the cerebral peduncle, the tegmentum, and the geniculate bodies. In some cases, their branches may enter the interpeduncular fossa.

The long circumflex arteries, also called quadrigeminal arteries,[26,35] usually arise from the P_1 or proximal P_2 segments, distal to the origin of the short circumflex arteries (Fig. 12.8). In 80% of cases, they originate from the P_1 segment.[33] These arteries lie medial to the PCA, pass around the cerebral peduncle and send branches to it and the geniculate bodies, then terminate on the quadrigeminal area where they anastomose with the collicular branches of the SCA.

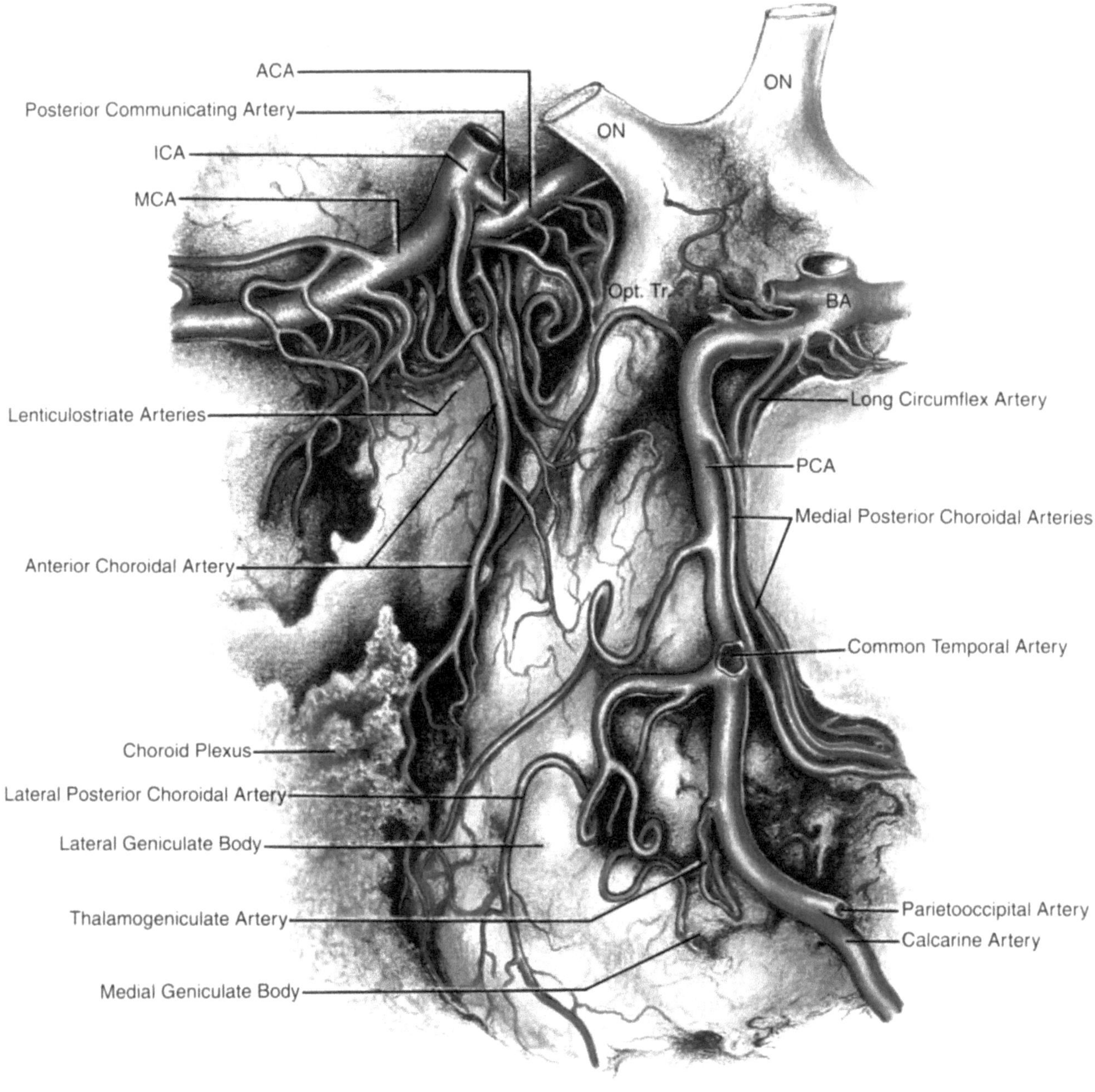

FIGURE 12.7. Basal view of the right cerebral hemisphere. The right temporal lobe has been removed to show the temporal horn. The right PCA encircles the brain stem and important branches enter the choroidal fissure.

The Posterior Choroidal Arteries

The medial posterior choroidal arteries (MPChAs) are usually multiple. They arise from the P_2 segment of the PCA, but they may originate from the other segments of the PCA (Fig. 12.9).

The arteries course medially to the parent artery, wind around the cerebral peduncle and reach the posterior surface of the midbrain where they enter the roof of the third ventricle from the lateral side of the pineal gland. They course anteriorly on the surface of the thalamus to reach the foramen of Monro, then pass through the foramen of Monro, and terminate on the choroid plexus of the lateral ventricle. At the posterior surface of the midbrain, the arteries may send branches to the pineal gland and the choroidal fissure.

The MPChAs supply the medial thalamus, the pulvinar, the pineal gland, the cerebral peduncle, the tegmentum, and the geniculate bodies.

The lateral posterior choroidal arteries (LPChAs), which usually arise as multiple arteries from the P_2 segment or major branches of the PCA, course laterally,

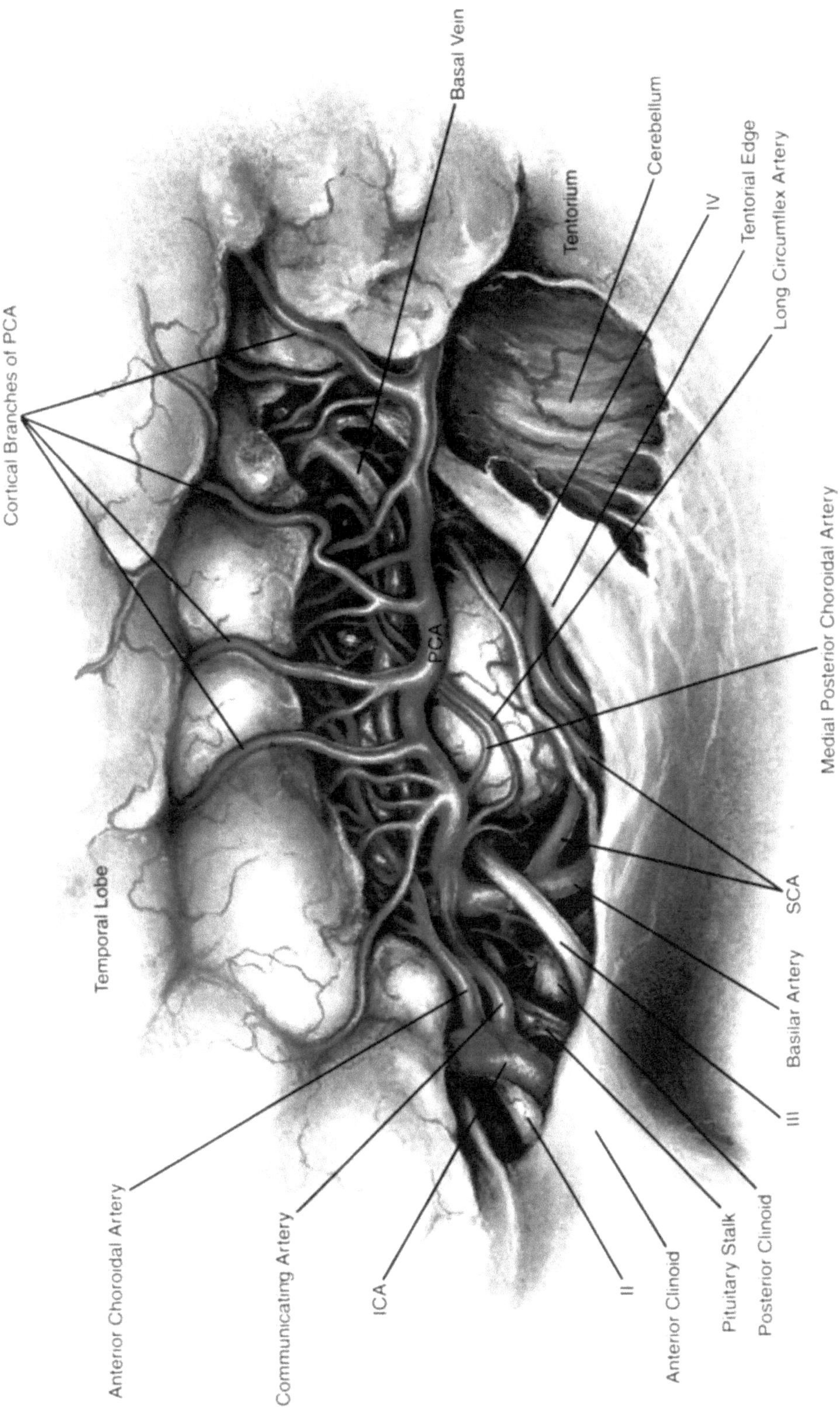

FIGURE 12.8. Extended left lateral view with the temporal lobe elevated to show the important branches of the left posterior cerebral artery. The tentorium has been partly opened to demonstrate the deep branches and their relationship to the cranial nerves.

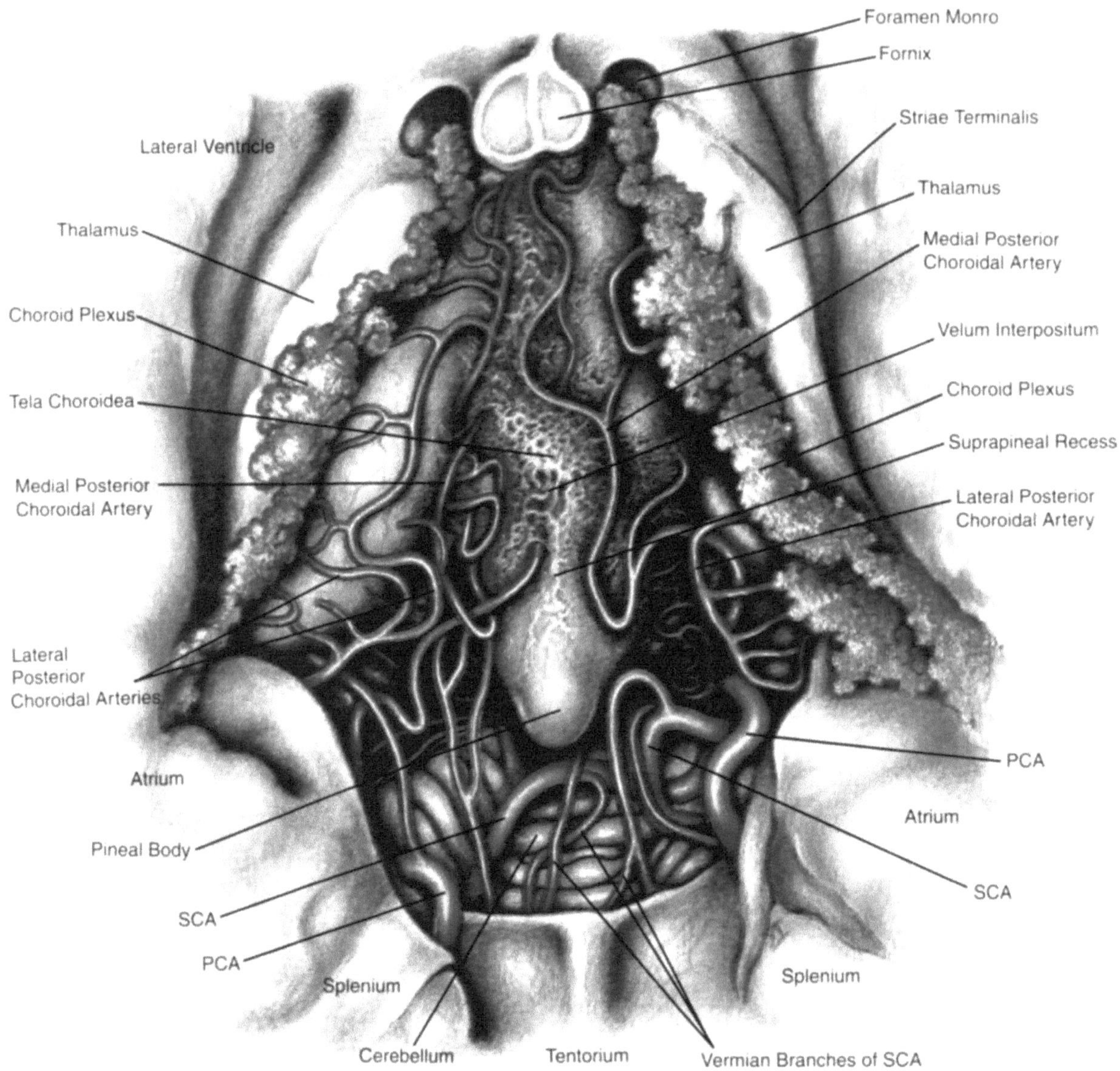

FIGURE 12.9. Posterior–superior view of the posterior incisural space. The occipital lobes, the splenium of the corpus callosum, and the posterior fornices have been removed. The branches that pass beneath the pulvinar to reach the temporal horn and atrium are shown.

enter the choroid plexus of the temporal horn and atrium of the lateral ventricle. The LPChAs supply the cerebral peduncle, the lateral geniculate body, the dorsomedial thalamic nuclei, the pulvinar, some part of the fornix, the posterior commissure, and the choroid plexus. They also anastomose with branches of the AChA.

The Cortical Branches of the PCA

Zeal and Rhoton[33] divided the cortical branches of the PCA into the inferior temporal group, the parietooccipital artery, and the calcarine artery (Figs. 12.10 and 12.11).

The inferior temporal group consists of the hippocampal artery, the anterior temporal artery, the middle temporal artery, the posterior temporal artery, and the common temporal artery.

1. The hippocampal artery is usually the first cortical branch of the PCA and supplies the hippocampal gyrus, the uncus, and the dentate gyrus.
2. The anterior temporal artery usually arises from the proximal P_2 segment and distributes to the anterior inferior surface of the temporal lobe.
3. The middle temporal arterial branch originates from the P_2 segment, and, if it exists, usually supplies the inferior surface of the temporal lobe.
4. The posterior temporal artery most commonly arises

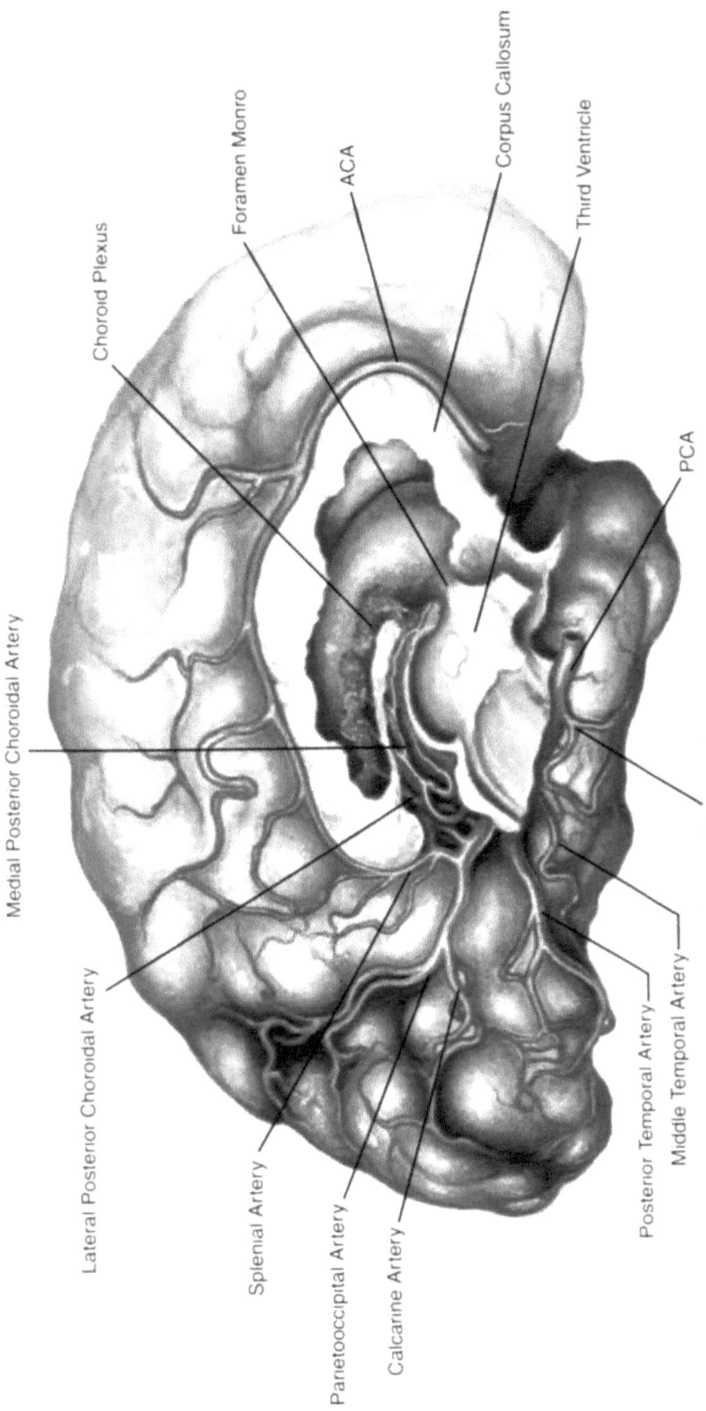

FIGURE 12.10. The right hemisphere has been removed in order to show the medial branches of the posterior cerebral artery.

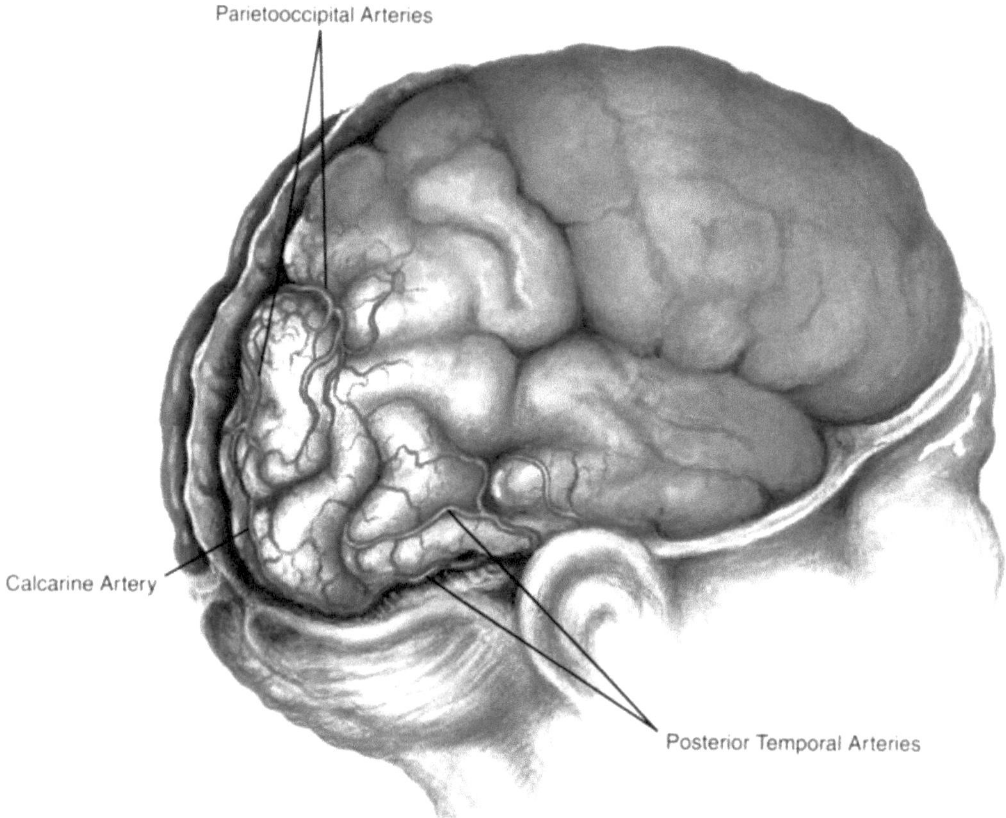

FIGURE 12.11. Right lateral and posterior view of the cortical branches of the posterior cerebral artery are shown.

from the P_2 segment and courses on the inferior surface of the temporal lobe through the occipital pole and the lingual gyrus. Occlusion of this artery may cause ischemia of the inferior surface of the temporal lobe and the lingual and falciform gyri.

5. The common temporal artery usually originates from the P_2 segment, passes laterally, and supplies the inferior surface of the temporal and occipital lobes.

The parietooccipital and calcarine arteries usually constitute the terminal branches of the PCA. *The parietooccipital artery* arises from the P_3 segment and courses through the parietooccipital fissure and distributes on the posterior portion of the medial surface of the cerebral hemisphere. This artery supplies the precuneus, the cuneus, and the lateral occipital gyrus. In some cases the parietooccipital artery may supply some parts of the precentral and superior parietal lobules.

The calcarine artery passes through the calcarine fissure and distributes to the occipital pole, the lingual gyrus, and the inferior cuneus.

The cortical branches of the PCA, particularly the posterior temporal and the parietooccipital arteries, usually send several branches to the lateral surface of the cerebral hemisphere.

The splenial artery originates mostly from the parietooccipital artery, but it may arise directly from the PCA or its other major branches.[33] This artery supplies the splenium of the corpus callosum and anastomoses with the terminal branches of the pericallosal artery.

Clinical Features

Unruptured vertebrobasilar aneurysms produce protean clinical features because many variables determine the symptoms and signs produced. Among these, the location of the aneurysm and its size are perhaps the most important. Small aneurysms, as a rule, produce no focal neurological symptoms prior to their bleedings. Even with small aneurysms, however, headaches have been reported, depending on the position of the head in relationship to the aneurysm. Large unruptured aneurysms may produce cerebellar, cerebellomedullary, and cerebellopontine signs. Cranial nerve dysfunction may appear, depending on the location of the aneurysm in relation to the nerve. The third cranial nerve may be affected when the aneurysm arises from either the SCA, the PCA, or the apex of the BA. Aneurysms originating on the basilar or vertebral arteries may affect caudal cranial nerves IX, X, XI, and XII. Isolated abducent nerve paralysis or fourth nerve paralysis may also be associated with aneurysms of the BA, especially those that are fusiform.

Giant aneurysms of the vertebrobasilar system produce findings similar to those encountered with intracranial neoplasms except that the onset is usually more insidious. In addition to cranial nerve dysfunction, aneurysms of the basilar apex also produce disorders of the cerebellar peduncle with hemiparesis, hemianesthesia, and gaze paralysis. Even upward gaze abnormalities have been seen with large aneurysms that compress the brain stem and tectum from a dorsal position. Involvement of the short perforating branches of the brain stem may produce signs compatible with brain stem infarction. Large and giant aneurysms also produce hydrocephalus when they obstruct CSF pathways. More commonly, this results from large aneurysms that block or distort the aqueduct of Sylvius in its upper or lower portions, or, occasionally, when large basilar apex aneurysms obstruct the foramen of Monro.

Ruptured Aneurysms

Fox[4] studied over 2800 aneurysms of the intracranial circulation. Of those occupying the SCA, all aneurysms encountered had previously ruptured. For those of the basilar bifurcation, 95% had already ruptured by the time they were found. For PICA aneurysms, 89% had caused SAH, and, of those arising from the VA, 83% had already bled when they were found. In the other cases, the aneurysm either presented as an intracranial mass or was discovered incidentally. Hook et al.[36] reviewed the consequences of ruptured aneurysms of the posterior cranial circulation. In his series, 43% of the patients who developed SAH due to an aneurysm of the posterior cranial circulation arrived in a comatose state. In 18% of the cases, dysarthria, dysphasia, nystagmus, and ataxia were present on admission. In 7%, there were gaze abnormalities and total homolateral ophthalmoplegia in 7%. Sixty-four percent presented with hemiparesis. Stehbens[37] reported that aneurysms in this location are associated not only with SAH but also frequently with small intracerebral hemorrhages. Large aneurysms of the basilar apex that project into the inferior wall of the third ventricle may be associated with intraventricular hemorrhage on rupture. Aneurysms of the PCA may produce hematomas in the thalamus, occipital lobe, the posterior aspect of the temporal lobe, and in the cerebral peduncle proper. In Stehbens' studies, aneurysms in this location accounted for 6.2% of all the subdural hematomas associated with aneurysms. Patients developing significant hematomas in the posterior cranial fossa apparently did not survive long enough for clinical presentation, and, in most, death occurred suddenly and unexpectedly.

The clinical course of patients with SAH from vertebrobasilar artery (VBA) aneurysms is closely related to the severity of the SAH and the route of propagation of the clots throughout the subarachnoid cisterns. Approximately, 15% to 20% of patients with SAH due to VBA aneurysms are in grade 1, 50% appear in grade 2 (grades 3 and 4 Hunt and Hess), and the remainder arrive in grade 3, deeply comatose (grades 4 and 5 Hunt and Hess). Peerless and Drake[38] underlined the increased frequency of vasospasm that occurs in the patients with aneurysms in this location, explaining why many patients with aneurysms in this location decompensate at the end of the first week or in the perioperative period.

Clinical signs associated with PICA aneurysms are not greatly different from those associated with SAH elsewhere. The headache accompanying PICA aneurysms is said to be localized in the neck and occipital region more often than that accompanying supratentorial aneurysms. Rarely, localizing symptoms may be present and these are usually due to involvement of the brain stem itself, the cerebellum, or the lower cranial nerves that pass over the aneurysm. A giant aneurysms in this region may present as a fourth ventricular or medullary tumor. They may also compress the trigeminal, abducent, facial, vestibular, glossopharyngeal, spinal accessory, and hypoglossal nerves in addition to the brain stem. They may obstruct CSF outflow and present as hydrocephalus.

Surgical Options

Aneurysms of the posterior cranial circulation have been approached by neurosurgeons with some trepidation. Operative morbidity and mortality have been high.

In the 1950s, the earliest operations were done for mass lesions. When aneurysmal growth or thrombus formation led to compressive signs, procedures were developed, usually to exclude the lesion from the circulation by some form of trapping maneuver. In 1961, Drake[39] described four cases in which aneurysms of the BA bifurcation were approached directly. By 1965, his series had enlarged to about seven patients.[40] Of these, four died, one was severely disabled, and only two had returned to their usual work. The importance of preservation of the short branches arising from the apex and P_1 was emphasized. During the past 20 years, many strides have been made in imaging these lesions. The microsurgical anatomy of the area has been outlined, and visualization of this anatomy has become commonplace through operating microscopes. Nevertheless, because of the location of these lesions adjacent to the brain stem and because of the many short perforating arteries that exit adjacent to them and from their walls, aneurysms in this location still carry high mortality and morbidity, much more so than those arising from vessels of the anterior circulation. This has led many endovascular surgeons and interventional neuroradiologists to seek another approach through the vascular system to these treacherous lesions. Endovascular methods such as coils and detachable balloons may now be used to treat virtually any aneurysm arising from the basilar or vertebral artery. Those having a fusiform shape or those with wide orifices, can often be excluded from the intracranial circulation by means of an endovascular trapping procedure after the functional significance of the vessel in question has been determined.

Because of the close relationship of VBA aneurysms to the brain stem, different and sometimes heroic methods must be used to present the lesion for favorable clipping. Although these are occasionally applicable to aneurysms in other locations, their use is especially appropriate for lesions of the basilar trunk, vertebrobasilar junction, and basilar apex. In many instances, the important perforating arteries have been incorporated into the neck of the aneurysm, usually on the posterior surface, since they originate from this area. Preservation of these perforating end arteries is critical to success of the operation and this requires folding of the aneurysm to either side for posterior inspection and dissection. This cannot be achieved with a turgid aneurysm. Temporary clipping of the basilar trunk permits collapse and mobilization of the large tense aneurysm. The use of temporary clips may lead to ischemic complications, and the temporal profiles of safe clipping have not, as yet, been defined for each vessel. However, anecdotal evidence suggests that a time limit of about 15 to 20 min causes few ischemic deficits. In some cases, Drake[39] has applied permanent occlusion effectively.

Hypothermia and/or pentobarbital anesthesia, or agents like etomidate, may also prolong safe occlusion times. Hypothermic cardiac arrest has been used successfully to collapse the aneurysm that is large and embedded in the brain stem. Cardiopulmonary bypass is achieved via the femoral vessels, and body temperature is reduced to less than 20°C. At a level of 22° to 23°C, fibrillation of the heart begins and the bypass is instituted. Heparinization is required. The dissection of the sac proceeds until total collapse of the aneurysm is needed, at which time, the pump is turned off and intracranial blood is allowed to drain toward the pump. Arrest times at 15°C ranged from 12 to 45 min with an average of 26 min in the Henry Ford Hospital series.[41] As body temperature is reduced to 15°C, metabolic requirements of the brain are 10% of the normothermic resting state. Experimental studies indicate that there is diffuse loss of neurons after 40 min and that intelligence test quotients diminish after this interval. After successful clipping, meticulous hemostasis must be obtained and the pump restarted and the patient rewarmed. Refibrillation usually occurs spontaneously, but electric shock methods should be available. The correction of clotting defects should start immediately with fresh platelets, ε-aminocaproic acid (EACA), and factor IX. The major complications of the method alone include intracranial bleeding, distal embolization, hepatic and renal deficiency, and deep vein thrombosis and pulmonary embolism. Several authors have reported risks for death or poor operative result with large difficult aneurysms of less than 20%. Stroke rates were also not unreasonable considering the complexity of the lesions treated. The method must be reserved for those lesions that are unclippable by other methods. The surgeon should evaluate potential occlusion times before direct operation to assess need for cardiac arrest. Possible deconstructive procedures and their consequences must be known by occlusion testing methods. If expected, occlusion intervals must extend beyond safe limits due to complexities of the lesion, then hypothermic cardiac arrest should be considered.

Some VBA aneurysms are unclippable by virtue of their contents. Clots that are poorly organized may be removed by suction. Organized clots may require the ultrasonic aspirator. The atheroma may require full dissection from the wall of the aneurysm and parent artery.

Based on the experience of the authors, Table 12.1 indicates the possible choices for various lesions that arise on the vertebrobasilar circulation.

Direct Approaches

Aneurysms of the Vertebral Artery and Posterior Inferior Cerebellar Artery

A paramedian suboccipital approach is preferred for approaching aneurysms in this location. Many positions have been suggested by different surgeons including sitting, park bench, and lateral decubitus, a prone position with the head turned slightly toward the side of the aneurysm, which is preferred. A question mark incision for right vertebral lesions or a reversed question mark incision for left aneurysms is used. This exposes the appropriate suboccipital region and directs the surgeon back to the midline for dissection of the paraspinal muscles and for the removal of the C_1 arch. The craniectomy is begun just medial to the mastoid process and extends into the foramen magnum. The exposure of a large area of the cerebellar hemisphere is not necessary. Likewise, exposing the VA in the arch of C_1 is usually unnecessary. The VA may be visualized just beneath the cerebellar tonsil. Far lateral exposure, however, is important because sometimes the aneurysm projects quite far laterally and the free edge of the cerebellum must be displaced medially. The VA pierces the atlantooccipital

TABLE 12.1. Operative alternatives for surgical management of vertebrobasilar aneurysms

Type of aneurysm	Direct operation	Endovascular operation	Test occlusion	Combined operation
Vertebral artery				
< 5 mm	+	−	−	−
> 5 mm	+	±	−	−
> 10 mm	+	+	+	−
Large or giant	±	+	+	±
Basilar artery and PCA				
< 5 mm	+	−	−	−
> 5 mm	+	±	−	−
> 10 mm	+	+	+	−
Large or giant	±	+	+	±

membrane at the level of C_1. Here the VA may be easily exposed for temporary clipping should it be needed at a later time. Temporary clipping also reduces pressure in the aneurysm during the time of dissection and before clipping.

Opening the cisterna magna may be useful for exposing those aneurysms that arise deep on the distal portions of the VA. Using small brain retractors, the VA is identified beneath the cerebellar tonsil after the dura and arachnoid have been opened. The vessel is followed cranially using a small retractor to displace the cerebellar tonsil upward and medially. In the acute period, it may be necessary to remove clots from the subarachnoid cistern surrounding the VA and the aneurysm. Cranial nerves IX, X, and XI usually lie dorsal to the VA and the PICA branch. The aneurysm usually lies beneath these nerve rootlets and must be dissected free and preserved. The surgeon will dissect between these nerves to find the neck of the aneurysm. To locate the PICA branch and the aneurysm, the VA should be followed cranially with inspection of each segment. Smaller aneurysms present less difficulty in this region than larger giant aneurysms (Fig. 12.12). They can usually be dissected free of the cranial nerves and a clip applied to preserve the parent arteries. Larger and giant aneurysms, on the other hand, often lack a well-differentiated neck, and some are fusiform. If the artery does not contain significant amounts of clot, Sugita fenestrated clips may be used effectively to create an arterial channel from a fusiform dilatation. Sometimes investment with muslin or other fabric is the only choice.

The Subtemporal Approach

The subtemporal approach to BA apex aneurysms was introduced by Drake[39] in 1961. Ordinarily, the operation is carried out on the nondominant hemisphere beneath the nondominant temporal lobe. Therefore, the patient is placed in a left lateral decubitus position with the head slightly flexed laterally toward the left. This allows the surgeon to view the subtentorial space on the right side. However, if the aneurysm projects predominantly toward the left side, if there is a left third nerve paresis, or if there is a right hemiparesis indicating peduncular compression, this aneurysm may be approached from the left subtemporal space. Either a straight or a curved scalp incision is possible. However, if a curvilinear incision is used, the frontalis branch of the seventh nerve must be preserved anteriorly. The curvilinear horseshoe shaped incision over the subtemporal area permits somewhat wider bone resection and exposure of the undersurface of the temporal lobe. The approach described by Pitelli et al.[42] is especially helpful in exposing the cranial base without sacrifice of the seventh cranial nerve. This allows a subtemporal approach in which the muscle does not obstruct the view of the microsurgeon.

Brain relaxation, according to Drake,[39] is the key to this approach. Spinal drainage and dehydrating agents are extremely useful but the anesthetic agent should be chosen for the objective of brain relaxation.

The zygoma interferes with inferior retraction of the temporal muscle. Therefore, it must be divided as far forward on its attachment to the orbital rim as possible and posteriorly, at its attachment to the temporal bone. A Gigli saw or a high-speed air drill may be used. After operation, the zygoma must be reattached with a small wire or heavy nylon suture. This permits the temporal muscle and the zygoma to be displaced inferiorly in order to expose more of the subtemporal area. The dura is opened as low as possible in the temporal area and reflected anteriorly to expose the anterior aspect of the base of the temporal lobe. The temporal lobe must be retracted superiorly and medially in order to expose the incisura of the tentorium. The vein of Labbé crosses the posterior portion of the defect and should be preserved. Damage may result in dysphasia or an aphasia in the dominant hemisphere. The temporal lobe is retracted upward, exposing the incisura of the tentorium. The

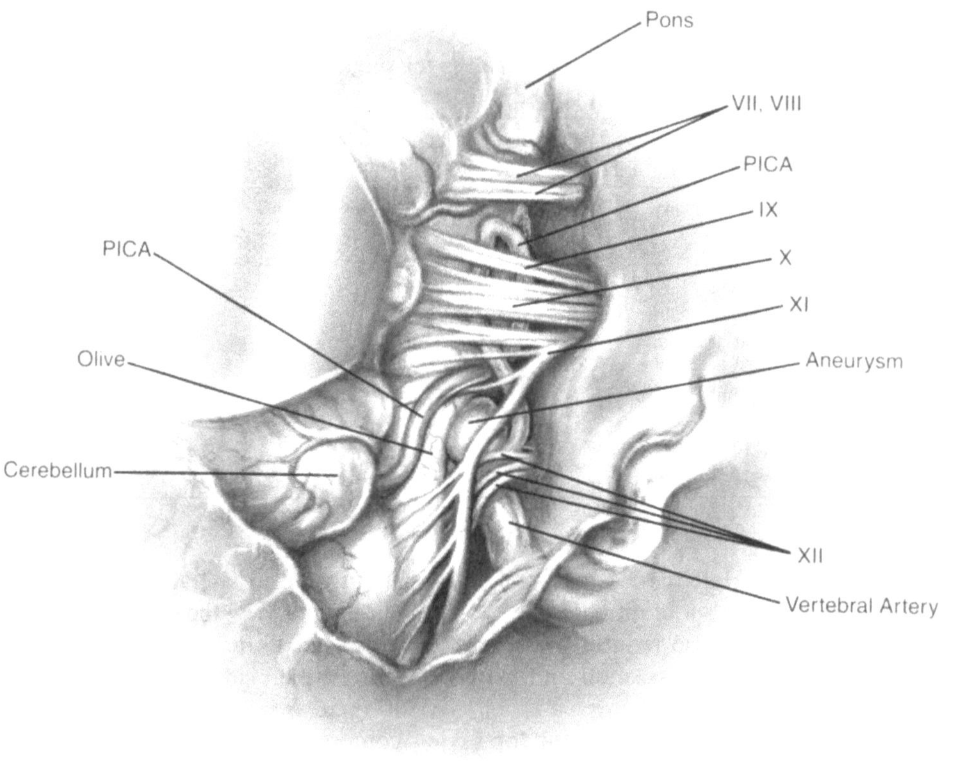

A

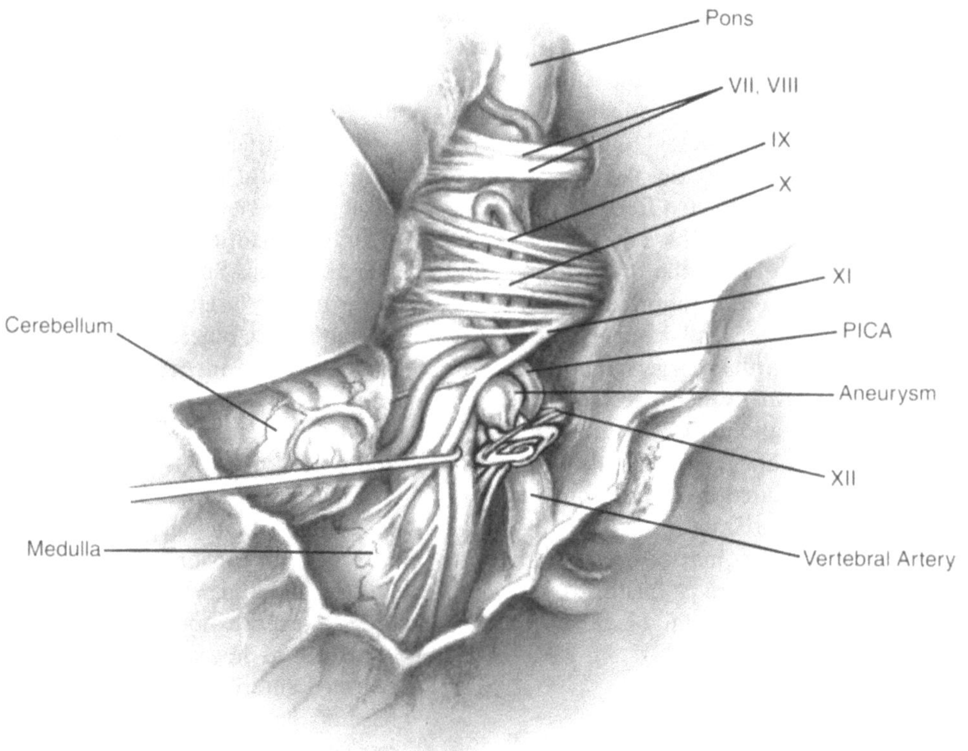

B

FIGURE 12.12. (A) Suboccipital approach for an aneurysm arising from the right vertebral artery at the PICA branch. The figure illustrates the aneurysm in relation to cranial nerves IX, X, and XI. Usually, the aneurysm is covered by the ninth and tenth nerves. (B) The accessory nerve has to be deflated, medially exposing the vertebral artery, and a clip has been applied to the aneurysm.

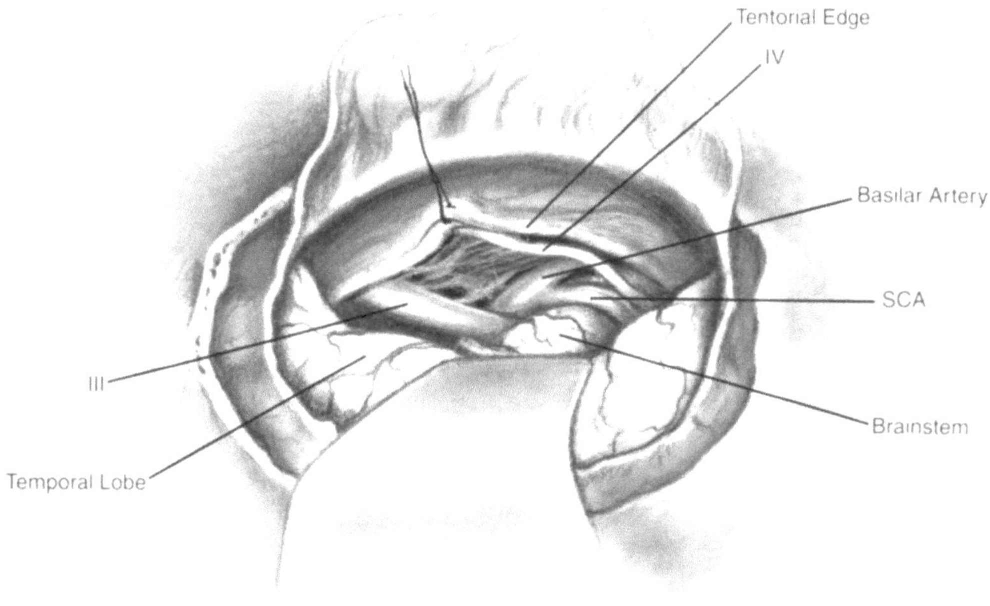

A

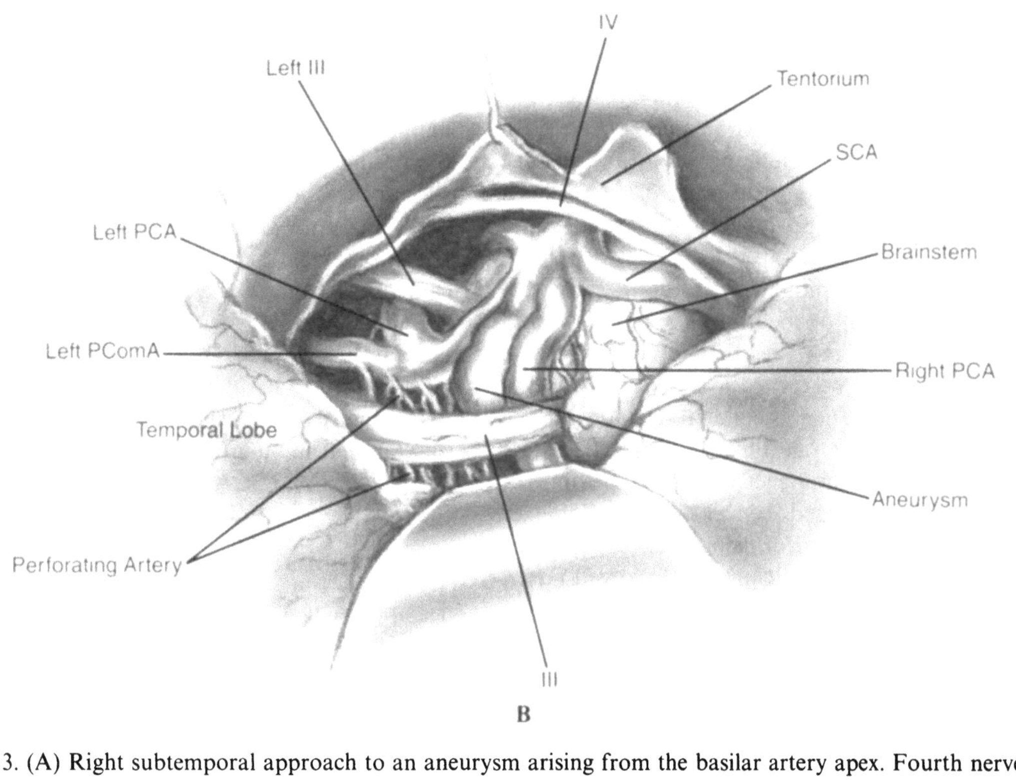

B

FIGURE 12.13. (A) Right subtemporal approach to an aneurysm arising from the basilar artery apex. Fourth nerve entrance into the edge of the tentorium is shown with the tentorium retracted by suture. (B) The posterior cerebral artery visualized and the aneurysm shown between the two posterior cerebral arteries. (C) The posterior cerebral artery has been retracted posteriorly to identify the important perforating vessels before a clip is applied to the basilar artery apex aneurysm.

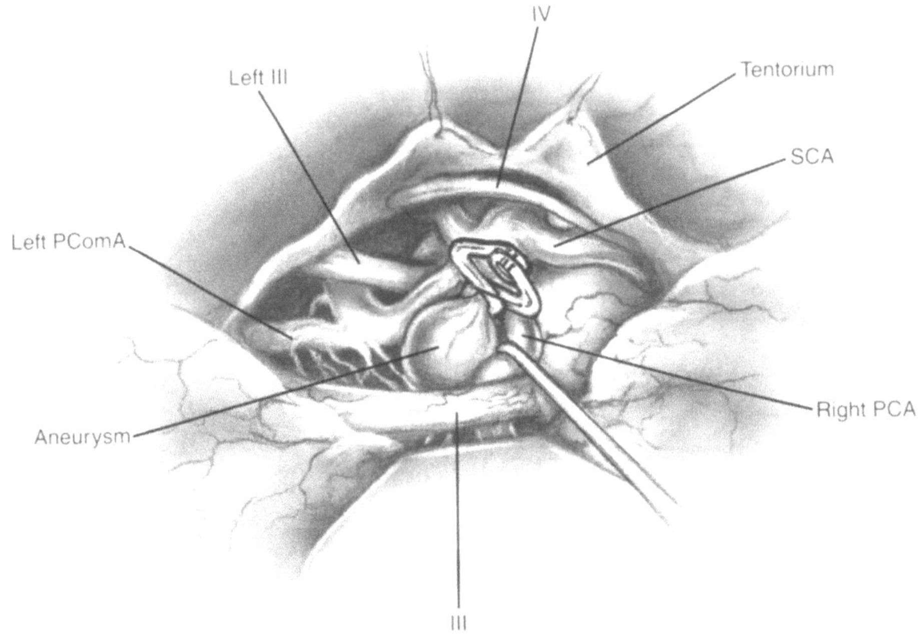

C

fourth cranial nerve also passes into the incisura at this level and must be identified and preserved.

The opening in the incisura must be made posterior to the entry of the fourth cranial nerve into the edge of the tentorial incisura. Stay sutures are placed in both the anterior and posterior portions of the incisura and these are brought out and tied to the dura of the middle cranial fossa. The arachnoidal membrane in the interpeduncular space is then opened and a small cottonoid strip is placed over cranial nerves IV and III to preserve them. The suction must be turned as low as possible to prevent injury should the nerves come in contact with the suction tip. At this point, the PComA is usually identified. The perforating branches that arise from the PComA must be recognized and preserved. Some of these branches enter the anterior diencephalon providing the major blood supply. The PComA is followed posteriorly, gently dissecting along the arachnoidal membrane until the PComA comes into contact with the ipsilateral PCA. This is the junction of P_1 and P_2. Additionally, P_1 may be elevated slightly to expose the opposite P_1, which courses also in the interpeduncular fossa to meet the P_1 on the opposite side. Only by visualizing both P_1s can the neck of the aneurysm be identified in relationship to the short arteries that exit from the basilar apex and from the P_1 segment.

To achieve proximal control, a temporary clip may be placed on the trunk of the BA. The complex relationship of both P_1s to the aneurysm must be appreciated at this time. A special curved clip or fenestrated clip may be needed to preserve the ipsilateral P_1. However, identification of the tips of the blades allows identification of the contralateral P_1 segment and its perforator. The subtemporal approach is limited by an inferior position of the basilar bifurcation in relation to the clivus. In these special cases, it may prove impossible to place a temporary clip on the BA, and, therefore, intraoperative hypotension may be the only alternative that may be used to cause shrinkage of the aneurysm. Aneurysms of the P_1 segment may also be clipped from an ipsilateral subtemporal approach (Fig. 12.13). However, it may be necessary to adjust the flap somewhat in order to achieve more posterior exposure. Figures 12.14 and 12.15 demonstrate the angiographic results of direct clipping of basilar apex and SCA aneurysms.

The Pterional Approach

To approach lesions of the basilar bifurcation and P_1 segment, Yasargil[6] recommended wide dissection in the sylvian fissure, separating the frontal and temporal lobes and coagulation of the many perforating and penetrating veins. Along with this, the cisterns surrounding the ICA and the chiasm must be exposed widely and opened. This approach shows the unique relationship between the optic nerve, the carotid artery, the third cranial nerve, and the edge of tentorium. Thus, there are three possible mechanisms evolved to visualize the basilar bifurcation using a pterional approach. In some circumstances, the space between the optic nerve and the ICA may be used. In addition, the space between the ICA and the third cranial nerve may be employed (Fig. 12.16). If there is

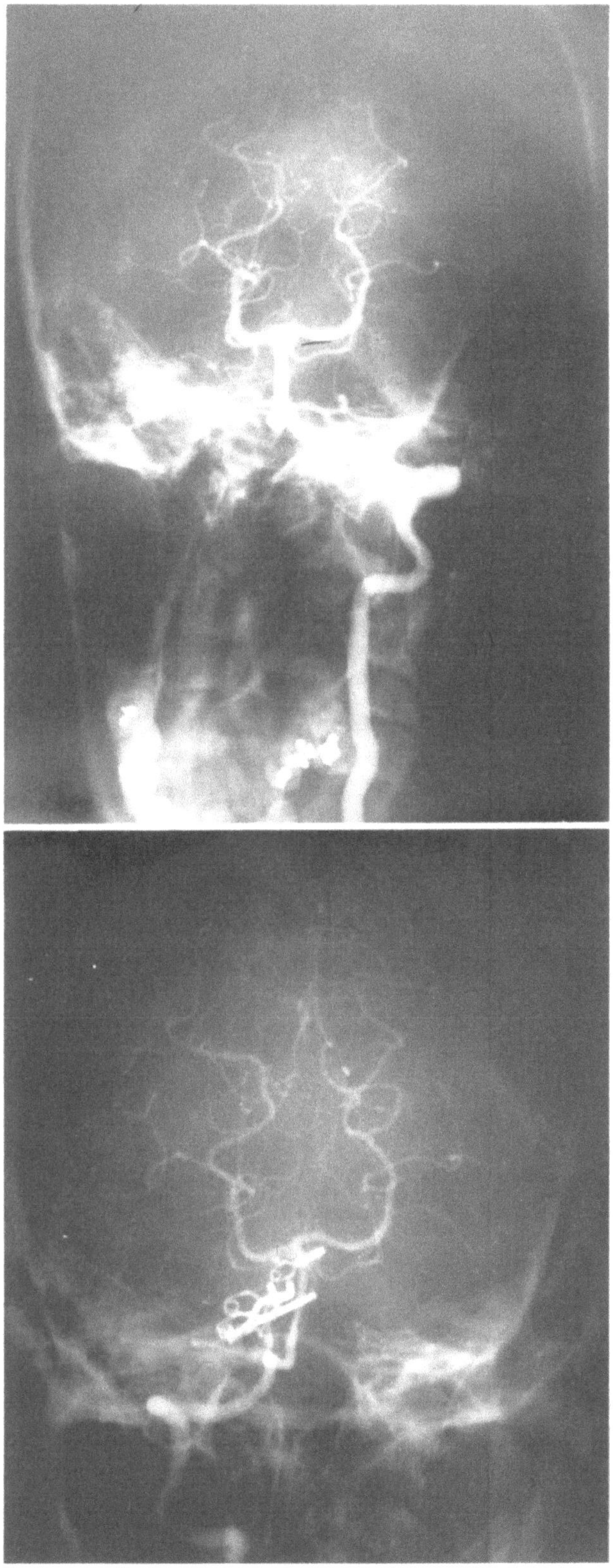

A

B

FIGURE 12.14. (A) Superior cerebral artery aneurysm in a patient with multiple intracranial aneurysms. (B) After clipping the aneurysm of superior cerebellar artery and anterior communicating artery aneurysms.

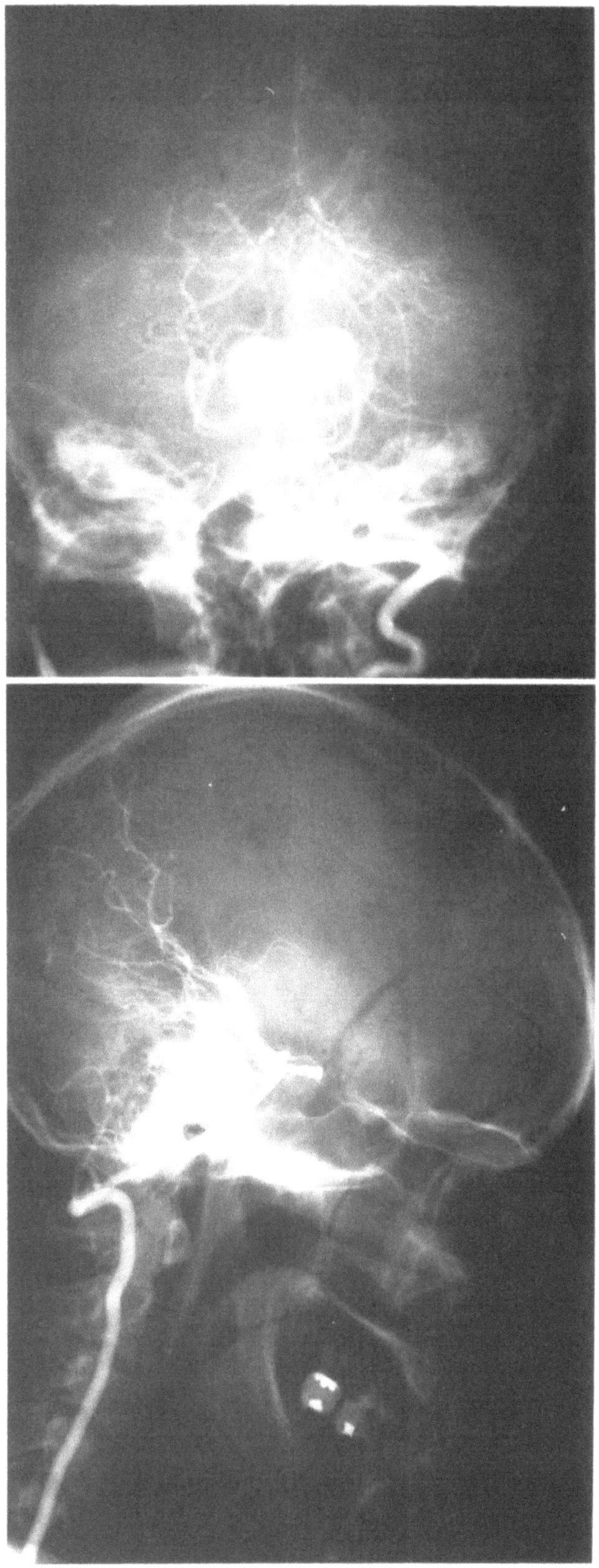

A

B

FIGURE 12.15. (A) Large bilobular aneurysm of the basilar artery apex. (B) After clipping via a pterional approach.

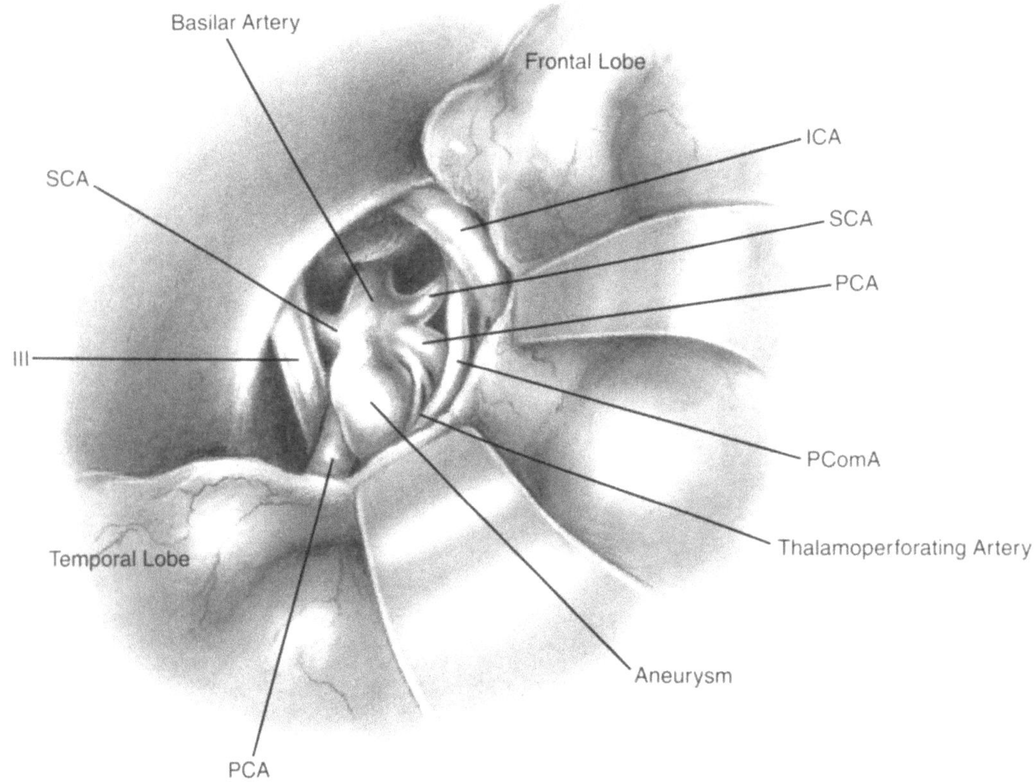

A

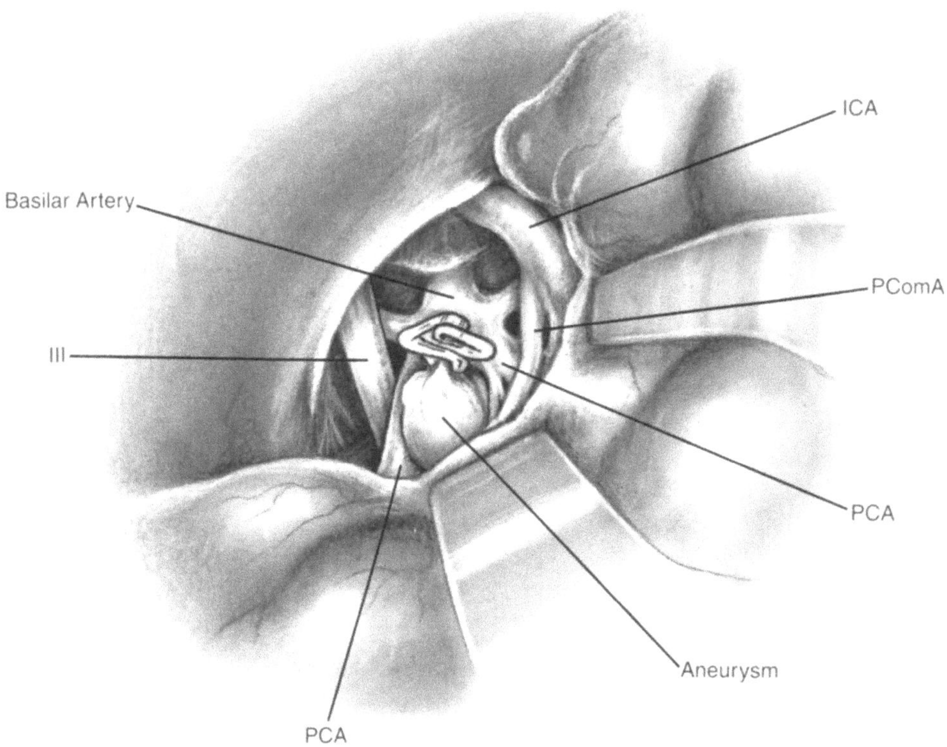

B

FIGURE 12.16. (A and B) This is a left pterional approach to an aneurysm arising from the basilar artery bifurcation. The left approach should be used for aneurysms that are displaced toward the left and are hidden behind the left side of the clivus. This figure shows the relationship of the aneurysm to the important perforating arteries and nerves.

inadequate exposure due to prefixation of the chiasm or a short carotid artery segment due to a low A_1 takeoff, the space between the carotid artery and the tentorium, after division and retraction, may be used to expose aneurysms in this location. Combining both of these spaces to visualize a large aneurysm of the basilar bifurcation may be necessary. This maneuver is especially useful to view adequately the relationship of the aneurysm to the short arteries that arise from the basilar apex and P_1 segments. Yasargil[6] recommended cutting the PComA (P_1), or the A_1 if these branches are hypoplastic. Sugita and Kobayashi[5] emphasized that it is unnecessary to divide these branches. We would add a third caution, that these branches should not be divided, even in the face of an adult-type circulation.

Sugita and Kobayashi[5] suggested an approach that is placed in the sylvian fissure but above the bifurcation of the carotid artery. In these cases, the location of the major perforating and short arteries from the A_1 and M_1 branches must be identified. All authors emphasize the difficulties in displacing the A_1 segment, especially if the approach is made in an elderly patient with arteriosclerosis. The artery may be torn easily from its attachment to the carotid artery. Because of these short penetrating branches with their unique and important area of supply, the approach to lesions in this location must be made with care and trepidation.

The safest approach to an aneurysm of the basilar apex is along the inferior surface of the P_1 branches. Few perforators exit from this side, and following this artery always leads to the BA. The PComA can always be identified because of its position exiting from the ICA. Retraction of the PComA superiorly exposes a few lateral perforating arteries to the uncal area of the temporal lobe. Further retraction discloses the entry point of the PComA through Liliequist's membrane, near to which is a safe area for opening. The PComA is followed to the P_1 branch and then along the medial and anterior surface of the P_1 to the BA. The posterior communicating branch should be retracted superiorly because important penetrating branches to the thalamus course dorsally and medially off this artery.

The arteries that arise near the aneurysm on the P_1 segment from the basilar apex and the occasional perforator that exits the fundus of the aneurysm *must be preserved at all costs*. The aneurysm that projects in a superior–posterior direction is especially treacherous because of perforating branches and because the superior mesencephalic arteries hug the posterior wall. Clipping these vessels will likely result in infarctions in the midbrain, and permanent coma may result. Aneurysms containing thrombus or atheroma are also difficult to manage using a direct clipping procedure. Clips placed upon these aneurysms tend to migrate either toward the fundus or toward the parent artery. Migration toward the fundus may expose weak portions of the aneurysm to later growth and rupture. Those that migrate toward the P_1 segments may occlude important short penetrating arteries.

Aneurysms that arise 1 cm or more below the level of the posterior clinoid process and those that hug the clivus may be difficult to visualize using a pterional approach. If the aneurysm projects toward one side or the other, the posterior clinoid process and part of the clivus may be drilled away in order to expose aneurysms that arise from these locations. If the aneurysm arises low, however, a pterional approach may not provide the exposure required to clip aneurysms in this location, especially if the perforating vessels are to be preserved.

The Anterior Subtemporal Approach

In this approach, the incision, either straight or curvilinear, is made in the anterior portion of the temporal fossa. The temporalis muscle is divided low, the zygoma sectioned and displaced inferiorly. This exposes the cranial base anteriorly, and the temporal lobe is elevated from the floor. Veins entering the sphenoparietal sinus must be coagulated and divided in order to elevate the temporal lobe from the floor of the middle fossa completely. This exposes the incisura of the tentorium and the third nerve entry into the cavernous sinus. The tentorium is divided at this point to allow visualization of the membrane of Liliequist beneath the third cranial nerve and between the carotid artery and third cranial nerve. The incisura is divided proximal to the entry of the fourth nerve, permitting the membrane of Liliequist to be opened. This exposes the BA bifurcation from an anterior subtemporal approach. The leaves of the incisura are retracted laterally. If the aneurysm arises high, i.e., greatly above the clinoid, its exposure may prove impossible from this approach. Also the fourth nerve prevents good visualization.

The Transtentorial Approach to the Basilar Trunk

BA trunk aneurysms may be approached by several different but equally effective means. If the aneurysm arises from the upper trunk, inferior to the SCA takeoff, a transtentorial incision may be elected. A standard subtemporal incision is made and the temporal lobe elevated and held in position by retractors. The temporal lobe is elevated until the veins of the temporal lobe are identified. The vein of Labbé should be identified and preserved.

The free edge of the tentorium is then isolated from the brain stem with nerve hooks and dissectors and followed anteriorly. The arachnoidal covering of the fourth nerve and the PCA should be preserved and suction should be reduced to prevent injury of the nerve.

At the petrous ridge, the tentorium is incised and the incision carried laterally to the cranial bone edge, being careful to preserve the subtentorial structures. The tentorium is incised along the cranial surface as far as possible; the triangular piece made up by the petrous portion, the free edge, and the base is attached. A suture is placed into the apex of the triangle and retracted to allow entry into the subtentorial compartment.

After the arachnoid has been opened, the greater petrosal vein and several smaller veins enter the petrosal sinus in the lateral position under cover of the fifth cranial nerve. The seventh and eighth nerves enter the petrous pyramid in a more perpendicular direction.

The SCA is often associated with the trochlear nerve as it passes around the cerebral peduncle. This vessel continues along the superior surface of the cerebellum but it usually bifurcates at the midbrain level and may touch the free edge of the tentorium. The basal vein and trochlear nerve are normally found superior to the arteries. In circling the midbrain, the SCA or one of its trunks may actually press against the trigeminal nerve. Following the vessels to their origination is a useful maneuver for locating the BA and the aneurysm, when they are not readily apparent. However, the SCA leads to a more anterior position that is uncomfortably achieved via a transtentorial approach.

A space between nerves V and VII allows a 5- to 6-mm brain retractor. The AICA is usually seen leaving the inferior, or sometimes middle, basilar artery trunk. The artery normally passes ventral to the abducent nerve but may pass over it. The artery makes an inferior loop in the cistern and often comes into contact with the inferior surface of the facial and vestibuloacoustic nerves. It usually has two or more trunks at this level and gives off several branches to the pons. The meatal loop may enter the canal and the IAA usually originates from this loop. The sixth cranial nerve runs along the clivus in a position usually lateral to the BA. A small retractor is used to gently elevate the pons until the BA comes into view. The artery may be tortuous to either side, however, and the approach should be taken to present the aneurysm most superficially. Usually, the dome of the aneurysm will be encountered first. The retractor must be used to compress the fundus, allowing the neck and origin from the BA to come into view. After isolation of the neck, the aneurysm may be seen in relation to the SCA above and the AICA below. During the retraction, the nerve is held elevated by the retractor.

For aneurysms that arise from the BA near the AICA, the dissection must begin more posteriorly. The tentorial incision may be extended further along the cranial base permitting entry between the seventh and eighth nerves superiorly and the ninth and tenth nerves inferiorly to expose the BA and the aneurysm. The AICA branch must be clear from aneurysm clips if hearing is to be preserved.

Combined Approaches

As the title suggests, both supratentorial and infratentorial approaches may be combined. The infratemporal posterior fossa approach is especially useful for large aneurysms occupying the BA trunk or for those arising from the vertebrobasilar junction. This approach provides wide exposure in which the perforating vessels from the basilar trunk can be seen and intercepted early (Fig. 12.17). The combined approach begins with a question mark incision beginning at the zygoma, and circling around the ear and descending 1 cm behind the mastoid process. Four burr holes are first made, two on each side of the transverse sinus. The burr holes flanking the lateral sinuses are connected using a rongeur; the others are connected using a high speed air drill (Fig. 12.18). The bone may adhere to the dura mater along the

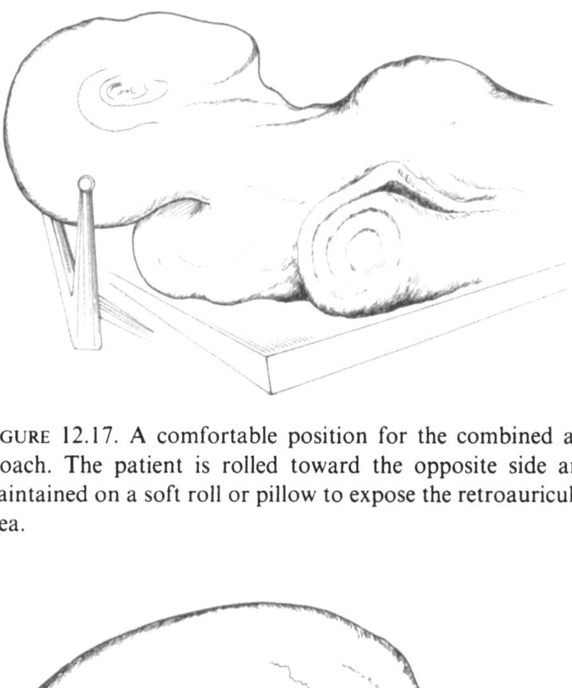

FIGURE 12.17. A comfortable position for the combined approach. The patient is rolled toward the opposite side and maintained on a soft roll or pillow to expose the retroauricular area.

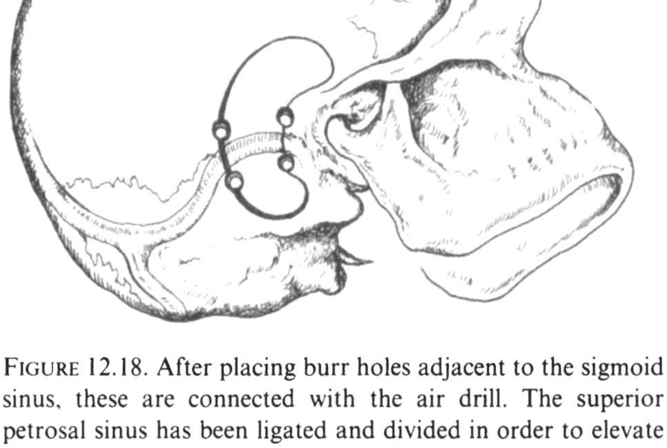

FIGURE 12.18. After placing burr holes adjacent to the sigmoid sinus, these are connected with the air drill. The superior petrosal sinus has been ligated and divided in order to elevate the brain stem. The lateral sinus has been preserved.

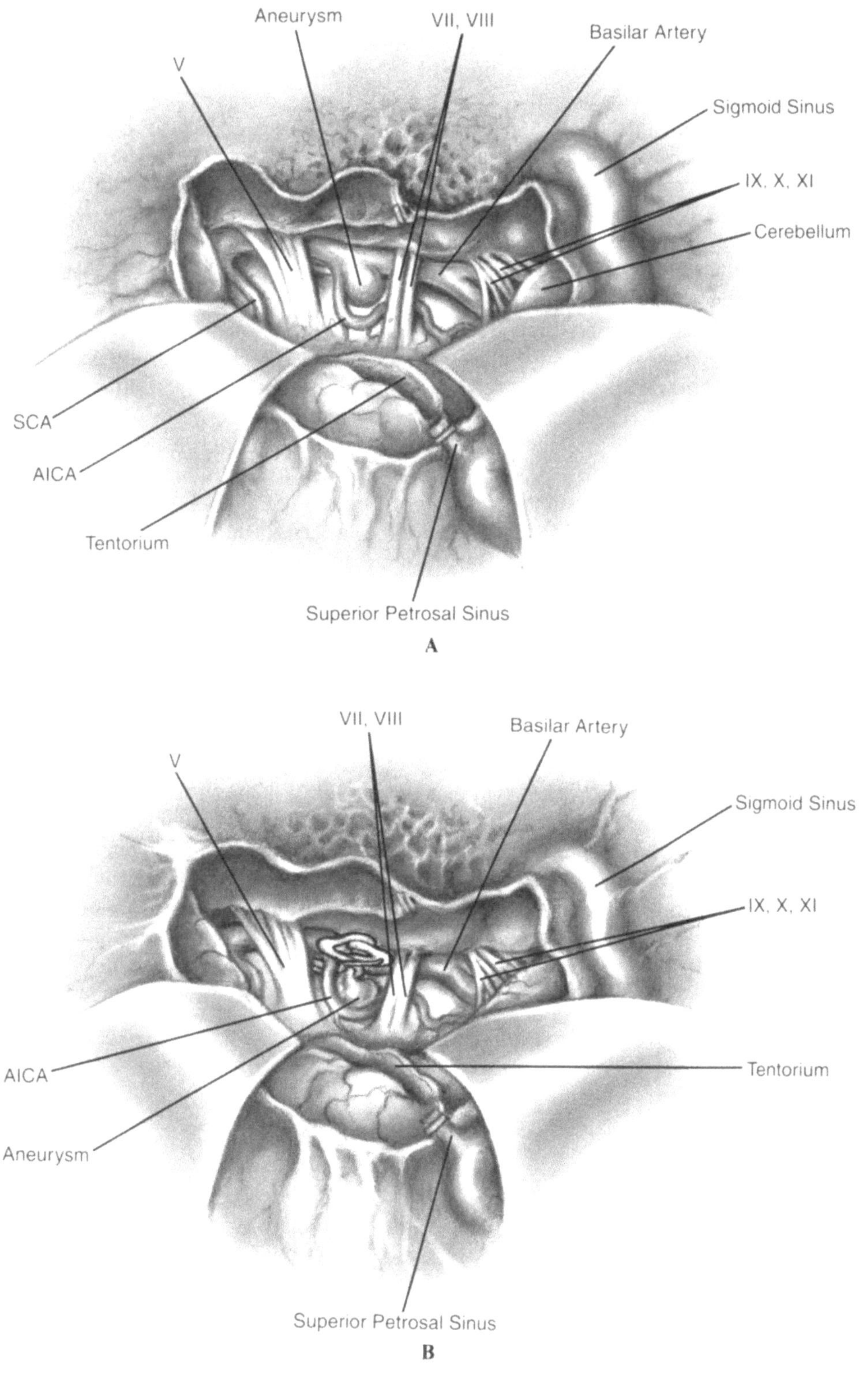

FIGURE 12.19. (A and B) Right lateral combined approach demonstrating the basilar artery and its relation to cranial nerves V, VI, VII, VIII, IX, X and XI. The aneurysm projects posterolaterally from the bifurcation of AICA and the basilar artery. The AICA has been retracted to permit application of a clip to the aneurysm. The clip blades should be applied parallel to the basilar artery when possible.

sinuses, and this must be dissected carefully. A mastoidectomy may also be performed using the high-speed air drill, but, unless the aneurysm extends far into the cerebellopontine angle, this drilling is usually unnecessary. If the lesion extends into the supratentorial compartment, the dura mater is opened along both sides of the sigmoid sinus. The supratentorial incision extends toward the temporal fossa. The vein of Labbé should be preserved if possible by dissection from the cortical surface allowing retraction of the temporal lobe without tension on the venous wall. The tentorium should be incised with care being taken to preserve the trochlear nerve. The trigeminal nerve rootlets usually mark the anterior extent of the dissection (Fig. 12.19).

Endovascular Approaches

The first endovascular operations for lesions of the BA were carried out by Serbinenko[43] in 1971. These early operations yielded only partial occlusion of the aneurysm with detachable latex balloons. In 1982, Romodanov and Shcheglov[44] published their results of 100 aneurysms, but only one of these was in the vertebrobasilar circulation at the PICA junction. In this case, the endovascular procedure was deconstructive, excluding the VA from the circulation. In 1984, Berenstein et al.[45] published two cases in which the VA and PICAs were approached using endovascular methods. In these cases, the aneurysm was excluded from the intracranial circulation with good results. In other cases, where the proximal VA was occluded with a balloon, late rebleeding and death occurred. In 1985, Zeumer et al.[46] described two cases managed with endovascular methods, the first of which involved the VA, and the second the trunk of the BA. In one case, in which a giant aneurysm involved the trunk of the BA, both VAs were occluded sequentially with balloons, one month apart. Using an axillary approach, these authors placed a latex balloon in a large basilar bifurcation aneurysm. The catheter and balloon were left in place with the balloon inflated over a 3-week period before removing it. Postoperatively, there was no change in the aneurysm size.

Hieshima et al.[47] and Higashida et al.[48] described the endovascular results achieved in the treatment of 25 patients with aneurysms of the BA. In 11 of these, the aneurysm was successfully occluded, thus preserving the parent artery. In nine, however, the parent artery was occluded in the occlusive process. In three, the results were excellent and/or good. In six, the results were poor. Further observation of this entire group of patients from a period of 2 to 43 months, however, was disappointing. Ten died during this interval—five from ruptured aneurysm and five from unrelated conditions. Fox[4] described results in seven cases with vertebrobasilar artery aneurysms. One of these involved the trunk of the VA, and one was a distal VA aneurysm. Only one patient developed ischemic complications after occlusion of the VA. In four patients, the aneurysm was completely obliterated after occlusion of the VA.

In 1991, Moret and co-workers[49] reported their results with 128 aneurysms at the Interventional Congress in Zurich. Thirty-nine involved the vertebrobasilar system. Thirty-one occurred on the BA, three on the PCA, five at the PICA junction, and three on the VA. Nineteen complications occurred in these 128 patients. In nine of these, death occurred and the remaining 10 suffered

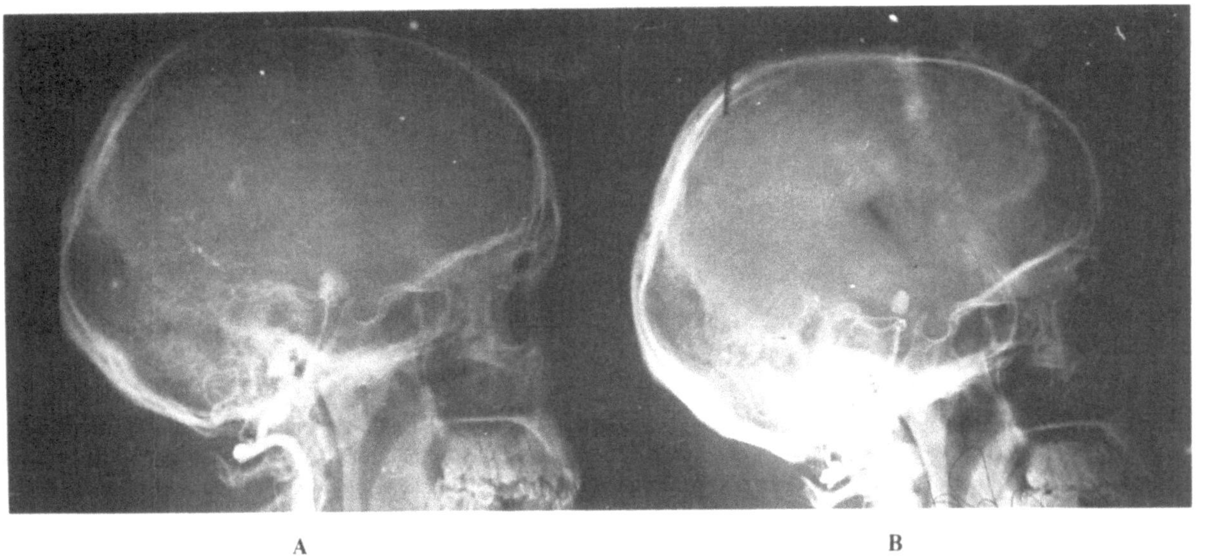

A B

FIGURE 12.20. (A and B) Basilar apex aneurysm before and 1 year after balloon occlusion with a latex balloon. The balloon has separated slightly due to shrinkage.

major neurological deficit. Eight of the nine deaths occurred in patients with aneurysms on the vertebrobasilar circulation. Three of these resulted from brain stem ischemia and five from rupture. At this conference, five reports appeared in which coils or other methods had been used to obliterate aneurysms of the vertebrobasilar system. Whether using coils or detachable balloons, each endovascular surgeon emphasizes the positive role of test occlusion. The concept of total occlusion of an aneurysm at its orifice using endovascular methods has not been addressed. Often, there is partial occlusion, separating the fundus from the major intracranial circulation with preservation of significant amounts of filling around the orifice Fox et al.[51] Partial occlusion, is often associated with late rebleeding from the dome.

Technique

Both transaxillary and transfemoral approaches have been used to gain access to the posterior cranial circulation. The transaxillary approach places the surgeon at a shorter distance from the lesion and therefore makes manipulation much easier in the vertebrobasilar circulation. Full four-vessel angiography is necessary for adequate decision-making about whether a balloon, clip, or coil is the most appropriate method to treat the lesion. The collateral circulation to the aneurysm, its location and takeoff position, and any perforating or short branches that surround the aneurysm must be identified. The approach depends upon the location of an aneurysm in relation to the VA. Aneurysms arising from the left VA must be approached from the left axillary artery. Conversely, those arising on the right VA should be approached from the right side. To pass a balloon catheter retrograde down a VA from the opposite one is a difficult task.

When the aneurysm arises at the vertebrobasilar junction or the BA per se, the nondominant VA that has the fewest curves and serpentine movements throughout its course should be selected. Preocclusion testing is important in making a decision about whether deconstructive or reconstructive procedures will be carried out. If the parent artery is to be sacrificed, the functional significance of this vessel must be determined using preliminary balloon occlusion for a 30-min test interval prior to its final detachment. Even if the balloon is to be placed into the aneurysm sac, a preliminary test period of 30 min should be carried out to ensure that any small perforating branches that may reside near the aneurysm fundus will not be compromised by the balloon. If the patient's condition does not change during the test interval of 30 min, permanent occlusion with the detachable balloon is possible. Again, with small aneurysms, a hardening material is preferred to fill the aneurysm prior to deflation. However, for large and giant aneurysms, a liquid

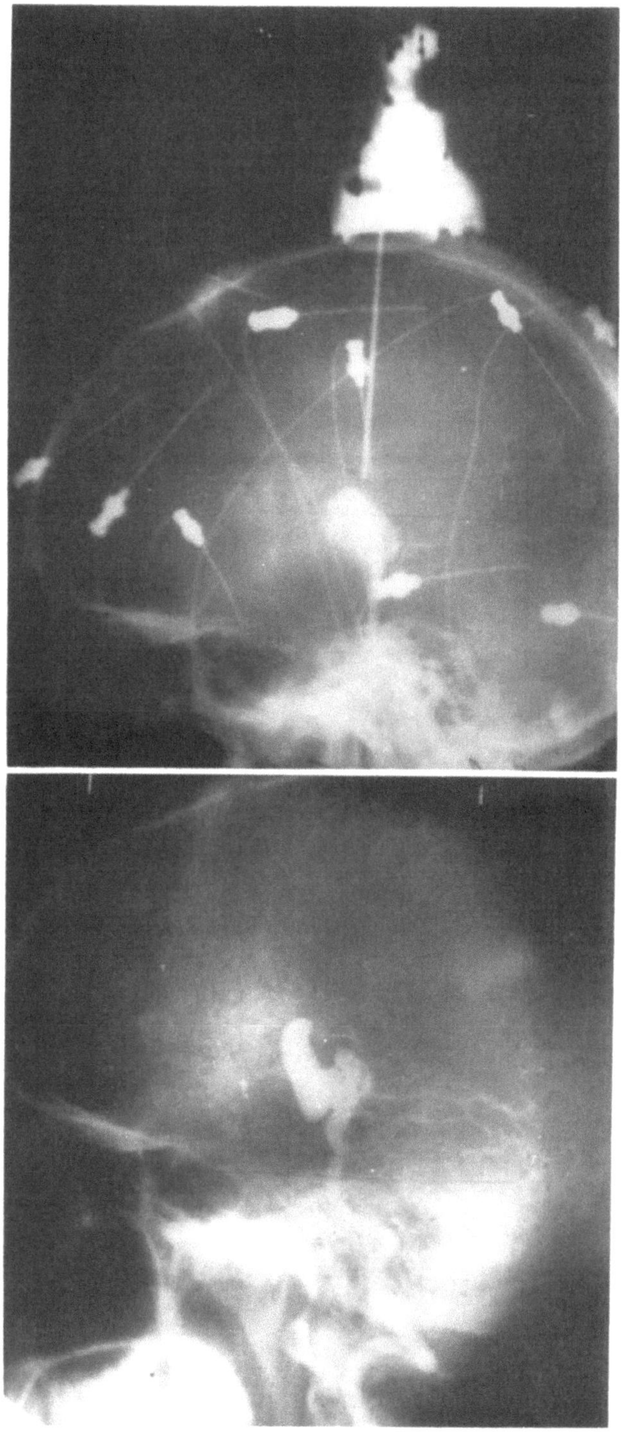

A

B

FIGURE 12.21. (A) Stereotaxic occlusion of a basilar artery apex aneurysm. The trocar has been introduced stereotaxically, indenting the dome of the aneurysm. (B) Two balloons have been introduced into the aneurysm, excluding it from the circulation.

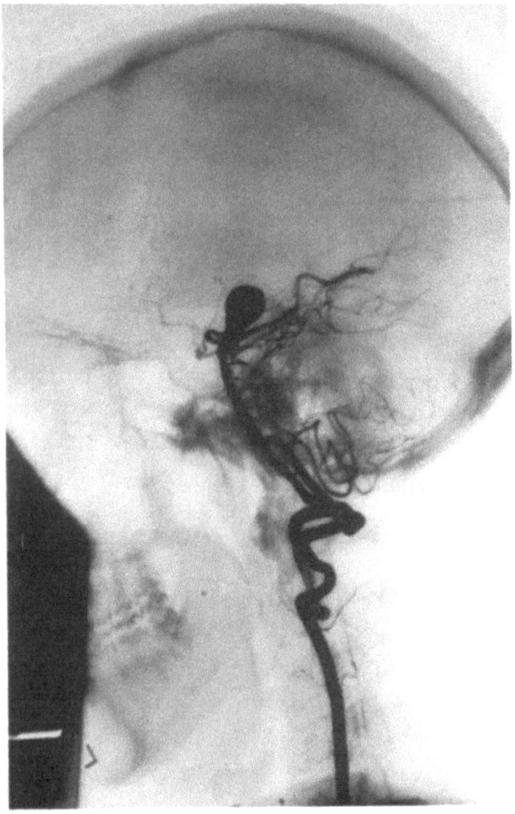

A

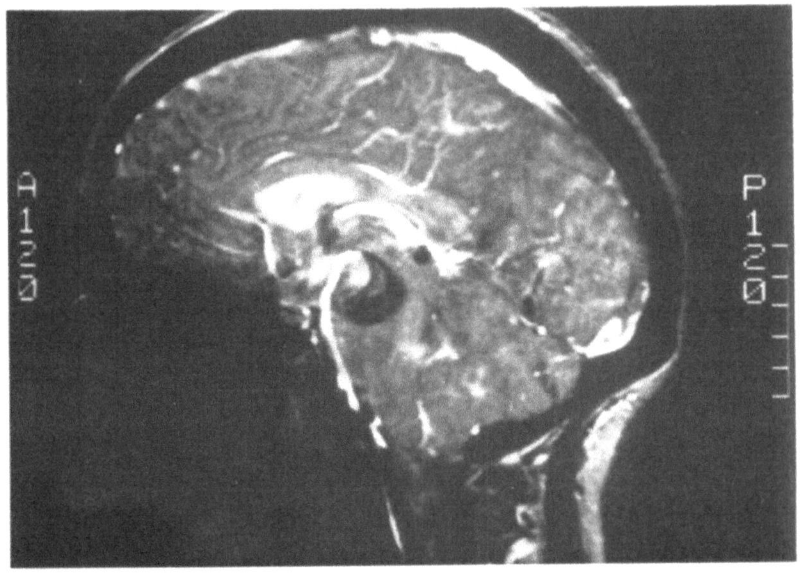

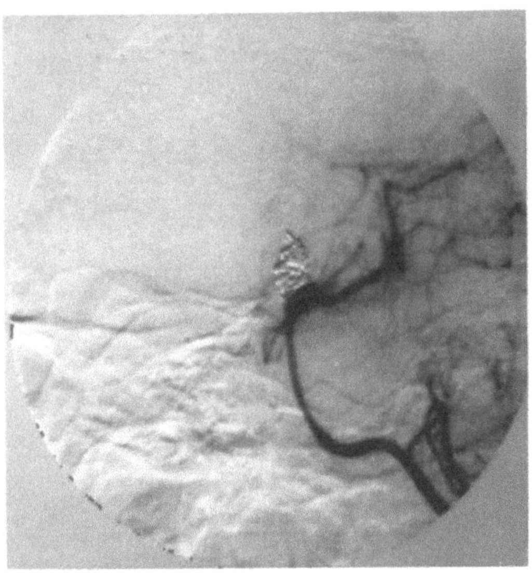

C

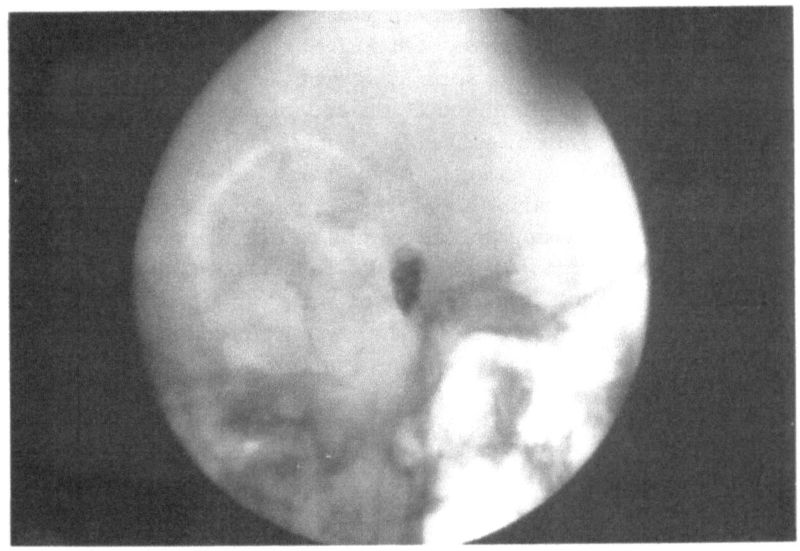

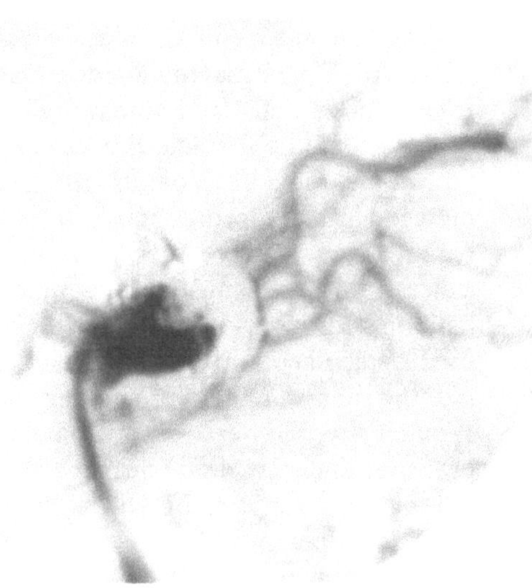

FIGURE 12.22. (A) Giant basilar apex aneurysm that contains atheroma and thrombus, and was unclippable because of migration of the clips. (B) Magnetic resonance imaging (MRI) showing basilar apex aneurysm with thrombus. (C) The dome of the aneurysm has been filled with platinum coils. The neck is still visible. (D) The platinum coils are impacted within the aneurysm. (E) One year later, the coils have been displaced into dome of the aneurysm and there has been growth from the neck.

inflating material is preferred because this will allow shrinkage of the aneurysm over time.

In patients with large and giant aneurysms, the decision must be made as to whether to place multiple balloons within the aneurysm sac in order to achieve complete obliteration. In these cases, it is preferable to place two, three, or more balloons within the aneurysm, adjust their volume and position under radiographic and clinical control, and then detach them together if occlusion seems favorable. Deconstructive operations, in which the parent artery is occluded, is not always possible, especially with aneurysms along the basilar trunk.

A

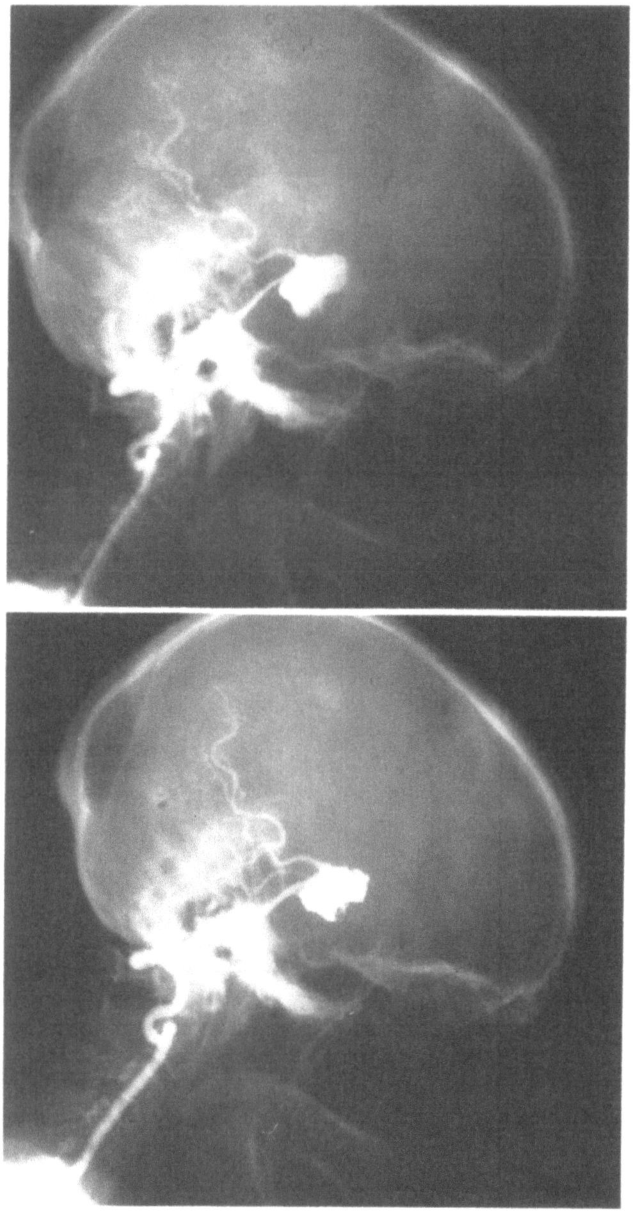

B

FIGURE 12.23. (A) Giant aneurysm of the basilar trunk. (B) This aneurysm was occluded using platinum coils.

Here, many short arteries penetrate the paramedian areas of the pons and midbrain to supply vital reticular and nuclear areas. In these cases, symptoms may appear upon inflation, and thus the balloon must be deflated and the operation aborted. Fox and Drake[50] emphasized the complications that may arise during temporary occlusion testing in this group of patients in whom short arteries must be compromised if a balloon is to be detached permanently in the BA.

Postoperatively, maintaining vascular homeostasis is essential. Blood pressure, viscosity, and coagulation must be monitored and controlled effectively. Figures 12.20 through 12.23 demonstrate the results of occlusion of large and giant aneurysms of the vertebrobasilar system using both coils and detachable balloons.

Conclusions

Vertebrobasilar artery aneurysms are regarded as the most difficult class for direct operative clipping. Many are giant; most lie adjacent to vital structures. Perforating arteries, thread-like on gross inspection, carry blood to small, but important areas of the brain. Infarction in their territories may lead to death or severe disablement. Likewise, endovascular methods are not simple. An axillary entry may be needed and because of the tortuosity of this system, manipulation of catheter and balloon may be tedious. Coils and other material may be placed into these lesions, but long-term effects using these methods have not been assessed. Even a remnant of neck can lead to recurrence and bleeding. Direct clipping is still the method of choice when it can be delivered with reasonable risk. The surgeon must be experienced in many methods, however, in order to provide the best treatment, at the best time, to the patient most appropriate for it.

References

1. Stehbens WE. The pathology of intracranial arterial aneurysms and their complications. In: Fox JL, ed. *Intracranial Aneurysms*. New York: Springer-Verlag; 1983;I:272–357.
2. Sahs AL, Perret GI, Lockley HB, Nishioka H. *Intracranial Aneurysms and Subarachnoid Hemorrhage: A Cooperative Study*. Philadelphia PA: JB Lippincott; 1969.
3. Drake CG. Basilar artery bifurcation aneurysms. In: Apuzzo MJL, ed. *Brain Surgery: Complication Avoidance and Management*. New York, Edinburgh, London, Melbourne, Tokyo: Churchill Livingstone; 1993;I.
4. Fox JL. *Intracranial Aneurysms*, vols. I and II. New York: Springer-Verlag; 1983.
5. Sugita K, Kobayashi S. *Microneurosurgical Atlas*. Berlin: Springer-Verlag, 1985.
6. Yasargil MG. *Microsurgical Anatomy of the Basal Cisterns and Vessels of the Brain, Diagnostic Studies, General Opera-*

tive Techniques and Pathological Considerations of the Intracranial Aneurysms. Microneurosurgery. Stuttgart and New York: Georg Thieme Verlag; 1984:I.
7. Duvernoy MH. *Human Brainstem Vessels.* New York: Springer-Verlag; 1978.
8. Grand W, Hopkins LN. The microsurgical anatomy of the basilar artery bifurcation. *Neurosurgery.* 1977;1:128–131.
9. Hardy DG, Rhoton AL. Microsurgical anatomy of superior cerebellar artery. *Neurosurgery.* 1980;6:10–28.
10. Lister JR, Rhoton AL, Matsushima T, Peace A. Microsurgical anatomy of the posterior inferior cerebellar artery. *Neurosurgery.* 1982;10:170–199.
11. Marinkovic S, Milisavljevic M, Kovacevic M. Interpeduncular perforating branches of the posterior cerebral artery. Microsurgical anatomy of their extracerebral and intracerebral segments. *Surg Neurol.* 1986;26:349–359.
12. Saeki N, Rhoton AL. Microsurgical anatomy of the upper basilar artery and the posterior circle of Willis. *J Neurosurg.* 1977;46:563–578.
13. Padget DH. The development of the cranial arteries in the human embryo. *Contrib Embryol.* 1948;32: 205–261.
14. Fisher CM. The circle of Willis: anatomical variations. *Vasc Dis.* 1965;2:99–195.
15. Stopford JSB. The arteries of the pons and medulla oblongata. Part I. *J Anat Physiol.* 1916;50:131–163.
16. Von Mitterwallner F. Variationstatistische unter Suchungen an den basalen Hirngefassen. *Acta Anat.* 1955;24:51–88.
17. Morris ED, Moffat DB. Abnormal origin of the basilar artery from the cervical part of the internal carotid artery and its embryological significance. *Anat Rec* 1956;125:701–711.
18. Nakajima K, Ito Z, Hen R, Vemurd K, Matsuoka S. Congenital anomalies of cerebral artery and intracranial aneurysms. *No To Shinkei.* 1976;28:197–201.
19. Carpenter MB. *Context of Neuroanatomy.* Baltimore, MD: Williams & Wilkins; 1991:438–461.
20. Margolis MT, Newton TH. The posterior inferior cerebellar artery. Gross and roentgenographic anatomy. In: Newton TH, Potts DG, eds. *Radiology of the Skull and Brain, Angiography.* St. Louis: C.V. Mosby; 1974:Vol. II(Book 2).
21. Salamon G, Huang YP. *Radiologic Anatomy of the Brain.* Berlin: Springer-Verlag; 1976:303–331.
22. Fuji K, Lenkey C, Rhoton AL. Microsurgical anatomy of the choroidal arteries: lateral and third ventricles. *J Neurosurg.* 1980;52:505–524.
23. Westberg G. Arteries of the basal ganglia. *Acta Radiol Diagn (Stockh).* 1966;5:581–596.
24. Krayenbuhl H, Yasargil MG. Radiological anatomy and topography of the cerebral vessels. In: *Cerebral Angiography,* 2nd ed. Philadelphia, PA: JB Lippincott; 1968.
25. Binet EF, Young RF. Bilateral persistent trigeminal arteries. *J Neurosurgery.* 1977;47:619–622.
26. Stephens RB, Stilwell DL. *Arteries and Veins of the Human Brain.* Springfield, IL: Charles C. Thomas; 1969.
27. Weir L. *Aneurysms Affecting the Nervous System.* Baltimore: Williams and Wilkins; 1987:308–344.
28. Martin RG, Grant JL, Peace D, Theiss C, Rhoton AL. Microsurgical relationship of the anterior inferior cerebellar artery and the facial-vestibulocochlear nerve complex. *Neurosurgery.* 1980;6:483–507.
29. Sunderland S. The arterial relations of the internal auditory meatus. *Brain.* 1945;68:23–27.
30. Fisch U. The surgical anatomy of the so-called internal auditory artery. In: *Proceedings of the Tenth Nobel Symposium on Disorders of the Skull Base Region.* Stockholm: Almqvist and Wiksell; 1968.
31. Mani RL, Newton TH, Glockman MG. The superior cerebellar artery: an anatomic roentgenographic correlation. *Radiology.* 1968;91:1102–1108.
32. Hardy DG, Rhoton AL. Microsurgical relationship of the superior cerebellar artery and the trigeminal nerve. *J Neurosurg.* 1978;49:669–678.
33. Zeal AA, Rhoton AL. Microsurgical anatomy of the posterior cerebral artery. *J Neurosurg,* 1978;48:538–559.
34. Percheron G. The anatomy of the arterial supply of the human thalamus and its use for the interpretation of the thalamic vascular pathology. *Z Neurol.* 1973;205:1–13.
35. Peele TL. *The Neuroanatomical Basis for Clinical Neurology.* 2nd ed. New York: McGraw-Hill, 1976.
36. Hook O, Norlen G, Guzman J. Saccular aneurysms of the vertebral–basilar arterial system: a report of 28 cases. *Acta Neurol Scand.* 1963;39:271–304.
37. Stehbens WE. *Pathology of the Cerebral Blood Vessels.* St. Louis: Mosby; 1972.
38. Peerless SJ, Drake CG. Posterior circulation aneurysms. In: Wilkins R, Rengachary S, eds. *Neurosurgery.* New York: McGraw-Hill, 1985,II:1422–1437.
39. Drake CG. Bleeding aneurysms of the basilar artery: direct surgical management in four cases. *J Neurosurg.* 1961;18: 230–238.
40. Drake CG. The treatment of aneurysms of the posterior circulation. *Clin Neurosurg.* 1979;26:96–144.
41. Thompson J, Chung RS. Giant cerebral aneurysm repair. Incorporating cardiopulmonary bypass and neurosurgery. *AORN J.* 1991;54:224–227, 230–233, 236–241.
42. Pitelli SD, Almeida GGM, Makagawa EJ, Marchese AJT, Cabral WD. Basilar aneurysm surgery: the subtemporal approach with section of the zygomatic arch. *Neurosurgery* 1986;18:125–128.
43. Serbinenko FA. Catheterization and occlusion of magistral brain vessels. *Proceedings of the First Congress of Neurosurgeons of USSR.* Moscow. 1971;1:121–123.
44. Romodanov AP, Shcheglov VI: Intravascular occlusion of saccular aneurysms of the cerebral arteries by means of a detachable balloon catheter. In: Krayenbuhl H, ed. *Advances and Technical Standards in Neurosurgery.* New York: Springer-Verlag; 1982:25–49.
45. Berenstein A, Ransohoff J, Kupersmith M, Flamm E, Graeb D. Transvascular treatment of giant aneurysms of the cavernous carotid and vertebral arteries. *Surg Neurol.* 1984;21:3–12.
46. Zeumer H, Bruckman H, Adelt D, Hacke AW, Ringelstein EB. Balloon embolization in the treatment of basilar aneurysms. *Acta Neurochirurg.* 1985;78:136–141.
47. Hieshima GB, Higashida RT, Wapenski J, Halbach VV, Cahan L, Bentson JR. Balloon embolization of a large distal basilar artery aneurysm. *J Neurosurg.* 1986;65:413–316.

48. Higashida RT, Halbach VV, Cahan LD, Hieshima GB, Konishi Y. Detachable balloon embolization therapy of posterior circulation intracranial aneurysms. *J Neurosurg*. 1989;71:512–519.
49. Moret J, Boulin A, Mawad M, Castaigne L. Endovascular treatment of berry aneurysms by endovascular balloon occlusion. *Neuroradiology* 1991;33(suppl):S135.
50. Fox AJ, Drake CG. Detachable balloon embolization for intracranial aneurysms. Letter-to-editor. *J Neurosurg*. 1990;73:157–158.
51. Fox AJ, Viuela F, Pelz DM, Peerless SJ, Ferguson GG, Drake CG, Debrun G. Use of detachable balloons for proximal artery occlusion in the treatment of unclippable cerebral aneurysms. *J Neurosurg*. 1987;66:40–46.

13
Results and Complications

Results

Many factors influence results after acute aneurysmal subarachnoid hemorrhage (SAH). The configuration, size, and location of the aneurysm as well as its relationship to intracranial structures are important. The clinicoanatomic form of the hemorrhage and the presence of vasospasm, hydrocephalus, intracranial hypertension, and rebleeding affect the outcome. The age of the patient, the associated systemic pathology, hypertension, heart disease, and other conditions associated with the ictal event (e.g., heart failure) are all significant. Neurological condition is a significant variable but yet an integral part of all other factors.

Decisions made by the surgeon also affect survival. The timing of operation, the choice of the operative approach, complications related to and accompanying any surgical treatment, and the tactics of the surgeon can all be modified to improve the outcome.

The Aneurysm

A significant difference in outcome is dependent on the size and configuration of the lesion being treated. Results associated with small aneurysms are much lower than those that accompany surgery for large or giant lesions. Likewise, reconstructive operations in which the vessel is spared and deconstructive procedures in which vessels are sacrificed cause different endovascular results. Ligation of the carotid artery in the cervical region results in overall operative mortality between 0% and 6%.[1]

After direct operations in patients with giant aneurysms, the mortality is high. Sengupta et al.[2] recorded a 38% mortality rate. Onuma and Suzuki[3] recorded 20.8%. Kesaev and Zubkov[4] used both direct and endovascular operations on giant aneurysms in 54 patients and noted a 20.3% mortality rate in this group. Using only endovascular methods, Lasarev[5] reported a 7.3% mortality rate. Montero[6] noted 11.4% of his patients died who had only endovascular procedures. Benashvili[7] reported an 8.3% mortality using both direct and endovascular methods on giant aneurysms.

Braun and co-workers[8] used intravascular metal coils to treat two patients with internal carotid artery (ICA) aneurysms. In one patient, the aneurysm was located in the cavernous sinus, and in the other in the extracranial carotid artery. In each case, the ICA was occluded successfully without causing deficits. Hilal and coauthors[9] used synthetic fiber-coated platinum coils for treating patients with aneurysms in the distal lenticulostriate arteries.

Graves et al.[10] studied the makeup of coils and their effects. Simple coils consisted of a single coil; complex coils were fabricated with and without silk fibers. They introduced these coils into artificial aneurysms formed on the carotid arteries of dogs onto which venous pouches were sutured. Complex coils with silk fibers formed into a complex configuration, such as a flower petal design, produced the most stable pattern, which lessened the chance of migration from the pouch. Dowd et al.[11] described three cases of posterior inferior cerebellar artery (PICA) aneurysms treated with coils to preserve the parent arteries. They used 0.018-in platinum coils interwoven with Dacron fibers (Hilal microcoils, Cook, Inc.)

During the past 3 years, the number of reports describing the use of coils and the number of patients treated with this method have increased tremendously. There is clear inference in recent reports that coils produce better results than microballoons. The authors report fewer complications and wider application of the technique. Guglielmi[12] described the results of treating 37 patients with intracranial aneurysms using this method. Intraaneurysmal thrombus developed in 70% to 100%, but complete thrombosis of the aneurysm occurred in only seven patients. In 16 patients, the aneurysm was 90% to 95% occluded. One patient developed temporary, and another developed permanent, neurological deficits. Four patients died: three in grade 5 (Hunt and Hess) and one in grade 4.

Berenstein and co-workers[13] described the treatment of 32 aneurysms using the Guglielmi detachable coil system. Complete obliteration of the aneurysm was achieved in only 53%. In 12 aneurysms, 95% occlusion was accomplished. In one aneurysm, the aneurysm was 90% obliterated, and in two 80% occlusion occurred. The total morbidity was 9.7% and there were no deaths. These authors concluded that this technique showed promise for aneurysm treatment. Lylyk and co-workers[14] described the use of this technique in 69 aneurysms. There were 41 complete occlusions (59%), 19 subtotal occlusions (28%), and 6 partial obliterations less than 70% (9%). The mortality rate was 10%. Tortuous vessels and vasospasm were described as remaining challenges to the technique.

The early results with this technique seem promising, as several users have indicated. However, major shortcomings include less than satisfactory occlusion of the aneurysm, the primary aim of therapy. The method often leaves significant rests from which growth and rupture may later occur. Electrothrombosis is not a simple process and regulation of the amount of clot that forms is difficult. Clot lysis is also greatly determined by the patient's fibrinolytic system. The system is currently under trial and may not be widely applicable because of its inherent complexity. Thus, the final chapter in this encouraging development must be written later.

Peerless and Drake[15] analyzed results of treatment of 1055 vertebrobasilar artery aneurysms. The differences in outcome primarily depended on location and size. Mortality for basilar apex aneurysms was 6%, superior cerebellar artery (SCA) aneurysms 5%, anterior inferior cerebellar artery (AICA) 11%, vertebral artery junction 6%, vertebral artery (VA) 6%, and for posterior cerebral artery (PCA), 8%. In patients with small aneurysms, the mortality was 4%, with large aneurysms 6%, and for giant lesions, 12%. Sundt and co-workers[16] reported a 5% mortality and 4% morbidity in 178 large and giant lesions.

From the combined University of Mississippi and Polenov Neurosurgical Institute series in St. Petersburg, 111 giant aneurysms of the anterior circulation were managed surgically. There were 14 deaths (13%). Most of these followed direct clipping and were associated with ischemic strokes due to prolonged temporary clipping. No deaths accompanied proximal artery occlusion, and excellent control of growth and rupture of the lesions was achieved by this method. Direct operative morbidity was high (28%) among 58 patients treated by direct craniotomy. Endovascular procedures and carotid occlusion were used in 34 patients with four deaths. Two were due to hemorrhagic complications and two were due to ischemic complications. Five patients died among 19 treated using combined methods (26%). One death was related to carotid artery dissection when an intravascular balloon was used for proximal control for an ophthalmic segment aneurysm. During the past 5 years, the mortality has fallen from 22% to 8.3% due to test occlusion, imaging, and better operative alternatives. The surgical treatment of these difficult lesions, when compared to nonsurgical treatment however, is always more favorable. Whittle et al.[17] reported a good result in 75% of surgical patients, but in those who did not have operative treatment, 86% either died or had significant morbidity. Onuma and Suzuki[3] recorded 62% good results with surgical treatment and 75% morbidity and mortality in nonsurgical patients.

Clinical Anatomic Forms

Many surgeons stress the importance of intracerebral hemorrhage in the outcome of the acute case. Size and location of intracranial hematomas greatly influence intracranial pressure (ICP). The presence of severe intracranial hypertension and herniation syndromes necessitates emergency clot evacuation, even though the results may not be good.[18,19] Pasqualin et al.[19] reviewed treatment results in 309 patients with intracranial hematomas subsequent to a ruptured intracranial aneurysm. Only 24% were finally considered as a good result, and 56% died. In the series reported by Inomori et al.,[20] 21 patients had middle cerebral artery (MCA) aneurysms and 81% of these had hematomas. Fourteen percent died with temporal lobe hematomas less than 4 cm in diameter. In patients with larger hematomas, the mortality was 50%. The overall mortality in this group was 33%. In our series, 158 patients had hematomas associated with arterial aneurysms, and good results were obtained more frequently in patients with less than 50 ml of hematoma volume. The highest mortality was seen in patients with hematomas exceeding 100 ml in size. All patients with hematomas of this size without surgical treatment died. All 82 patients with large intraventricular hematomas died, regardless of treatment. Thus, the outcome in patients with intracerebral and intraventricular hematomas is determined before the patient enters the hospital, perhaps in the first few minutes after aneurysm rupture.

Also following small SAHs, in which only a small amount of blood has accumulated in the subarachnoid space, the outcome is much better than when thick hematomas surround the brain stem and cerebral vessels. Vasospasm may have a significant influence on the choice of treatment and the tactics to be used, although the point is not settled. Bollander et al.[21] suggested that the surgical treatment of any intracranial aneurysm was possible only after vasospasm had run its course. Mizukami et al.,[22] George et al.,[18,23] and Krilov et al.[24] preferred operative treatment before the development of vasospasm. Hugenholtz and Elgie[25] concluded that it made little difference whether the surgical treatment proceeded prior to the development of vasospasm or was applied after it had terminated. However, many, if not most, investigators have underscored the relationship of vasospasm to the operative complication rate. Most have found clear correlation between operative complications and the presence of vasoconstriction, seen on the preoperative angiogram.[26-28] In our series of 358 patients, the surgical mortality rate was twice that in those with vasospasm than in those without vasospasm. The presence of intracranial hypertension and hydrocephalus is also detrimental.

In our study of 80 patients without hydrocephalus and 100 with severe hydrocephalus, the mortality rate was 6.3% and 44% ($p < .005$), respectively.

Rebleeding is also important. Patients undergoing a second hemorrhage, even 20 years after the first, have significantly more morbidity and mortality than those who have experienced only one hemorrhage. The most recent hemorrhages have the greatest influence, especially if they have occurred between 1 and 4 weeks of admission.

Age is a factor in risk assessment.[29] Sahs et al.[30] reported a 66% mortality and morbidity rate in patients older than 66 years. Noterman et al.[31] suggested that age was only obliquely involved, but they recommended surgical treatment in these patients no earlier than 3 weeks after onset of SAH. Ausman et al.[32] reported that 72% of their low-grade patients had good results from direct aneurysmal surgery. In patients less than 60 years of age, however, 81% had good results. Many of the complications occurred after 7 days from intervening systemic complications. Pazstor[29] suggested that patients older than 60 years should be shifted into the next higher Hunt and Hess grade if their age exceeded 60. This point of view was shared by Deruty et al.[33] and Jomin et al.[34]

Many surgeons regard arterial hypertension as a significant deterrent to successful outcome. Eskesen et al.[35] underlined the possibility for hyperactivity of vessels and reactive vasospasm. Their worst results occurred in those patients who were hypertensive but on no therapy. Of 18 patients, 10 died in this latter group. In 96 normotensive patients, only five died. Among 19 treated hypertensive patients, two died. These authors concluded that hypertension, treated or untreated, has a significant negative influence on the outcome. Our results are similar. Of 147 patients operated in grade 1, 5.7% of the normotensives versus 17% of the hypertensives died during the postoperative period ($p < .001$). In 119 patients in grade 3, 38.2% of the normotensives died versus 53% of those with hypertension ($p < .001$).

Postoperative morbidity and mortality in high-grade patients has been reported to be 30% to 80%.[36-39] In grade I or II Hunt and Hess or in grade 1 Zubkov and Smith (compensated), rates between 0% and 13% have been described.[40,41] The reported results indicate that it is theoretically possible to operate at any time interval after SAH with acceptable mortality and morbidity. In patients in grade III Hunt and Hess (subcompensated, Zubkov, Smith, and Tarassoli), there is great variability. DaPian et al.[40] reported a morbidity rate of 32% (54% in grade 4). In 1981, Weir and Aronyk[41] reported 40% mortality in grades III and IV patients (Hunt and Hess). Early operation in the intermediate group is still highly controversial. For this group, recognizing and treating complications with delayed surgery may be more advantageous.

In decompensated (grades IV and V Hunt and Hess) patients, mortality approaches 90% and surgical treatment is rarely satisfactory. Lebedev and coauthors[42] and DaPian and coauthors[43] independently came to the conclusion that the decision is not when to operate these patients, but whether to proceed with an operation at all. A good result occurs in this group only rarely in the patient harboring an intracerebral clot that is evacuated. The risk of operation in higher grades of patients exceeds that associated with rebleeding during the waiting interval. For this reason, treatment must be based on the pathogenesis of the underlying disorder that places the patient in the high clinical grade.

Comparisons between direct and endovascular operations are probably not accurate at present because endovascular procedures are just developing in some centers, and complication rates seem unduly high. Only aneurysms that are inoperable are being referred to endovascular therapists, and thus the results of these difficult lesions are incomparable to those that can be managed easily by more conventional methods. In addition, the procedures may have been performed by different specialists, i.e., neurosurgeons and radiologists. For the endovascular surgeon, the most important indication has been "unclippable aneurysms"; who decides when an aneurysm is clippable or not depends greatly on the experience of the individual who performs the evaluation. During the past years, the indications for endovascular treatment have flourished. Yet, many neurosurgeons still hold the view that few aneurysms are "unclippable" if the costs in terms of complications are justified.

Originally, endovascular treatment applied primarily to the "cold period." More recently, endovascular procedures have been extended to the "hot period" and to aneurysms that have recently ruptured. These carry additional risks, and indications for treatment have not been well defined. There is diverse opinion among specialists in the field regarding the appropriate application of endovascular therapy and many have used these procedures as a panacea. Endovascular therapy is not a panacea. It must be applied to the patient and the aneurysm in a specific way and in a specific time interval.

In the reports of Moret et al.,[44a,b] 124 patients who had 128 intracranial aneurysms were operated. Among these, 22 were operated during the first 48 hours of hemorrhage. Forty-five were operated after 10 days of SAH, and 61 patients with aneurysms had not sustained SAH. Nineteen complications were encountered in this group of 128 aneurysms treated (15%). Nine patients died from these complications, and 10 had serious neurological deficits. The cause of death was brain stem ischemia in 13, rupture of the aneurysm in five, and embolization in one. Guglielmi and Vinuela[45] reported endovascular electrothrombosis of intracranial aneurysms in 28 patients. All, excluding two, were in Hunt and Hess grades I and II. Thrombosis occurred in 70% to 100% using soft detachable platinum coils varying between 4 and 40 cm in length. In 26 patients, there was good flow through the parent vessel after coil placement. Two patients in stage 5 died and one developed homonymous hemianopsia.

In the literature, the overall mortality associated with direct operation during the various phases of the hemorrhagic period have been well documented. Jensen et al.[46] analyzed the course of 1045 patients with arterial aneurysms in 24 clinics in Germany. Fifty-four percent entered the hospital after acute SAH. The overall mortality was 18%. DaPian et al.[47] operated two groups of patients, one within 2 weeks and the second group later. The results of surgical treatment were approximately equal. The mortality was 35% and good results occurred in 50%. In the series reported by Bollander et al.,[21] 162 patients were operated during the hemorrhagic period; 33% of these patients died. Ljunggren and co-workers[48] presented their data on 281 patients in grades I to III Hunt and Hess; 31% of these patients died. Kassell et al.[49–51] presented the cooperative investigation of 68 centers and reported the mortality among 3600 patients. In grades II and III Hunt and Hess, 22% died. Auer et al.[52] also presented the postoperative mortality in different patients treated early. The mortality was 17.5% in all groups, but vasospasm was present in less than 20%. Hugenholtz and Elgie[25] described a 22% mortality rate but de-emphasized the relationship of vasospasm during the postoperative period. Benedetti et al.[53] operated patients with intracranial aneurysms during the first 3 days after rupture. Mortality in grades I and II was 22.5%, but all patients in higher grades died. In a series of publications, Lebedev and coauthors[42,54] analyzed the results of treatment in patients during the hemorrhagic period. The mortality in operative patients was 31%, but in nonoperative patients the mortality was 87% during several months of follow-up.

Several variables determine the results of any aneurysm series. For any management team, the outcome also depends upon the type of hospital to which patients are admitted. Patients arriving soon after hemorrhage to a primary center are at greater risk than those who are referred remotely to distant tertiary centers. Apparently, however, mortality would not be different if measured from ictus. Patients selected for referral because of special risks or conditions influence the mortality and morbidity statistics of the center to which they are referred. There is a common agreement among surgeons that operative mortality has fallen during recent years due to technology and training for the surgeon. Whether overall management mortality and morbidity has lessened is a question that has not been answered. The combined mortality for all patients with acute aneurysmal SAH treated during the past 5 years at the Polenov Neurosurgical Institute, St. Petersburg, and at the University of Mississippi Medical Center, Jackson, Mississippi, is listed in Table 13.1.

TABLE 13.1. Combined mortality for all patients treated 1987–1993*

Patient grade	Number	Mortality
Grade 1	158	5.1%
Grade 2	69	15.9%
Grade 3	19	57.8%
Total	246	12.2%

*Zubkov, Smith, and Tarassoli (see Chapter 4)

Mortality for all grades of patients during the years 1980 to 1986 was 22% and during the years 1987 to 1993 was 12.2%. For the combined series, the surgical results are listed in Table 13.2.

TABLE 13.2. Surgical results in 246 patients operated 1987–1993*

Results	Grade 1	Grade 2	Grade 3	Total
Good	100	29	2	131
Satisfactory	35	16	1	52
Poor	15	13	5	33
Dead	8(5.1%)	11(15.9%)	11(57.9%)	30(12.2%)
Total	158	69	19	246

*Giant and complex aneurysms are reported separately.

Complications

Complications of the perioperative period fall into two categories, those associated with the operation and those relating to the disease. Disease-related issues have largely been covered in previous chapters. Modern surgical approaches require wide opening of the cranial base. This provides additional working space for the surgeon and multidirectional views of the difficult aneurysm, but it exposes the patient to trauma of vessels and nerves near the surface and in the scalp and cerebral tissues. Large bony openings lead to postoperative epidural, subdural, and scalp hematomas and create opportunities for damage to the surrounding brain due to retraction, drying, and bleeding.

Preservation of the neuron and its connections must be the primary concern of every aneurysm surgeon. The patient's external appearance, or cosmetic result, should not be the factor dictating the form of the operation, but attention to small details can make the operation cosmetically acceptable, and inattention can, just as easily, lead to preventable injury to superficial nerves and other tissues. The superficial nerves most commonly affected are the frontalis branch of the seventh facial nerve and the ophthalmic division of the fifth nerve. Both lie in positions where they are vulnerable, but both can be preserved by careful dissection. The frontalis branch lies in the fatty subdivision of the deep fascia anterior to the temporal muscle and can be reflected forward with the scalp flap and preserved. For preservation of the ophthalmic branch, the incision must be placed posteriorly in the scalp as far as possible and the nerve reflected forward with the scalp. The temporal muscle and its nerve supply, the temporal branch of the fifth cranial nerve must be protected from drying and excessive retraction to prevent atrophy. The bony opening should fit well anteriorly to prevent facial dyssymmetry. The pterional bone flap tends to migrate inward with time, creating temporal flattening. This can be prevented by placing a ledge on the anterior surfaces of the connection in closing so that the removed bone cannot migrate inward. Small fine sutures should be used to close the scalp and removed in a timely fashion to prevent a disfiguring scar.

Temporary proximal clipping may be needed to occlude some aneurysms. The interval of temporary clipping during the operative procedure should be closely monitored and controlled. Although safe occlusion times for every vessel are not known, prolonged clipping times have been associated with ischemic deficits and poor results. Tolerance for clipping is highly variable and depends on collateral circulation. In patients in whom vasospasm is not a factor, clipping times of 40 to 60 min in some vessels have been tolerated without infarction. After SAH, only 15 to 20 min occlusion times are acceptable. Interval release of the temporary clips seems to be protective, but this method is controversial. Temporary clips may also occlude blood supply into one or more short branches supplying the brain stem and are poorly accepted.

Increased ICP is a serious complication and is critical during induction of anesthesia. Small increases in intracranial volume may lead to herniation syndromes, recognized upon opening the cranium. Regulation of systemic arterial pressure is essential because of the effect on intracranial volume in the autoregulatory impaired patient. Aneurysms are also susceptible to rupture during arterial pressure peaks.

Brain swelling is a major detriment to good outcome. Ventricular puncture and drainage may create a new subset of problems. Postoperatively, hypoxia, hypercarbia, intracranial bleeding, and hydrocephalus must all be managed appropriately to reduce intracranial volume. Elevated ICP may not be a problem solely restricted to the patient whose aneurysm has ruptured. In both direct and endovascular procedures in which vessels are occluded permanently or for prolonged intervals, ischemic zones lead to swelling and increased ICP. ICP monitoring during the operation and the perioperative period allows early treatment of excess volume.

Infections following aneurysm surgery are uncommon, but unusual circumstances expose the patient to higher risk.[55,56] Prolonged craniotomy creates risk for meningitis and brain abscess. CSF leakage and prolonged ventricular drainage exposes the patient to intracranial infection. Large cranial base exposure, in which the air sinuses are opened, may lead to infection, especially in the patient with preexisting sinusitis or mastoiditis. Patients in higher grades with evidence of brainstem and hypothalamic dysfunction are also predisposed to develop infections that occur in 9% to 20% of patients undergoing craniotomy for direct aneurysm clipping.[38] The more serious of these are meningitis, meningoencephalitis, and ventriculitis; both morbidity and mortality are increased. The value of prophylactic antibiotics in craniotomy for aneurysm clipping has not been established, but if a known contaminant is present, prophylactic coverage with broad spectrum or appropriate antibiotics may be indicated. In the presence of postoperative infection, the treatment must be appropriate and specific. Wound, blood, and fluid cultures with sensitivity studies combined with appropriate antibiotic therapy are necessary. Central nervous system infections are serious and always lead to unfavorable outcomes if not treated aggressively.

Specific Complications

Cavernous Aneurysms

Cranial nerve injury is the most frequent complication of direct cavernous sinus aneurysm surgery, occurring in the majority of cases operated. Fortunately, most of these are temporary (Fig. 13.1). If the nerve has not been divided, recovery usually follows in about 3 to 6 months. Aberrant regeneration occurs following third cranial nerve injury. This is usually manifest by lid elevation on medial gaze. In one of our four cases, a bruit was present postoperatively and was attributed to a small fistula involving a cavernous branch.

Injury to the optic nerve is a serious complication that

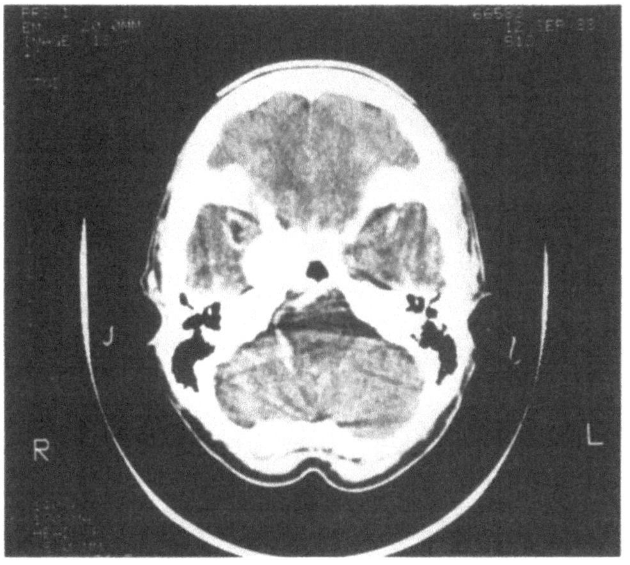

FIGURE 13.1. Large aneurysm in the cavernous sinus that thrombosed following carotid artery occlusion. With thrombosis, the patient developed transient ophthalmoplegia and sensory loss in the V_1 and V_2 distribution.

may result in significant permanent visual loss. Ohmoto et al.[57] described one case after operation in seven patients. Apparently, this complication occurs during drilling around the optic strut. Whenever the drill comes in contact with the nerve or adjacent bone, constant saline irrigation must be used. These deficits probably arise because of heat rather than direct compression.

If the intracavernous aneurysm must be opened and endaneurysmectomy performed, several complications may arise. Ischemic complications may occur due to prolonged clipping or occlusion of the artery. These may affect the entire or partial territory of the ICA. Usually, with low-flow ischemia, the lesions are found in the territory of the penetrating arteries that arise along the MCA trunk.

The lesion due to distal embolization is more difficult to characterize. It usually occurs in the MCA, and distribution involves cerebral cortex and deep white matter tracts. The lesion produces motor and sensory deficits in the affected hemisphere and/or visual field loss.

CSF leaks have occurred infrequently in our patients. This apparently results when air cells are encountered in the sphenoid bone or clinoid process. Leakage has stopped spontaneously in each case.

Supraclinoid Aneurysms

Complications that arise after direct surgery for aneurysms of the supraclinoid segment are, in many respects, similar to those encountered after operative exposure of aneurysms in other locations. Certain peculiarities in local anatomy may, however, produce unique complications.

Complications may arise after retracting the optic nerve that is already stretched by a large aneurysm. Inadequate drilling of the optic foramen so that the nerve can be displaced easily may be responsible for this complication. The falciform ligament binds the nerve laterally and attempts to displace the nerve over the aneurysm, possibly producing inferior and lateral visual field defects. Excess heating of the diamond drill bit may injure the nerve at any location on its superior surface, but the relation near the optic strut is usually the place of maximum tightness. Damage to the ophthalmic artery or clipping of the ophthalmic artery may lead to ipsilateral blindness.

From our 35 cases in which an orbitocranial operation was carried out for ophthalmic aneurysms, one case of CSF rhinorrhea occurred. This leak subsided spontaneously with elevation of the head and antibiotics. The openings are quite small, and spontaneous closure should be expected in most cases. Visual impairment resulting from direct trauma to the optic nerve also occurred in one patient. The orbital roof fracture apparently occurred near the optic canal rather than in the orbital roof. Several patients have had ptosis that cleared spontaneously within a period of 3 to 6 months. There were no cases of retinal artery occlusion in our series. Third nerve palsy with pupillary sparing occurred in one case.

Injury to the third cranial nerve may occur during dissection of an aneurysm involving the cranial base or from the exposure of aneurysms originating near the junction of the posterior communicating artery and carotid artery. It may also occur after drilling the lateral aspect of the anterior clinoid process, especially if the dissection enters the upper anterior aspect of the cavernous sinus. There may be pupillary sparing in the latter condition but ptosis is usually evident and the patient may complain of diplopia. The ptosis is usually self-limiting, clearing in 3 to 4 months.

The carotid artery is the major nutrient vessel for the entire hemisphere, excluding the territories supplied by collateral channels from the anterior and posterior cerebral arteries from the opposite carotid and vertebral system. Thus, infarcts from permanent occlusion may affect the territories of middle, posterior, and anterior cerebral arteries, along with the deep distribution of these vessels (Fig. 13.2). Usually, less severe lesions are actually seen.[58]

From temporary occlusion, low-flow infarcts are more often seen. These occur in the terminal territory of the penetrating vessels of the MCA and anterior cerebral artery (ACA) and involve major motor pathways as well as white matter tracts of the cerebral hemispheres.[58] The superior hypophyseal arteries arise from the proximal portion of the supraclinoid ICA to supply the

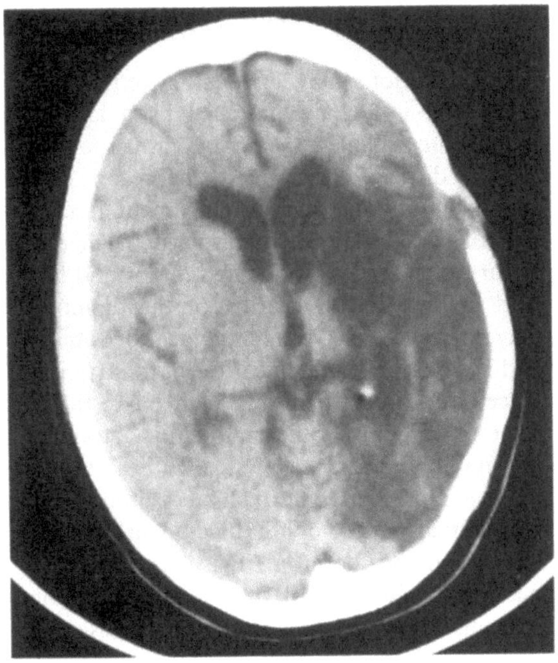

FIGURE 13.2. Large infarct in the middle cerebral artery distribution resulting from carotid artery occlusion by a displaced aneurysm clip.

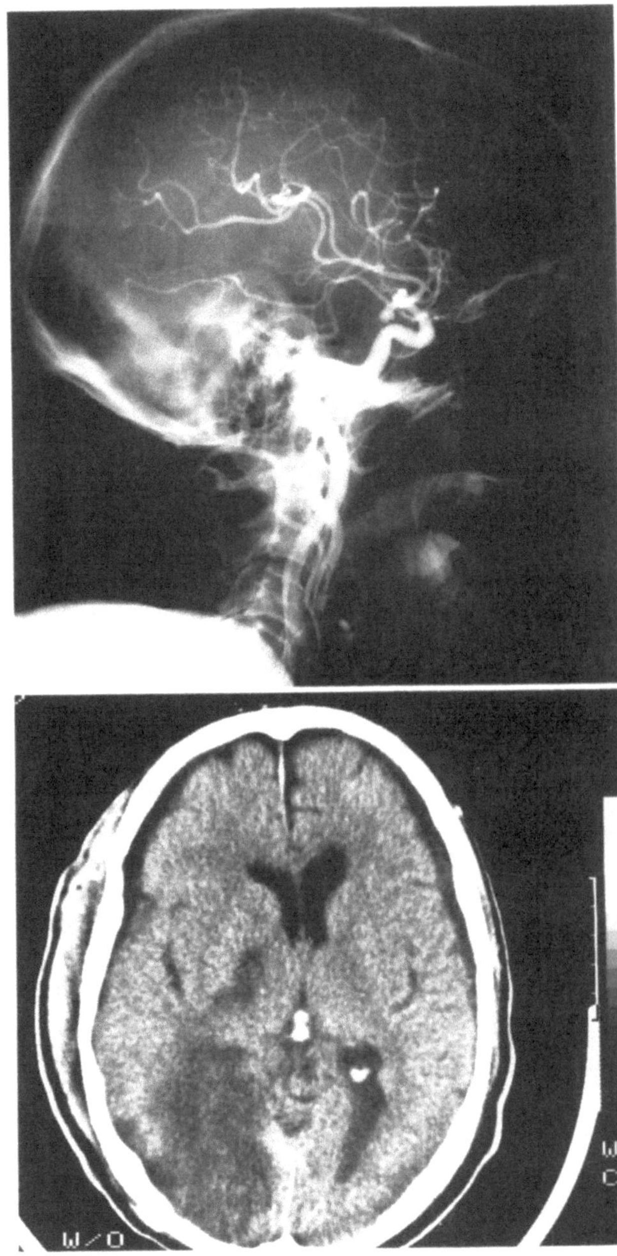

FIGURE 13.3. (A) Posterior communicating artery aneurysm. The posterior cerebral artery filled from both the anterior and posterior circulation injection. (B) Infarct involving the posterior thalamus and occipital lobes. This was associated with a contralateral pain and hemianopsia syndrome when the aneurysm clip occluded the posterior communicating artery.

pituitary stalk and gland. An infundibular artery may arise from the medial surface of the posterior communicating artery (PComA). This vessel may be injured in approaching aneurysms, especially ophthalmic aneurysms, that arise from the medial surface of the ICA at the superior hypophyseal branch. Endocrinologic dysfunction or visual disturbances may follow injury to this vessel. Diabetes insipidus and amenorrhea have been reported after injury to the hypophyseal vasculature.

Fox[56] and others emphasize the safety of occlusion of the *posterior communicating artery* (PComA), especially if the posterior circulation is independent of this collateral channel. However, sparing of this artery from clips should always be attempted. Varying degrees of ischemia and infarction may appear after occlusion of this vessel, even when collateral pathways seem anatomically adequate (Fig. 13.3). The most benign complications are those affecting the visual system of the occipital lobe, and these may be transient, clearing completely over the course of a few days. The most severe complications result in infarction of the occipital lobe, thalamus, and midbrain. Hemisensory loss, hemiplegia, involuntary movements, gaze paresis and hemianopsia may result. A thalamic pain syndrome may also occur.

Helgason[59] described a hypesthetic ataxic hemiparesis with infarction in the contralateral posterior limb of the internal capsule with anterior choroidal artery (AChA) occlusion. In 15 patients, the infarct extended superiorly into the adjacent paraventricular region, and into the lateral thalamus in seven patients. The lesion correlated with the region of supply at the posterior medial superior territory of the AChA. Hwang et al.[60] noted that with occlusion of the AChA, the most common finding was hemiparesis, but anesthesia may be transient. Some patients develop hemianopsia and quadrantanopsia. Bruno et al.[61] found that some patients with AChA syndromes have carotid artery stenosis.

Some believe the AChA to be the source of most lacunar infarctions resulting in ataxic hemiparesis. Mohr et al.[62] studied 16 infarcts involved with the AChA. All involved the posterior limb of the internal capsule. The medial pallidum was involved in 75% of the cases and the cerebral peduncle in 44%. The thalamus was involved in 37% and the medial temporal lobe in 38%. None extended outside these areas (Fig. 13.4). The clinical picture was characterized by motor deficits with varying degrees of visual field and sensory impairments. Only two showed hypesthetic ataxic hemiparesis, and ataxic hemiparesis occurred infrequently.

A lesion of the lateral geniculate body produces congruent visual field defects. The lateral geniculate body has a dual blood supply from the AChA and from the lateral choroidal artery, a branch of the PCA.[63]

A

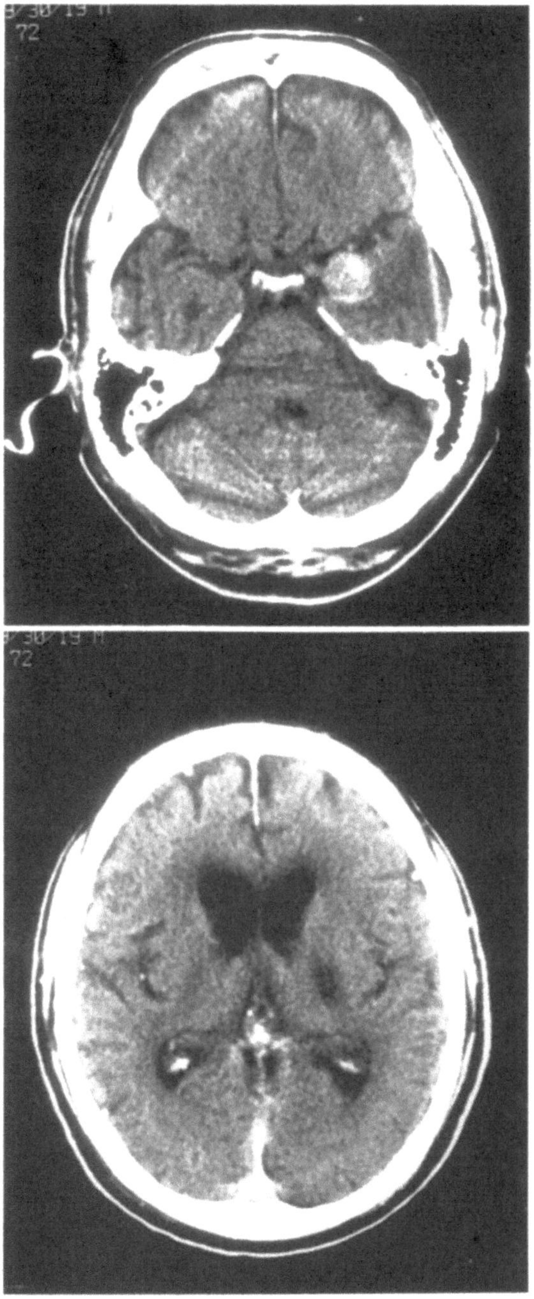

B

FIGURE 13.4. (A) Giant aneurysm of the internal carotid artery at the anterior choroidal junction. (B) The aneurysm occluded the anterior choroidal artery causing the infarct in the internal capsule and medial globus pallidus.

Anterior Cerebral Artery–Anterior Communicating Artery Aneurysms

The complications of treatment of these aneurysms, whether direct methods or endovascular techniques are used, are not unlike the complications of other craniotomies or catheter-related procedures. Bleeding, infection, and embolization must all be considered. Some complications are unique to the areas that harbor the aneurysms and to the arterial system from which these lesions arise. Surgical treatment of the rare aneurysm of the A_1 or of the anterior communicating or pericallosal arteries that produce infarcts may lead to disturbances in memory, behavior, speech, bladder function, and motor activity. Infarcts that involve the knee of the corpus callosum have been associated with aneurysms of the AComA and with surgery in this area (Fig. 13.5). An amnestic syndrome and severe learning deficit associated with severe forgetfulness has been described with ruptured aneurysms in a wide distribution along this arterial

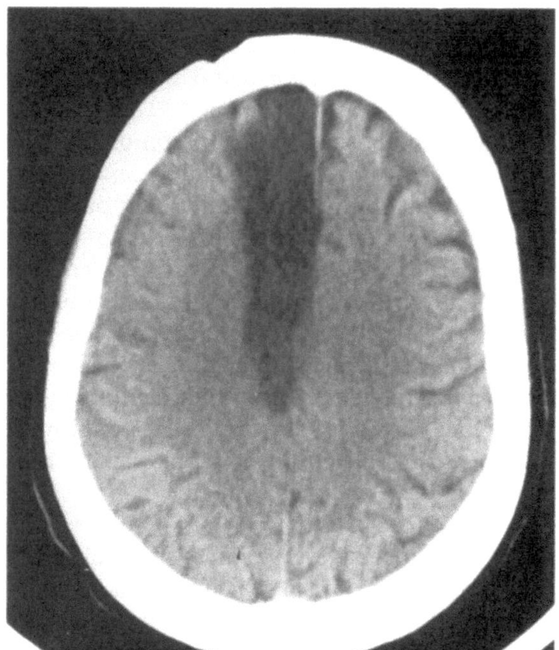

FIGURE 13.5. Infarction resulting from an aneurysm clip that involves the A_2 branch.

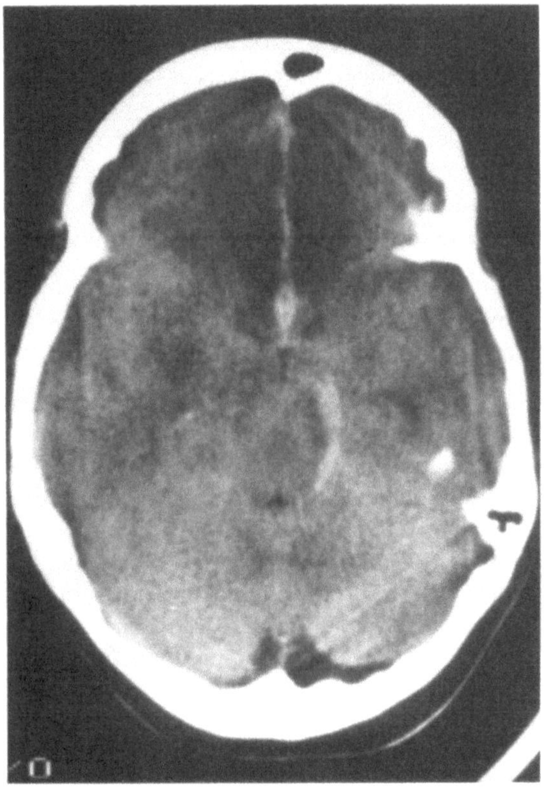

FIGURE 13.6. Paramedial infarction resulting from vasospasm associated with an anterior communicating artery aneurysm.

system. Among the patients who have AComA aneurysms, a confabulatory-amnestic syndrome has also been described.[48] In these cases, infarcts in the territory of both ACAs involving the rostral part of the anterior cingulate gyrus and the bilateral fornices have been noted (Fig. 13.6).

Akinetic mutism is a dysfunction of the mesial basal frontal lobe. It consists of indifference, docility, inattention, and inappropriate urination. The patient may hold food in the mouth, and there seems to be inability or dyspraxia of oral activity. The rostral part of the anterior cingulate gyrus and medial prefrontal cortex are usually involved with lesions in the underlying white matter. This lesion may also extend into the fornices. It may accompany bilateral infarctions of the anterior cingulate gyrus only, but the lesions may spill over into the medial parts of the frontal lobe involving supplementary motor areas in part. Loss of general interest in lofty pursuits has been described.

Many patients develop akinesis of oral activities with frontobasal lesions, in which normal function of the mouth and throat are impaired. Thus, they may appear to understand but be unable to speak. They may also hold food in their mouths without chewing adequately. When the fornix is affected, memory loss may be a predominant deficit and may be the most persistent. Aneurysms that originate from the frontopolar artery, or hemorrhage or vasospasm in the territory that this vessel supplies, may cause abnormal bladder function and control. Usually, this is manifest by an inability to avoid automatic emptying of the bladder. The greatest problems arise in patients in whom the aneurysm ruptures intraoperatively.

Memory dysfunction is harder to characterize. In some patients, the inability to concentrate overshadows the amnestic syndrome. Lindqvist and Norlen[64] identified a subgroup with Korsakoff's syndrome after operation for AComA aneurysms. Small perforating arteries exit the AComA and penetrate the anterior hypothalamus. Thus, infarcts here may simulate those lesions associated with vitamin deficiencies and alcoholism. Both antegrade and retrograde amnesia may be present when the fornices are affected.

Occlusion of the left pericallosal artery affects the cingulate gyrus, the precentral lobule, and the precuneus of the left hemisphere along with corpus callosum. It is characterized by right hemiparesis with predominant crural involvement, a disconnection agraphia, and a left unilateral disconnection tactile naming deficit.

The cingulum contains projections from all parts of the frontal lobe and sends fibers toward the interrhinal areas and hippocampus. Therefore, a partial disconnection syndrome may result from pericallosal artery occlusion. An alien hand syndrome has also been reported in patients with AComA aneurysms. In this syndrome, one hand will pick up objects and move them into the path of

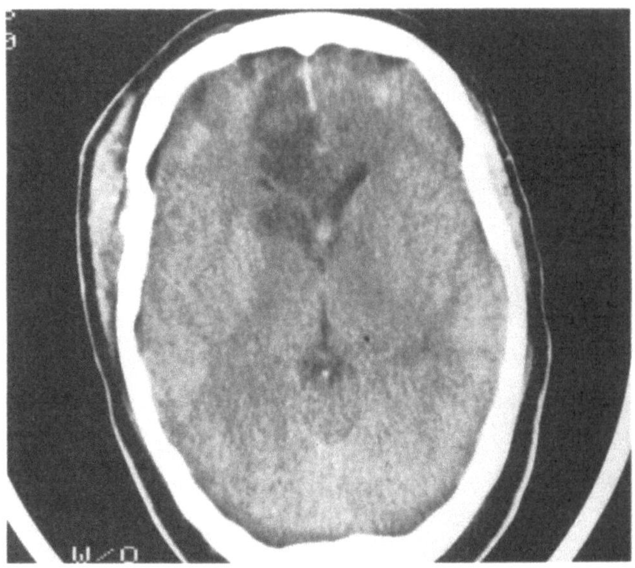

FIGURE 13.7. Infarction resulting from prolonged temporary clipping of the A_1 branch. There is infarction in the territory of A_2 and the caudate distribution of Heubner's artery.

the other, which was carrying out a different task. In this case the lesion extends into one side of the genu of the corpus callosum.

A capsulopallidal infarct involving the capsule and caudate nucleus is associated with occlusion of the internal lenticulostriate branches of the ACA, or Heubner's artery. The lesion involves the distribution of this striate branch, the lower anterior parts of the head of the caudate nucleus, the lower frontal pole of the putamen, the frontal pole of the globus pallidus, and the anterior limb of the internal capsule, up to the dorsal limit of the globus pallidus (Fig. 13.7). Occasionally, transcortical motor aphasia occurs after AComA surgery. Usually, this is associated with territory infarct in the A_2 distribution on the left side.

Middle Cerebral Artery Aneurysms

The complications associated with aneurysms of the MCA are similar to those that occur with aneurysms elsewhere. Unique clinical syndromes, however, occur with MCA occlusion or occlusion of the branches. MCA occlusion can be divided into four types based on the level at which the occlusion takes place. Type I occlusions occur before the origins of the lenticulostriate branches. Type II lesions occur distal to these branches. Type III occlusions are at the main trunk bifurcation; when peripheral branches are involved, Bozzao et al.[65] classified the occlusion as type IV. Involvement of the lentiform nucleus is constant with type I and with ICA occlusion. Butcher et al.[66] noted that proximal lesions caused larger infarcts of the cortex and striatum.

Weiller et al.[58] looked at low-flow lesions of the carotid and MCA territories. These were found more often in the white matter in the territories of the lenticulostriate, anterior choroidal, or Heubner's arteries. Aphasia and neglect were found only in patients with persistent occlusion of the M_1. These subcortical infarcts are the lesion expected with prolonged temporary clipping of the M_1 segment. Angeloni et al.[67] found internal border zone watershed infarcts in patients with proximal MCA branch occlusions. The collateralization pattern from the ACA and PCA determine, to a great extent, the size of the infarct to be expected with MCA trunk occlusion. The presence of a pial anastomotic pattern reduced the size of the cortical component but not the deep lesion.

Obstruction of the cortical branches of the MCA causes contralateral motor weakness due to involvement of the corticospinal tract in the central gyrus, motor aphasia due to involvement of the posterior inferior surface of the frontal lobe in the dominant hemisphere, mental and personality impairment due to involvement of the prefrontal area, sucking and grasping reflexes due to involvement of the premotor area, visual field defect (from damage to the geniculocalcarine tract and the temporal, parietal, and occipital lobes), reduction in discrimination due to involvement of the parietal lobes, receptive aphasia due to disturbance of the temporoparietal area in the dominant hemisphere, and finger agnosia, right–left disorientations, acalculia, and agraphia (Gerstmann's syndrome) caused by disturbance of the parietooccipital junctional area in the dominant hemisphere.

Occlusion of the angular artery in the dominant hemisphere has been associated with hemiparesis, facial weakness, hemianopsia, acalculia, dysphasia, visuospatial agnosia, and constructional apraxia. An acousticoamnestic syndrome has also been noted. Temporal lobe hematomas, occurring both preoperatively and postoperatively, are the most frequent complication of these aneurysms (Fig. 13.8).

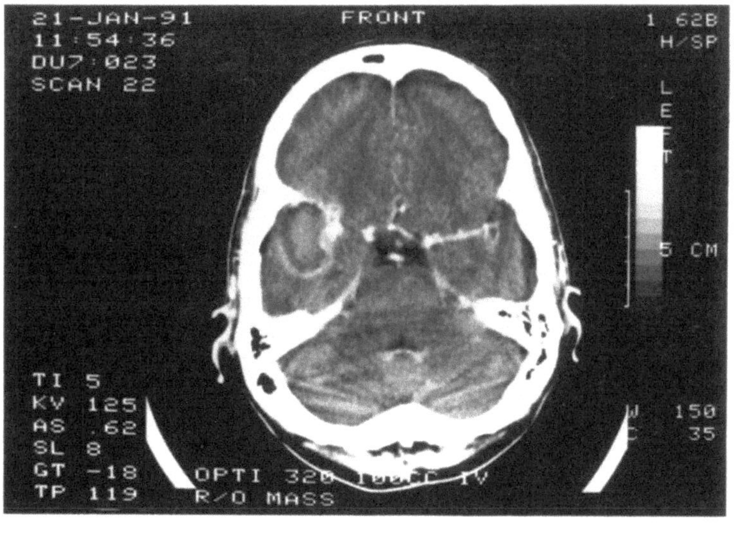

FIGURE 13.8. Resolving hematoma of the right temporal lobe associated with right MCA aneurysm that ruptured 3 weeks previously.

Vertebrobasilar Aneurysms

Understanding the relationship between the major arterial trunks and their perforating vessels is the key to successful aneurysm surgery at the basilar artery (BA) bifurcation. Here, numerous small but important arteries penetrate the brain stem, and their preservation is vital to a successful outcome. Beginning on the PComA, an anterior polar artery may supply the anterior portion of the contralateral thalamus. A premamillary artery or anterior thalamoperforating artery may also be found. There is some confusion over nomenclature in this area, and the anterior polar artery and the anterior thalamoperforating artery may actually be one and the same. Occlusion of the long circumflex arteries produces conjugate gaze dysfunction, contralateral hemianesthesia, ipsilateral cerebellar dysfunction, and nystagmus.

On the P_1 branch, the most consistent important perforators are the arteries of Percheron, or posterior thalamoperforators (PTPs), that exit approximately 5 mm from the BA apex and ascend through the posterior perforating substance to supply the anterior and medial thalamus and the upper mesencephalon. Occlusion of the PTP arteries may produce rubral tremor with ipsilateral third nerve paresis (Nothnagel's syndrome), cerebellar ataxia, contralateral hemiplegia; hemiballismus will also be present if the subthalamic area is involved (Fig. 13.9). Bilateral occlusion of this artery may produce memory impairment and a variety of Korsakoff's syndrome. Castaigne and co-workers[68] accurately defined the clinical syndromes produced by occlusion of these arteries.

Lethargy and disturbances of consciousness are perhaps the most consistent postoperative finding. However, memory disturbance, mood disorders, abnormalities of extraocular muscle function, and a peculiar pain syndrome (dysphoria) may be late sequelae from infarctions in the anterior medial thalamus. Some patients develop severe movement disorders that appear months after the infarct has matured. Four or five perforating arteries, called the superior mesencephalic arteries, exit from the dorsal surface of the BA apex to supply the upper mesencephalon and cranial nerve nuclei. Occlusion of these branches results in coma and extraocular muscle dysfunction including pupillary nonreactivity. Autonomic disturbances follow occlusion of the premamillary arteries and those that supply the anterior thalamus and hypothalamus.[68]

When the infarct extends into the peduncle, sudden initial coma is present (Fig. 13.10). Hypersomnia, with abnormalities of ocular motility, are seen in survivors.

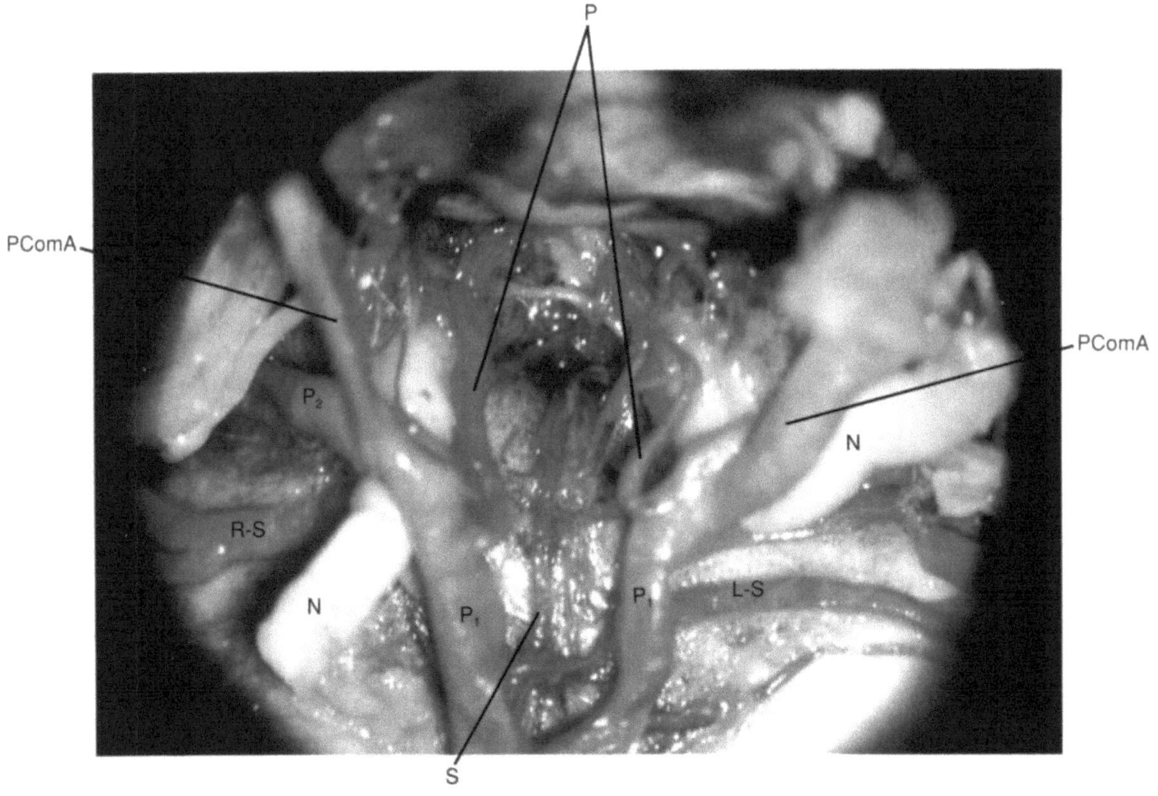

FIGURE 13.9. This injected anatomical specimen illustrates the important perforators from the basilar artery apex. (P) Percheron's arteries; (S) superior mesencephalic arteries; (PComA) posterior communicating artery; (N) third cranial nerve; (LS) left superior cerebellar artery arises from P_1.

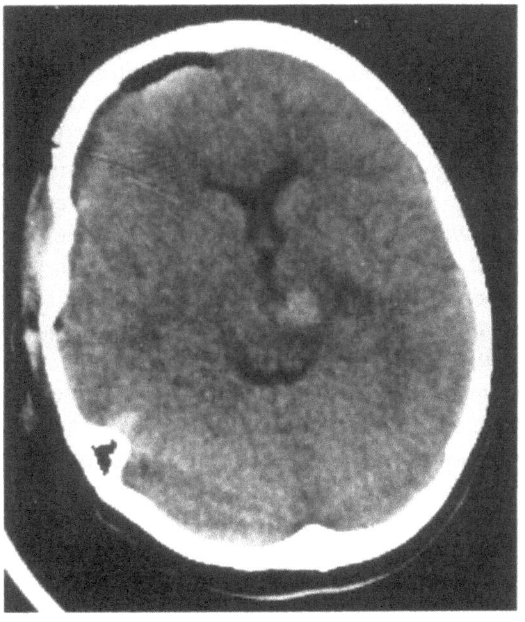

FIGURE 13.10. Infarct involving the contralateral peduncle and thalamus from the inclusion of Percheron's artery in an aneurysm clip.

Third nerve palsy may be unilateral or bilateral and may be associated with sixth nerve paralysis also. Abnormal movements appear. They are always delayed and have predilection for the arm and face. Thalamic and midbrain infarcts are rarely isolated; they predominate in the midbrain and may involve the motor system. There may be amnesia, attention deficits, mood disturbances, poverty of motor initiative, and memory difficulties. Many patients complain of dysphoria, a peculiar painful reaction. The lesion that results from occlusion of one artery of Percheron is variable. When there is only one arterial pedicle arising from the P_1 segment and it supplies both thalami, the thalamic infarct is always bilateral, and the clinical signs are much more severe.[68] Occlusion of the thalamogeniculate arteries produces a variety of clinical features of the thalamic syndrome, including the loss of superficial and deep sensation in the contralateral side, contralateral hypersensibility, and homonymous hemianopsia, as well as hyperpathy to pain, touch, and temperature stimuli.

Infarcts involving the AICA usually affect the middle cerebellar peduncle. Occasionally, the lesion may extend to the flocculus. The larger infarcts extend to the anterior and lateral aspects of the cerebellum, especially if the PICA is hypoplastic. Several cranial nerves may be involved. There may be facial paralysis, trigeminal sensory impairment, deafness (sometimes associated with tinnitus), a vestibular syndrome, or lateral gaze palsy. There may be cerebellar signs and motor weakness. Contralateral pain and temperature loss may be present. Horner's syndrome and skew deviation occur rarely.

Aneurysms of the SCA are rare, but they occur at the junction of the BA or, even more rarely, on the periphery as the vessel courses over the superior surface of the cerebellar hemisphere. Occlusion of the main trunk may cause infarction in the superior cerebellar hemispheres and in the major midline nuclear groups. This results in severe truncal ataxia. Infarction in the superior colliculus causes disturbances in oculomotor function, and occlusion of the geniculate branches may cause visual field changes. Occlusion of the collicular arteries may produce Parinaud's syndrome due to ischemia of the posterior commissure and of the Cajal and the Darkshevich nuclei.[69]

The SCA supplies the superior surface and deep cerebellar structures, the pons, and some parts of the mesencephalon. Occlusion of the SCA will produce various clinical syndromes caused by infarction of a portion of the cerebellum, the dentate nucleus, the brachium conjunctivum, and the long sensory pathways in the tegmentum of the rostral pons.

The SCA syndromes consist of dizziness, vomiting, ataxia, ipsilateral intention tremor due to the dentate nucleus and the superior cerebellar peduncle, ipsilateral Horner's syndrome due to impairment of the descending oculosympathetic pathway, nystagmus due to involvement of the medial longitudinal fasciculus and cerebellar pathways, loss of pain and temperature sensation on the contralateral side, and contralateral hearing impairment.

Unilateral ptosis and limitations of supraadduction but with normal pupillary reactivity have also been reported. The aneurysm was located at the junction of the superior cerebellar artery and posterior cerebral artery. This caused flattening and compression of the interpeduncular oculomotor nerve from below. The superior division of the oculomotor nerve supplies exclusively the superior rectus muscle and levator palpebrae superioris. An aneurysm involving this branch does not affect the pupillary constrictor fibers. An aneurysm of the intercavernous carotid artery may also affect the superior division selectively.

The tolerance time for temporary occlusion of the SCA is not known. Ogawa et al.[69] analyzed their cases undergoing STA (superficial temporal artery)–SCA anastomosis for posterior fossa ischemia disease. In only one case was there a small infarction in the pons. Two deaths, however, were related to cardiac disease. Occlusion of the BA resulted in infarctions in the SCA territory in 17 of 19 cases. It involved the PICA in only 10. The occlusion of the medial branch of the SCA may result in a small infarct in the left paravermial zone of the rostral cerebellum (lobulus simplex and similunaris superior). This may be associated with cerebellar dysarthria. The main clinical features of lateral branch occlusion are lateropulsion, dysarthria, and ipsilateral dysmetria. Bilateral occlusion of the AICA and the midportion of the BA results in bilateral hearing impairment associated with tinnitus at the onset. There is usually bilateral, lateral inferior pontine syndrome associated with gaze paralysis and upgaze palsy.

In isolated SCA occlusion there may be an infarction in the paramedian territory in the brain stem only. Hemiparesis is rare but may occur with edematous cerebellar infarction.

Occlusion of the PICA causes an infarct in the lateral medulla, dorsal to the inferior olivary nucleus. The syndrome includes ipsilateral numbness of the face due to injury of the spinal tract of the fifth nerve. Loss of pain and temperature sensation on the contralateral half of the body occurs due to involvement of the spinothalamic tract. Also, dysphasia, dysarthria, and hoarseness develop due to weakness of the palate and vocal cord, and there may be a weakness of the sternocleidomastoid muscle. The lesion may involve the nucleus ambiguus. Ataxia, dizziness, vertigo, nystagmus, and cerebellar signs on the ipsilateral side occur due to damage of the vestibular nuclei and cerebellar tracts in the brain stem. Ipsilateral Horner's syndrome also may occur. In Fisher's[70] series, 75% of the cases were associated with VA occlusion and only 12% with PICA occlusion. If paresis of the trunk, limb, or tongue occurred or if visual loss with involvement of the calcarine cortex were found, then usually VA occlusion, rather than PICA occlusion, had occurred. Involvement of cranial nerve VI, VII, or VIII also suggests VA occlusion. The distal branches of PICA supply the cerebellar hemisphere, and acute occlusion may result in massive fatal cerebellar infarction. This is most often seen in patients in whom the AICA and superior cerebellar branches are deficient. With PICA occlusion, the infarct usually involves the medial branch of PICA; these may cause a pure vestibular syndrome or a typical Wallenberg's syndrome. When the rostral BA is affected and occlusion also involves the SCA, coma with tetraplegia and cerebellar and vestibular signs predominates. Tonsillar herniation occurs rapidly with infarction in the inferior cerebellum.

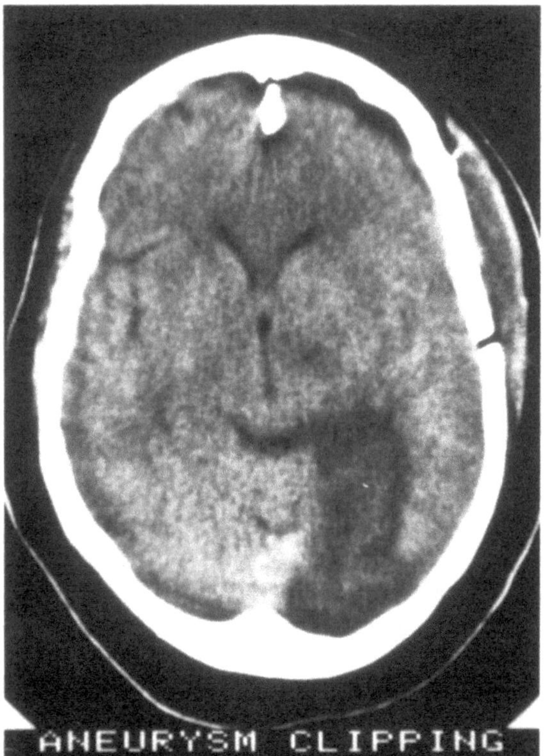

FIGURE 13.11. Large occipital lobe and posterior thalamic infarction associated with occlusion of the posterior cerebral artery.

In 1906, Dejerine and Roussy[71] described the thalamic syndrome, and, in 1927, Foix and co-workers[55] identified the vascular supply to the thalamic area. With occlusion of the PCA in the dominant hemisphere, memory disturbances, dysphasia, and homonymous hemianopsia to the opposite side may be produced (Fig. 13.11). Occlusion produces homonymous-type visual impairment with macular sparing, sometimes with Anton's syndrome, which is a peculiar denial of blindness and confabulatory behavior. Ischemia of the occipital pole in the dominant hemisphere, combined with ischemia of portions of the splenium of corpus callosum, which is supplied by the splenial arteries, may cause dyslexia without dysgraphia.

Summary

The results of aneurysm surgery are improving. From our combined data, it also seems that overall management mortality may also be improving. Much work needs to be done to verify these findings and to reduce the morbidity further after SAH and both direct and endovascular surgery. These are serious problems for the patient affected; they may mean the difference between functionality and dependent care. The surgeon must know the possible consequences of occlusion of any intracranial artery and weigh these against those likely with an aneurysm left in situ to bleed again or to grow in size. Recognition of safe temporary occlusion limits, evaluation of cerebral blood flow (CBF) and velocity recordings, preocclusion testing data, and surgical experience can help the patient through this most difficult time.

References

1. Miller JD, Jawad K, Jennett B. Safety of carotid ligation and its role in the management of intracranial aneurysms. *J Neurol Neurosurg Psychiatry*. 1977;40:64–72.

2. Sengupta RP, Gryspeerdt GL, Hankinson J. Carotid-ophthalmic aneurysms. *J Neurol Neurosurg Psychiatry.* 1976;39:837–853.
3. Onuma T, Suzuki J. Surgical treatment of giant intracranial aneurysms. *J Neurosurg.* 1979;51:33–36.
4. Kesaev SA, Zubkov YN. Clinical features and surgical treatment of large and giant intracranial aneurysms. In: *Arterial Aneurysms of the Brain* [in Russian]. Leningrad, Russia: 1983;32–35.
5. Lasarev VA. *Endovascular Surgery of Arterial Aneurysms of the Internal Carotid Artery* [in Russian]. Moscow, 1983. Thesis.
6. Montero KI. *Diagnostic and Endovascular Treatment of Giant Aneurysms of the Brain Vessels* [in Russian]. Kiev, 1986. Thesis.
7. Benashvili GM. *Treatment of Giant Intracranial Aneurysms.* Leningrad, Russia: 1990. Thesis.
8. Braun IF, Hoffman JC Jr, Casarella WJ, Davis PC. Use of coils for transcatheter carotid occlusion. *AJNR.* 1985;6: 953–956.
9. Hilal SK, Khandji A, Solomon RW, Chi L. Obliteration of intracranial aneurysms with preshaped thrombogenic coils. Presented at the 1989 Annual Meeting of the Radiological Society of North America, November 26–December 1, 1989; Chicago IL.
10. Graves VB, Partington CR, Rufenacht DA, Rappe AH, Strother CM. Treatment of carotid artery aneurysms with platinum coils: an experimental study in dogs. *AJNR.* 1990;11:249–252.
11. Dowd CF, Halbach VV, Higashida RT, Barnwell SL, Hieshima GB. Endovascular coil embolization of unusual posterior inferior cerebellar artery aneurysms. *Neurosurgery.* 1990;27:954–961.
12. Guglielmi G. Embolization of intracranial aneurysms with detachable coils and electrothrombosis. In: Vinuela F, Halbach VV, Dion JE, eds. *Interventional Neuroradiology: Endovascular Therapy of the Central Nervous System.* New York: Raven Press; 1992:63–65.
13. Berenstein A, Choi IS, Setton A, Kupersmith M, Jafar J. Endovascular treatment of cerebral aneurysms using the Guglielmi detachable coil: the NYU experience. Presented at the 1993 Annual Meeting of the American Association of Neurological Surgeons, April 24–29; 1993; Boston, MA.
14. Lylyk P, Guglielmi G, Vinuela J, Petrocelli S, Basso A. Endovascular neurosurgery in intracranial aneurysms with G.D.C. coils: Buenos Aires Experience. Presented at the 1993 Annual Meeting of the American Association of Neurological Surgeons. April 24–29, 1993; Boston, MA.
15. Peerless SJ, Drake CG. Posterior circulation aneurysms. In: Wilkins RM, Rengachary SS, eds. *Neurosurgery.* New York: McGraw-Hill; 1985;II:1167–1917.
16. Sundt TM, Kobayashi SK, Fode NC, Whisnant JP. Results and complications of surgical management of 809 intracranial aneurysms in 722 cases: related and unrelated to grade of patient, type of aneurysm, and timing of surgery. *J Neurosurg.* 1982;56:753–765.
17. Whittle JR, Dorsch NW, Besser M. Giant intracranial aneurysms: diagnosis, management and outcome. *Surg Neurol.* 1984;21:218–230.
18. George B, Roux FX, Beque T, Muzard O, Dematons C. Arguments pour une intervention precoce dans les aneurysmes intra-craniens. A partir d'une serie de 33 aneurysmes avec hematome. *Neurochirurge.* 1984;30:31–34.
19. Pasqualin A, Bazzan A, Cavazzani P, Scienza R, Licata C, Da Pian R. Intracranial hematomas following aneurysmal rupture: experience with 309 cases. *Surg Neurol.* 1986;25:6–17.
20. Inomori S, Ilu K, Ueda S, Shinsa D. Ruptured aneurysms of the middle cerebral artery with intracerebral hematoma: CT findings and outcome. *Neurol Med Chir.* 1984;24:573–579.
21. Bollander HG, Kourtopoulos M, West KA. Retrospective analysis of 162 consecutive cases of ruptured intracranial aneurysms. Total mortality and early surgery. *Acta Neurochir.* 1984;70:31–41.
22. Mizukami M, Kawase T, Usami T, Tazawa T. Prevention of vasospasm by early operation with removal of subarachnoid blood. *Neurosurgery.* 1982;10:301–307.
23. George B, Muzard O, Beque T, Roux FX, Goldstein A, Raqueneau JL. Efficacite d'un traitement medical (isoproterenol-auinophylline) du spasme des ruptures aneurysmes. *Neurochirurgie.* 1984;30:273–276.
24. Krilov VV, Lebedev VV, Shelkovski VN, Kuksova NS, Zakharov HG. Surgical treatment of intracranial aneurysm in acute period with vasospasm [in Russian]. *Vopr Neurozhir.* 1987;2:3–8.
25. Hugenholtz M, Elgie RG. Consideration in early surgery on good risk patients with ruptured intracranial aneurysms. *J Neurosurg.* 1982;56:180–185.
26. Hijdra A, Van Gijn J, Stetanko S, Van Dongen KJ, Vermeulen M, Van Cravel M. Delayed cerebral ischemia after aneurysmal subarachnoid hemorrhage: clinico-anatomic correlations. *Neurology.* 1986;36:329–334.
27. Kraus E, Scheil F. Influence of age, hypertension, vasospasm and other factors on the results of aneurysm surgery. *Acta Neurochir.* 1984;72:139–140.
28. Lebedev VV, Bikovnikov LD. *Textbook of Urgent Neurosurgery.* Moscow: Medicina; 1987:335.
29. Pazstor E. *Essentials of Neurosurgery* [in Russian]. Budapest Hungary: 1985.
30. Sahs AL, Perret GE, Locksley HB, Nishioka H, eds. *Intracranial Aneurysms and Subarachnoid Hemorrhage. A Cooperative Study.* Philadelphia, Toronto: JB Lippincott; 1969.
31. Noterman J, Mouawad E, D'Haens J, Dant T, Nuborgh Y, Telerman-Toppet N. Les indications et les conditions operatoires des anevrysmes chez les gens ages. A propos de trois cas [English Abstract]. *Acta Neurol Belg.* 1978;78:80–85.
32. Ausman JI, Diaz FG, Malik GM, Fielding AS, Son CS. Current management of cerebral aneurysms: is it based on facts or myths? *Surg Neurol.* 1985;24:625–635.
33. Deruty R, Bret P, Lecuire J, Duquesnel J, Chacornac R, Capdeville J, Manoclian G. Le traitment chirurgical de l'aneurysma de l'artere communicante anterieure. *Lyon Med.* 1980;244:147–151.
34. Jomin M, Lesoin F, Lozes G. Prognosis with 500 ruptured and operated intracranial arterial aneurysms. *Surg Neurol.* 1984;21:13–18.
35. Eskesen V, Rosenorn J, Ronde F, Schmidt K. The prog-

nostic significance of pre-existing hypertension in intracranial aneurysms. *Acta Neurochir.* 1986;79:155.
36. Friedrich M, Seifert V, Stolke D. Experience in aneurysm surgery: early versus late surgery. In: Auer LM, Kassell NF, eds. *Timing of Aneurysm Surgery.* Berlin, New York: DeGruyter; 1985:133–143.
37. Hori S, Suzuki J. Early intracranial operations for ruptured aneurysms. *Acta Neurochir.* 1979;46:93–104.
38. Nishimoto A, Kiyotake U, Onbe M, et al. Nationwide cooperative study of intracranial aneurysm surgery in Japan. *Stroke.* 1985;16:48–52.
39. Yasui N, Ho Z, Ohta M, Suzuki A. Surgical problems and pathophysiology in severe cases with ruptured aneurysms in the acute stage. *Acta Neurochir.* 1982;63:163–174.
40. DaPian R, Pasqualin A, Scienza R, Licata C, Cavazzani P. A preliminary report of early surgery for bleeding intracranial aneurysms. *J Neurosurg Sci.* 1983;27:1–8.
41. Weir B, Aronyk K. Management of supratentorial aneurysms. *J Neurosurg.* 1981;54:146–150.
42. Lebedev VV, Shelkovski VN, Krilov VV. Effect of temporary clipping of the major brain vessels on outcome of the surgical treatment of intracranial aneurysms [in Russian]. *Vopr Neurochir.* 1986;3:8–12.
43. DaPian R, Pasqualin H, Scienza R, Cavazzani P, Mazza C. Subarachnoid hemorrhage: influence of surgical timing on overall results of management. *Acta Neurochir.* 1984; 73:77–152.
44a. Moret J, Boulin A, Mawad M, Castaings L. Endovascular treatment of berry aneurysms by endosaccular balloon occlusion. First Congress of the World Federation of Interventional and Therapeutic Neuroradiology. *Neuroradiology.* 1991;33(suppl):S135–S136.
44b. Moret J. Endovascular treatment of berry aneurysms by endosaccular occlusion. (International Symposium, Vienna, Austria, May 21–25, 1990). *Acta Neurochir Suppl (Wien).* 1991;53:48–49.
45. Guglielmi G, Vinuela F. Endovascular electrothrombosis of intracranial aneurysms. Experimental research and initial clinical applications. First Congress of the World Federation of Interventional and Therapeutic Neuroradiology. *Neuroradiology.* 1991;33(suppl):S137.
46. Jensen MP, Kraus E, Scheil F. Surgical results in 1045 cases of intracranial aneurysms. *S Afr J Surg.* 1984;22: 3–11.
47. DaPian R, Pasqualin H, Scienza R, Cavazzani P. Early surgery for intracranial aneurysms: Influence of clinical and operative finding on final results. In: Auer LM, Kassell NF, eds. *Timing of Aneurysm Surgery.* Berlin, New York: DeGruyter; 1985:115–125.
48. Ljunggren B, Brandt L, Kagstrom E, Sundbarg G. results of early operations for ruptured aneurysms. *J Neurosurg.* 1981;54:473–479.
49. Kassell NF, Boarini DJ, Adams HP, Sahs AL, Graf CJ, Torner JC, Gerk MK. Overall management of ruptured aneurysm: comparison of early and late operation. *Neurosurgery.* 1981;9:120–128.
50. Kassell NF, Torner JC. The international cooperative study on timing of aneurysm surgery: an update. *Stroke.* 1984;15:566–571.
51. Kassell NF, Torner JC, Jane JA. The international cooperative study on the timing of aneurysm surgery. In: Auer LM, Kassell NF, eds. *Timing of Aneurysm Surgery.* Berlin, New York: DeGruyter; 1985:277–278.
52. Auer LM, Schneider GH, Auer T. Computerized tomography and prognosis in early aneurysm surgery. *J Neurosurg.* 1986;65:217–221.
53. Benedetti A, Curri D, Volpin L, Cervellini P. Our experience in early aneurysm operation. a preliminary report. *Neurochirurgia.* 1986;29:25–27.
54. Lebedev VV, Krolov VV, Shelkovski VN, Kholodov SA. Diagnosis and treatment of patients in acute period of subarachnoid hemorrhage after rupture of intracranial arterial aneurysms [in Russian]. *J Neurology Psychiatry* 1985;8:1143–1146.
55. Foix C, Chavany JA, Levy M. Syndrome pseudothalamique d'origine parietale. *Rev Neurol.* 1927;35:68.
56. Fox JL. *Intracranial Aneurysms.* New York, Berlin, Heidelberg, Tokyo: Springer-Verlag; 1983;II.
57. Ohmoto T, Nagao S, Mino S, Ito T, Homna Y, Fujiwara T. Exposure of the intracavernous carotid artery in aneurysm surgery. *Neurosurgery.* 1991;28:317–324.
58. Weiller C, Ringelstein EB, Reiche W, Thron A, Buell V. The large striacapsular infarct. *Arch Neurol.* 1990;47:1085–1091.
59. Helgason CM. A new view of anterior choroidal artery territory infarction. *J Neurol.* 1988;235:387–391.
60. Hwang SH, Huh K, Kim SM, Suh JH. Two cases of anterior choroidal artery territory infarction. *Yonsei Med J.* 1989;30:314.
61. Bruno A, Graff-Radford NR, Biller J, Adams HP Jr. Anterior choroidal artery territory infarction: a small vessel. *Stroke.* 1989;20:616–619.
62. Mohr JP, Steinke W, Timsit SG, Sacco RL, Tatemichi TK. The anterior choroidal artery does not supply the corona radiata and lateral ventricular wall. *Stroke.* 1991;22:1502–1507.
63. Luco C, Hoppe A, Schweitzer M, Vicuna X, Fantin A. Visual field defects in vascular lesions of the lateral geniculate body. *J Neurol Neurosurg Psychiatry.* 1992;55: 12–15.
64. Lindqvist G, Norlen G. Korsakoff's syndrome after operation on ruptured aneurysm of the anterior communicating artery. *Acta Psychiatr Scand.* 1966;42:24.
65. Bozzao L, Bastianello S, Fantozzi LM, Angeloni U, Argentino C, Fieschi C. Correlation of angiographic and sequential CT findings in patients with evolving cerebral infarction. *AJNR.* 1989;10:1215–1222.
66. Butcher SP, Bullock R, Graham DI, McCulloch J. Correlation between amino acid release and neuropathologic outcome in rat brain following middle cerebral artery occlusion. *Stroke.* 1990;21:1727–1733.
67. Angeloni A, Bozzao L, Fantozzi L, Bastianello S, Kushner M, Fieschi C. Internal border zone infarction following acute middle cerebral artery occlusion. *Neurology.* 1991;90: 1196–1198.
68. Castaigne P, Lhermitte F, Buge A, Escourolle R, Hauw JJ, Lyon-Caen O. Paramedian thalamic and midbrain infarcts: clinical and neuropathologic study. *Ann Neurol.* 1981;10: 127–148.

69. Ogawa A, Kameyama M, Muraishi K, Yoshimoto T, Ito M, Sakurai Y. Cerebral blood flow and metabolism following superficial temporal artery to superior cerebellar artery bypass for vertebrobasilar occlusive disease. *J Neurosurg.* 1992;76:955–960.

70. Fisher CM. Clinical syndromes in cerebral thrombosis, hypertensive hemorrhage and ruptured saccular aneurysm. *Clin Neurosurg.* 1975;22:117–147.

71. Dejerine J, Roussy G. Le syndrome thalamique. *Rev Neurol (Paris).* 1906;14:521–532.

Index

MIX
Papier aus verantwortungsvollen Quellen
Paper from responsible sources
FSC® C105338

If you have any concerns about our products,
you can contact us on
ProductSafety@springernature.com

In case Publisher is established outside the EU,
the EU authorized representative is:
Springer Nature Customer Service Center GmbH
Europaplatz 3, 69115 Heidelberg, Germany

Printed by Libri Plureos GmbH
in Hamburg, Germany